Chronic Health-Related Disorders in Children

Chronic Health-Related Disorders in Children

COLLABORATIVE MEDICAL AND PSYCHOEDUCATIONAL INTERVENTIONS

EDITED BY

LeAdelle Phelps

American Psychological Association
Washington, DC

Published by
American Psychological Association
750 First Street, NE
Washington, DC 20002
www.apa.org

To order
APA Order Department
P.O. Box 92984
Washington, DC 20090-2984
Tel: (800) 374-2721; Direct: (202) 336-5510
Fax: (202) 336-5502; TDD/TTY: (202) 336-6123
Online: www.apa.org/books/
E-mail: order@apa.org

In the U.K., Europe, Africa, and the Middle East, copies may be ordered from
American Psychological Association
3 Henrietta Street
Covent Garden, London
WC2E 8LU England

Typeset in Goudy by Stephen D. McDougal

Printer: Edwards Brothers, Inc., Ann Arbor, MI
Cover Designer: Go! Creative, Kensington, MD
Technical/Production Editor: Dan Brachtesende

The opinions and statements published are the responsibility of the authors, and such opinions and statements do not necessarily represent the policies of the American Psychological Association.

Library of Congress Cataloging-in-Publication Data

Chronic health-related disorders in children : collaborative medical and psychoeducational interventions / [edited by] LeAdelle Phelps.
    p. cm.
  Includes bibliographical references and index.
  ISBN 1-59147-408-6
  1. Pediatric psychopharmacology. 2. Child psychopathology. 3. Adolescent psychopathology. I. Phelps, LeAdelle.
  [DNLM: 1. Mental Disorders—drug therapy—Child. 2. Mental Disorders—drug therapy—Adolescent. 3. Psychopharmacology—methods—Child. 4. Psychopharmacology—methods—Adolescent. 5. Needs Assessment. WS 350 C5566 2006]
  RJ504.7C477 2006
  618.92'89—dc22
                                               2005029614

British Library Cataloguing-in-Publication Data
A CIP record is available from the British Library.

Printed in the United States of America
First Edition

I am indebted to Ron Teeter for his careful editing and helpful suggestions and to Dave Weston for being my personal trainer, best friend, and partner in play. This book is dedicated to Clint F. for his enthusiasm and willingness to cycle many miles in spite of having paramythoria.

CONTENTS

CONTRIBUTORS

K. Angeleque Akin-Little, PhD, University of California, Riverside

Rowland P. Barrett, PhD, Emma Pendleton Bradley Hospital, East Providence, RI

Jessica Blom-Hoffman, PhD, Northeastern University, Boston, MA

Melissa A. Bray, PhD, University of Connecticut, Storrs

Eleas J. Chafouleas, MD, Northeastern Nephrology Associates, Vernon, CT

Sandra M. Chafouleas, PhD, University of Connecticut, Storrs-Mansfield

Michael K. Cruce, Lincoln Public Schools, Lincoln, NE

Richard J. DioGuardi, PhD, Iona College, New Rochelle, NY

James P. Donnelly, PhD, State University of New York, Buffalo

Kristal Ehrhardt, PhD, Western Michigan University, Kalamazoo

Piero Garzaro, MD, The Permanente Medical Group, Stockton, CA

Michael Hixson, PhD, Central Michigan University, Mt. Pleasant

Melissa Janik, University of Kansas, Lawrence

Thomas J. Kehle, PhD, University of Connecticut, Storrs-Mansfield

Deborah King Kundert, PhD, State University of New York, Albany

Steven W. Lee, PhD, University of Kansas, Lawrence

Steven G. Little, PhD, University of California, Riverside

David E. McIntosh, PhD, Ball State University, Muncie, IN

Frederic J. Medway, PhD, University of South Carolina, Columbia

Megan M. Morse, MA, Ball State University, Muncie, IN

Heather L. Peck, PhD, University of Connecticut, Storrs

LeAdelle Phelps, PhD, State University of New York, Buffalo

Alan Poling, PhD, Western Michigan University, Kalamazoo

Thomas J. Power, PhD, The Children's Hospital of Philadelphia, Philadelphia, PA

Henry T. Sachs III, MD, Emma Pendleton Bradley Hospital, East Providence, RI

David E. Sandberg, PhD, Women & Children's Hospital of Buffalo, Buffalo, NY

Jonathan Sandoval, PhD, University of California, Davis

Terry A. Stinnett, PhD, Oklahoma State University, Stillwater

Lea A. Theodore, PhD, The City University of New York, Queens College, Flushing

Carrie L. Trimarchi, PsyD, Ravena-Coeymans-Selkirk Central School District, Albany, NY

Eric G. Waldon, PhD, University of the Pacific, Stockton, CA

David L. Wodrich, PhD, Arizona State University, Tempe

Lauren Zurenda, BA, Women & Children's Hospital of Buffalo, Buffalo, NY

Chronic Health-Related Disorders in Children

INTRODUCTION

LeADELLE PHELPS

It has been estimated that at least one in five youth have developmental, physical, or mental disabilities (U.S. Department of Health and Human Services, 2005). This results in approximately 1 million children in this country who have a chronic illness that affects their daily functioning (Thompson & Gustafson, 1996). The identification and treatment of children and adolescents with such disorders is a major health incentive in the United States. For example, U.S. Surgeon General Richard H. Carmona released *The Surgeon General's Call to Action to Improve the Health and Wellness of Persons With Disabilities* on July 26, 2005 (full text is available at http://www.surgeongeneral.gov). One of the goals of this initiative is to increase the knowledge of health care professionals for the improvement of services for this population.

In direct alignment with this goal, the primary purpose of this text is to provide diagnostic and treatment information on selected chronic health-related disorders that are first diagnosed in childhood. Chronic conditions are those that have a protracted course of treatment and often result in compromised physical, cognitive, and psychosocial functioning. The prevalence of chronic medical conditions in children has nearly doubled in the last several decades (Tarnowski & Brown, 2000). This increased prevalence has been attributed to improved medical care and early diagnosis, resulting in a significant decrease in infant mortality, as well as the amplified incidence of more recent diseases such as AIDS.

Because many childhood chronic health-related disorders continue throughout the adult years, it is imperative that children receive early and appropriate services. Although direct medical care by pediatricians has long

3

been a common practice, it has only been in the last 2 decades that the importance of psychological and educational support services for these children has been addressed (Phelps, 1998). Yet few primary care physicians have specific knowledge and training in the myriad psychosocial concerns that a chronic health problem can instigate. Child psychologists have come to play a critical role in collaborating with other health care professionals to ensure that children with health issues receive appropriate mental health and educational support services. Likewise, there is a strong movement in the field toward identifying and using multimodal evidence-based interventions for the promotion of effective treatment planning (Weisz, Sandler, Durlak, & Anton, 2005). Such information is intended to improve the support and intervention services such children need. Hence, specific knowledge of the probable psychosocial and educational outcomes of pediatric health problems as well as efficacious interventions is especially timely.

The specific disorders covered by this volume were selected because they represent the primary and more common health issues in this population. The first part of the book includes two chapters that enhance collaborative practices and service delivery. The second section of the book is dedicated to providing concise and current reviews of 14 specific disorders. Each of the disorder-focused chapters follows a common structure. The chapters begin with an *Overview* section that defines the disorder, reviews etiology and risk factors, and provides prevalence data. The *Outcomes* section outlines the behavioral, medical, psychoeducational, and socioemotional consequences of the disorder. The final segment (*Implications*) presents recommended evidence-based interventions that are intended to mitigate the negative outcomes of the disorder and improve the lifelong functioning of children with chronic health-related disorders.

Throughout each chapter, every effort has been made to define unusual medical terms. It is hoped that this user-friendly format will provide health care providers and school-based professionals the knowledge to improve the long-term functioning of children and adolescents affected by these disorders.

REFERENCES

Phelps, L. (1998). *Health-related disorders in children and adolescents: A guidebook for understanding and educating.* Washington, DC: American Psychological Association.

Tarnowski, K. J., & Brown, T. (2000). Psychological aspects of pediatric disorders. In M. Hersen & R. T. Ammerman (Eds.), *Advanced abnormal child psychology* (pp. 131–152). Mahwah, NJ: Erlbaum.

Thompson, R. J., & Gustafson, K. E. (1996). *Adaptation to chronic childhood illness.* Washington, DC: American Psychological Association.

U.S. Department of Health and Human Services. (2005). *Call to action on disability: A report of the Surgeon General.* Washington, DC: Author.

Weisz, J. R., Sandler, I. N., Durlak, J. A., & Anton, B. S. (2005). Promoting and protecting youth mental health through evidence-based prevention and treatment. *American Psychologist, 60,* 628–648.

1

COLLABORATIVE PRACTICES FOR MANAGING CHILDREN'S CHRONIC HEALTH NEEDS

THOMAS J. POWER

Chronic health problems can have an effect on children in virtually every domain of their lives. Individuals from a wide range of systems influence the course of development for children with chronic medical conditions, including family members, neighbors, and community residents, as well as professionals in the health and educational systems. Child development is strongly influenced not only by interactions that occur within systems (e.g., parent–child relationship, physician–child relationship), but also by the quality of interactions between systems (e.g., family–health provider relationships, parent–teacher relationships; Kazak, Rourke, & Crump, 2003; Pianta & Walsh, 1996). Collaborative practices among professionals and family members can be critical in planning interventions and sustaining effective care for children with chronic health needs (Power, DuPaul, Shapiro, & Kazak, 2003). This chapter describes numerous impairments associated with chronic health conditions and systemic factors that influence the level of competence and impairment experienced by these children. The chapter highlights the importance of understanding cross-system linkages and promoting collaborative practices among professionals, family members, and community leaders when addressing the needs of children with medical conditions. A multisystemic framework is applied to understand the challenges of collaborative practice in addressing cross-cutting issues in pediatric health care, such as pain, adherence, school reintegration, and medication management.

PERVASIVE EFFECTS OF CHRONIC HEALTH CONDITIONS

Chronic health conditions can contribute to functional impairments in essentially every domain of a child's life, including academic performance, peer relationships, and family functioning. The following is a description of the challenges children with health problems may experience across these domains.

Academic Performance

A wide range of chronic health conditions, particularly those affecting the central nervous system (e.g., brain tumors, strokes associated with sickle cell disease, traumatic brain injury) can have an impact on academic performance. Diseases of the central nervous system often have a direct effect on brain structure and physiology, leading to cognitive impairments in linguistic, visuospatial, executive, or sensorimotor functioning that result in impaired educational functioning (e.g., see Armstrong & Briery, 2004; Bonner, Hardy, Ezell, & Ware, 2004; Clark, Russman, & Orme, 1999). Also, iatrogenic effects of treatments for brain tumors can have a further impact on cognitive functioning and academic performance (Armstrong & Briery, 2004). Illnesses that typically do not have direct effects on the central nervous system may also be associated with educational impairments (e.g., asthma, leukemia, gastrointestinal disorders) by increasing absenteeism from school or by interfering with a child's ability to sustain effort and concentration (e.g., see Armstrong & Briery, 2004; Arnett, 2004; Walker & Johnson, 2004).

Peer Relationships

Chronic health conditions can have an impact on how children interact with their peers. In general, research has failed to support the hypothesis that children with chronic illnesses have trouble being accepted by their peers (Reiter-Purtill & Noll, 2003). There are some notable exceptions to this generalization, however. A common finding in the literature is that chronic medical conditions can restrict the activities of children and reduce the opportunities of children to interact with peers (e.g., Noll et al., 1999, 2000). Also, alterations in physical appearance related to chronic health problems can have an effect on peer relationships. Child self-perceptions of unattractiveness have been shown to contribute to socially anxious, withdrawn behavior among chronically ill children (Spirito, DeLawyer, & Stark, 1991). Furthermore, children have been shown to initiate contact with peers who have craniofacial conditions less frequently than with peers who do not have a medical condition (Pope & Ward, 1997). The subgroup of children with chronic illnesses who appear to be at greatest risk for peer relationship problems are those with central nervous system involvement. Neurological impairments may contribute to deficits in social perception or executive functioning, resulting in behavior that leads to aggression and social rejection (see Nassau & Drotar, 1995).

Family Functioning

Although coping with chronic health conditions can be highly challenging for families, research has consistently demonstrated that families with chronically ill children typically are just as adaptive and functional as families with healthy children. Families of children with medical conditions generally are highly resilient when faced with the challenges of coping with illness (see Kazak, 2001). Characteristics that may promote resilience in families coping with illness are adhering to family rituals (e.g., family meals, religious activities) and parental behavior that is warm, caring, and authoritative, particularly with children in the preadolescent years (Davis et al., 2001; Fiese & Wamboldt, 2000).

Nonetheless, these families often experience high levels of stress. Research has shown that parents of children coping with health conditions, such as cancer and physical injuries, often experience symptoms of posttraumatic stress disorder, which may contribute to impairments in their functioning (DeVrie, Kassam-Adams, & Cnaan, 1999; Kazak et al., 1997). Families of lower socioeconomic status appear to be at greater risk for experiencing family conflict in response to having a child with a chronic illness (Holmbeck, Coakley, Hommeyer, Shapera, & Westhoven, 2002). Also, there is evidence that level of family stress and conflict may vary depending on the developmental level of the child (Coakley, Holmbeck, Friedman, Greenley, & Thill, 2002).

ECOLOGICAL FRAMEWORK FOR UNDERSTANDING CHRONIC HEALTH CONDITIONS

The developmental ecological model, advanced by Bronfenbrenner (1979), is a useful framework for understanding the developmental challenges of children with chronic illnesses. This model is unique in that it accounts not only for dynamics within systems but also for interactions between systems (e.g., the extent of the connection between primary care practices and schools) and is highly useful in understanding how contextual factors contribute to risk and promote resilience. This model has been adapted to ac-

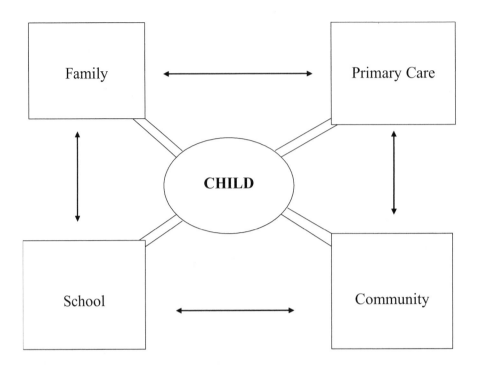

Figure 1.1. Important systems and intersystemic connections for promoting children's health. Parallel lines represent caring, mentoring relationships between adults in each system and the child, and arrows depict partnerships among the systems. Adapted from *Promoting Children's Health: Integrating School, Family, and Community* (p. 154), by T. J. Power, G. J. DuPaul, E. S. Shapiro, and A. E. Kazak, 2003, New York: Guilford Press. Copyright 2003 by Guilford Press. Reprinted with permission.

count for systemic variables that have an effect on the developing child with a chronic illness (Kazak et al., 2003; Power, DuPaul, et al., 2003). The following is a description of key elements of the model (see Figure 1.1 for an illustration of this framework).

Developing Child

The course of development for each child is highly unique. For example, more than 100 years of research in psychology has documented the presence of multiple domains of cognitive functioning (e.g., verbal, visuospatial, memory) and a broad range of individual variability in each domain. As another example, temperament research has identified numerous dimensions of emotionality and behavior (e.g., activity level, attention span, mood, adaptability) and demonstrated that children can vary greatly on each of these dimensions (Chess & Thomas, 1996). Developmentalists have cogently demonstrated how unique characteristics of the child transact with characteristics of the environment in complex ways over an extended period of time to shape human behavior (Sameroff, Bartko, Baldwin, Baldwin, & Seifer, 1998).

Illness can also be conceptualized as a set of characteristics that are unique to the child and that influence the course of development. Rolland (1994) has differentiated illnesses according to their onset (e.g., gradual vs. abrupt), course (e.g., consistent vs. cyclic), severity, level of incapacitation, and outcome (e.g., mild vs. severe developmental disorder). Of course, these dimensions can be highly influenced by psychosocial variables, but factors intrinsic to the disease itself have a strong bearing on the illness profile.

Systems

A person's environment can be conceptualized as a set of relatively discrete, yet overlapping, contexts or systems. Although a child's development is influenced by numerous systems, this chapter focuses on three that are particularly salient for a child with a chronic illness.

Family

The system that has the strongest influence on the developing child, particularly during the early childhood years, is the family. Strong attachment to one or more caregivers is critical to healthy child development; this has been shown to have an influence on a child's motivation to succeed academically, as well as the ability to self-regulate emotions and ability to engage in successful relationships with peers and adults outside the family (Cicchetti, Toth, & Lynch, 1995; Pianta, 1999). Effective parenting skills are critical in managing challenging family situations in a way that maintains order and stability in the family, demonstrates respect for the child, builds warm parent–child relationships, and teaches effective problem-solving skills (Patterson, Reid, & Dishion, 1992). Caregivers who are engaged in mutually supportive relationships with their partners and who can work creatively to resolve challenges presented by their children are more effective than caregivers who engage in conflictual dyadic relationships. Furthermore, parents who are extensively involved in social networks and can derive emotional and instrumental support from extended family, friends, and professionals typically are more effective in promoting their children's development than parents who are isolated (Wahler & Dumas, 1989).

Although families generally are remarkably adaptive in responding to the needs of children with chronic illness, the onset of a disease can be highly disruptive for families. For example, the parents and child may need to exert considerable effort to reestablish an attachment that has been disturbed by a traumatic injury. Furthermore, parents may need to make a concerted effort to understand the emotional needs of children whose siblings have been diagnosed with a brain tumor.

School

The school environment is critical in the development of self-regulation and social skills. Successful performance in school depends in part on a supportive, caring relationship between teachers and children (Pianta, 1999). Effective instruction obviously is essential for children to learn. Children need to be instructed in materials that ensure high rates of success yet involve a challenge (Shapiro, 1996). Teachers who are successful typically structure the classroom day and plan instructional sessions so that the amount of time devoted to instruction and student engagement in learning are high (Gettinger & Seibert, 2002). In addition, school is a laboratory for children to develop their social skills. Schools that are successful in promoting the social development of children provide effective supervision and guidance to children not only in the classroom, but also in the lunchroom and playground (Leff, Costigan, & Power, 2004).

Children with chronic illnesses often face significant challenges in school. These children may be difficult for teachers to understand, leading to relationships that are distant or lacking in support. Children with medical conditions, particularly those with central nervous system involvement, may have cognitive and motor problems that require specialized instruction. Further, the social challenges experienced by some children with illnesses may require a level of support and guidance that are difficult for schools to offer.

Primary Health Care and Other Community Systems

In general, children remain healthier and develop better when they are engaged in a continuous relationship with a primary care provider (Kelleher et al., 1997). The managed care movement has emphasized the critical role of primary care in the delivery of health services, but this approach typically limits the range of providers available to children and families and restricts access to specialized care (Roberts & Hurley, 1997). There are numerous barriers to effective health care for children, but perhaps the most significant obstacle is lack of health insurance, a problem that is increasing at an alarming rate in this country. Children who are uninsured or underinsured may not receive preventive care and may only receive health care when medical conditions become severe. Furthermore, medical care for these children often is provided in emergency department settings where opportunities for follow-up are limited.

Children with specialized chronic health conditions often face substantial difficulties getting their needs addressed within the health system. Primary care providers available to them may not be sufficiently knowledgeable about their health needs to be strong advocates for them (Brown, 2004). The managed care environment may limit access to specialists who have expertise related to their health care needs. Inadequate care may result in overuse of the health system, frequent visits to the emergency department, and the need for highly expensive services.

Health and social services also may be available through systems embedded in the community, such as after-school programs, recreational clubs, and faith-based organizations. Although these agencies may be limited with regard to the level of medical expertise and technology available, they have the potential to be highly influential in that some families are more likely to seek help through these systems than they are through more formal health settings (Tucker, 2002).

Connections Between Systems

The development of children within systems is highly influenced by the relationships existing between systems (Power, DuPaul, et al., 2003). Three critical intersystem connections for children with chronic health needs are the family and health system, the family and school, and the school and health system.

Family and Health System

It is widely recognized that the relationship between family and health system is essential for the effective care of children. The family-centered care movement, among other advocacy efforts, has been effective in educating health care providers about the importance of building linkages between these systems, particularly for children with chronic health conditions (Johnson, 2000). As a result many pediatric hospitals have established policies encouraging strong family involvement in the provision of health care, forums for parents and youth to express their needs and concerns, and resource centers for the dissemination of useful educational materials. Nonetheless, the relationship between family and provider has received little research attention. Research efforts to understand family trust in their health providers are noteworthy contributions that may be useful in developing strategies to improve this connection (Hall, Camacho, Dugan, & Balkrishnan, 2002). Higher levels of trust appear to be associated with increased satisfaction with providers and greater willingness to adhere to medical recommendations (Hall, Zheng, et al., 2002).

Family and School

Establishing a collaborative family–school relationship is important in promoting the academic and social success of children. The quality of this relationship can have an effect on the teacher-child relationship, which in turn influences adjustment in school (Pianta, 1999). Effective family involvement in education can provide children with increased opportunities to learn and practice academic skills. Furthermore, forming a family–school alliance and working through the steps of problem solving has been shown to be highly effective in addressing academic and social difficulties that arise in school (Sheridan, Eagle, Cowan, & Mickelson, 2001). Children with complex health problems present unique challenges to the family–school relationship. Teachers may not understand the special needs of these children, requiring that parents educate school personnel and serve as child advocates. Teachers' efforts to educate these children may not be successful, which can lead to frustration and conflict between parents and teachers. In many cases, professional consultation is needed to facilitate this interaction and assist with intervention (Power, DuPaul, et al., 2003).

School and Health System

The school and health systems typically are poorly linked. Although this may not be a problem for the child who is functioning competently, it can be a significant barrier to effective care for children with impairments. To work effectively with children who have impairments, school professionals need to understand the child's medical condition and the unique ways in which it has an effect on academic and social performance. Furthermore, health professionals need information from school professionals to understand how the child is coping in the community and responding to interventions, such as varying doses of medication (Power, DuPaul, Shapiro, & Parrish, 1995). Parents are often placed in the difficult position of mediating the relationship between school and health system, but this often does not promote effective care. There is a pressing need for professionals who can link these systems and advocate for the health and psychological needs of chronically ill children in the school setting. One initiative developed to address this need is the partnership between Lehigh University and the Children's Hospital of Philadelphia, which is designed to prepare doctoral students in school psychology to manage children's chronic health problems and to promote healthy behavior in the school context (Power, Shapiro, & DuPaul, 2003).

Cultural, Social, and Political Factors

System dynamics and intersystem relationship patterns are strongly influenced by cultural, social, and political variables. These factors influence systems in complex ways that can have a dramatic effect on the course of development for children with health conditions. For example, a change in employment for a single parent (because of large-scale layoffs at a previous job) that results in a loss of health insurance or decreased coverage can have a significant impact on the ability of the family to access appropriate medical care for a child with a chronic illness. The same situation could necessitate a change in primary health care provider that severs the relationship between family and a health care provider that had developed over many years.

As another example, a family may perceive stimulant medication as an unacceptable form of treatment for their child who has sustained a traumatic head injury and acquired attention-deficit/hyperactivity disorder (ADHD). An interview with the family uncovers that the family is embedded in a social network of extended family members and friends who believe that inattention and overactivity are generally caused by parenting and teaching style and that a change in disciplinary technique is needed to address the problems. As a further illustration, a change in policy at a state level that narrows the inclusion criteria for special education eligibility under the category of Other Health Impaired may prevent some children with medical conditions from receiving specialized services within the school.

MULTILEVEL PREVENTION AND INTERVENTION

As described in the previous section, understanding child functioning requires not only an analysis of how the child is developing within a system and how multiple systems are interacting but also an assessment of cultural, social, and political variables impinging on contexts that are critical in supporting the maturing child (Kazak et al., 2003). Such an analysis may be useful in detecting barriers to care or factors contributing to developmental risk, some of which may be amenable to change (Power, Eiraldi, Clarke, Mazzuca, & Krain, 2005). Also, this assessment is useful in identifying systems resources or protective factors that promote competence and resilience in the face of developmental challenges.

Although almost all children with chronic health conditions require medical intervention of some sort, they vary greatly with regard to their need for specialized care. The needs of these children vary on a continuum ranging from minimal need to high need for specialized services. Factors that may influence the level of intervention needed are the following: (a) the health condition of the child, including the severity and complexity of the child's medical problems; (b) the adaptability and functionality of the major systems in a child's life; and (c) the level of collaboration among these systems (Power, DuPaul, et al., 2003). The following is a description of the levels of prevention and intervention that may be suitable for children of varying degrees of need. These levels have been adapted from the model of prevention outlined by the Institute of Medicine (1994).

Universal Prevention

Most children with chronic health conditions are competent individuals who function reasonably well in school and the community. Although these children typically require more medical attention than their peers, their health problems may be minimally impairing. Also, although they may be more anxious than their peers, these children may not require specialized mental health services. All children with health problems can benefit from efforts to support family members and school professionals and strengthen the resources of these systems to promote successful development. Also, all children with medical conditions can benefit from efforts to establish and maintain collaborative relationships among family, school, and health system. Efforts directed at strengthening systems and intersystemic connections promote healthy behavior and reduce the probability that risk factors will emerge.

Indicated Prevention

Some children with health problems are at risk for developing significant functional impairments in the family, school, or community. Factors pertaining to the child, the systems in which the child is developing, or interactions among systems may place the child at risk for impairment. For example, the natural course of an illness may be to cycle through periods of stability and instability. In these cases, a child's illness may suddenly become more severe without any apparent stressor in the environment. Also, a disruption in the parents' marriage may contribute to inconsistent monitoring of adherence to a medical regimen, which could result in reduced intervention effectiveness. As another example, a child's changing schools may disrupt the relationship between school and primary care practice, which could lead to inconsistent medication monitoring in school and unsuccessful attempts to titrate medication level accurately. The emergence of one of more risk factors is a signal to professionals that preventive efforts are needed to keep the child performing at a competent level and to prevent the emergence of impairments.

Intervention

Some children with health problems experience significant impairments in one or more domains of functioning during the course of their development. These children require intervention to minimize impairment and restore functioning to an adaptive level. Although it may be appropriate to target intervention efforts at the level of the child (e.g., physical therapy to improve mobility and strength; cognitive rehabilitation to improve memory and problem-solving skills), the optimal approach to intervention includes a focus on system and intersystem dynamics (Power, DuPaul, et al., 2003). Applying an ecological framework, it is recommended that professionals examine family, school, and health system dynamics that may be contributing to unhealthy patterns of behavior. Also, it is important to understand the relationships among family, school, and health system to determine whether intersystem factors are compromising the child's health.

CROSS-CUTTING CHALLENGES
INVOLVING COLLABORATIVE PRACTICE

There are several issues in pediatric health care that cut across medical conditions and involve multiple systems. The following is a discussion of some of these themes with a particular focus on challenges for collaborative practice.

Recurrent Pain

Recurrent pain conditions, such as abdominal pain, musculoskeletal pain, and headaches, are common among children and frequently pose challenges to school professionals. Children with recurrent pain typically visit the school nurse on a frequent basis. Although physiological processes contribute to the pain in most cases (Dahlquist & Switkin, 2003; Sherry, 2000), it is often difficult for physicians to detect a specific organic cause of the symptoms and to resolve the condition. The contribution of cognitive and emotional processes to the perception and experience of pain is widely recognized among experts. Typically, the challenge of intervention is to alleviate the symptoms and to prevent secondary problems, such as school avoidance, social withdrawal, anxiety, and overdependence on parents. Strategies to reduce pain may include relaxation techniques, physical exercise, involvement in high-preference activities, and, at times, medication. A critical component of treatment is to eliminate reinforcement for avoidant behavior and to provide reinforcement for adaptive behavior (Dahlquist & Switkin, 2003; Walker & Johnson, 2004). It is essential that the family and school work effectively together to promote adaptive behavior and remove opportunities for the child to be reinforced for avoidant, withdrawn behavior. Effective management also requires that school professionals, health providers, and families collaborate to develop a plan to alleviate pain symptoms while the child is working on challenging academic and social tasks (Walker, 1999).

Adherence

A major challenge in the treatment of illness is the problem of nonadherence, which may compromise the effectiveness of intervention. Rates of nonadherence among families coping with chronic health conditions typically are high (Lemanek, 2001). In general, the more chronic the disorder and the more complex the medical regimen, the greater the likelihood of nonadherence (La Greca & Bearman, 2003). Adherence has traditionally been conceptualized as compliance with the directives of a physician or health care team. The problem with this model is that it fails to acknowledge the critical role that the family, school, and community serve in implementing an intervention plan. Failure to account for family preferences and issues of feasibility may result in intervention plans that are unreasonable and perhaps culturally insensitive.

Recently, collaborative models for designing intervention programs, which involve families and professionals from multiple systems, have been proposed (Power, DuPaul, et al., 2003). These models, which are based on developmental–ecological theory, reframe adherence as the implementation of a set of strategies that have been designed in collaboration with the major stakeholders of intervention, which typically include the parents and child, health providers, school professionals, and often community members.

School Reintegration

Pediatric health conditions, such as traumatic brain injury, cancer, heart and lung disease requiring transplantation, and stroke associated with sickle cell disease, often disrupt schooling and pose significant challenges on reentry to school (Madan-Swain, Katz, & LaGory, 2004). School reintegration may be particularly difficult when children have a medical condition that involves the central nervous system and has an impact on cognitive and academic functioning. Models of intervention that involve the health system, family, and school in an ongoing problem-solving process appear to be the most effective approaches to promoting successful school reintegration (Worchel-Prevatt et al., 1998). For example, Power, DuPaul, et al. (2003) proposed a model with the following sequence of phases: Phase 1—establishing a partnership between the health care team and family to strengthen the family's ability to cope with the child's medical condition; Phase 2—preparing the family to collaborate effectively with the school; Phase 3—preparing the school to collaborate effectively with the family and health team; and Phase 4—engaging the family, school, and health team in a collaborative process to plan, implement, and modify the intervention plan. A hallmark of this proposed model is building the capacity of these systems to promote health and competence, in addition to linking systems to resolve problems and reduce risk.

Medication Management

Pharmacotherapy is often a critical component of an intervention plan to treat children's medical conditions. Medications may be used to treat underlying physiological processes (e.g., insulin analogues for diabetes), alleviate physical symptoms (e.g., analgesics for pain), or treat emotional and behavioral problems that may co-occur with medical conditions (e.g., stimulants for attention disorders). Medications are typically used to regulate functioning and behavior over the course of an entire day, including the hours spent in school. Medication management generally is more effective when it is conducted in a systematic manner and incorporates data from multiple adult informants, in particular parents and teachers, to monitor effects and side effects (DuPaul, McGoey, & Mautone, 2003; Phelps, Brown, & Power, 2002). Collaboration between health provider and family and between health provider and school professionals is useful in identifying the most appropriate medication and the best dosage level. Failure to link the school and health systems in the management of medication may place families in the challenging position of having to translate the perceptions of school professionals to health providers, which may lead to inadequate care.

CONCLUSION

Chronic pediatric conditions have pervasive effects on the developing child and can affect functioning in the family, academic, and social domains. The developmental–ecological model is highly useful for understanding the processes that contribute to competence and impairment among children with chronic health problems. This model describes how dynamics within and between systems influence the course of development. For a child with a chronic health condition, critical systems include the family, school, and health system, and essential connections include the family–health provider relationship, the family–school relationship, and the school–health provider interaction. Understanding factors that contribute to developmental risk and factors that promote resilience requires an ecological assessment of critical contexts (systems) of development and interaction among systems. Also, this assessment involves an understanding of cultural, political, and economic factors that influence systems and transactions between them.

The developmental–ecological model also can be highly useful in plotting a course of prevention and intervention for children with chronic health conditions. Given that most children with chronic conditions are relatively competent, a universal prevention strategy that focuses on strengthening systems and intersystemic transactions is a highly appropriate course of action for all children with health problems. For children with health conditions who display signs of risk, an indicated prevention approach targeted to reduce risk and promote competence is recommended. For individuals manifesting impairments in one or more critical domains, intervention targeted at the systems and system interactions that are dysfunctional is the recommended approach.

Although each medical condition poses unique challenges to children and the systems in which they develop, there are cross-cutting themes in pediatric health care that span a wide range of illnesses and are associated with a similar pattern of challenges. These themes include pain, adherence, school reintegration, and medication management. A consideration of each theme highlights the need for professionals from multiple disciplines and systems to form collaborative relationships with families to manage health conditions and to promote healthy development.

REFERENCES

Armstrong, F. D., & Briery, B. G. (2004). Childhood cancer and the school. In R. T. Brown (Ed.), *Handbook of pediatric psychology in school settings* (pp. 263–281). Mahwah, NJ: Erlbaum.

Arnett, R. D. (2004). Asthma. In R. T. Brown (Ed.), *Handbook of pediatric psychology in school settings* (pp. 149–168). Mahwah, NJ: Erlbaum.

Bonner, M. J., Hardy, K. K., Ezell, E., & Ware, R. (2004). Hematological disorders: Sickle cell disease and hemophilia. In R. T. Brown (Ed.), *Handbook of pediatric psychology in school settings* (pp. 241–262). Mahwah, NJ: Erlbaum.

Bronfenbrenner, U. (1979). *The ecology of human development.* Cambridge, MA: Harvard University Press.

Brown, R. T. (2004). Introduction: Changes in the provision of health care to children and adolescents. In R. T. Brown (Ed.), *Handbook of pediatric psychology in school settings* (pp. 1–19). Mahwah, NJ: Erlbaum.

Chess, S., & Thomas, A. (1996). *Temperament: Theory and practice.* New York: Guilford Press.

Cicchetti, D., Toth, S. L., & Lynch, M. (1995). Bowlby's dream comes full circle: The application of attachment theory to risk and psychopathology. In T. H. Ollendick & R. J. Prinz (Eds.), *Advances in clinical child psychology* (Vol. 17, pp. 1–75). New York: Plenum Press.

Clark, E., Russman, S., & Orme, S. (1999). HIV/AIDS among children and adolescents: Implications for the changing role of school psychologists. *School Psychology Review, 28,* 228–241.

Coakley, R., Holmbeck, G., Friedman, D., Greenley, R., & Thill, A. (2002). A longitudinal study of pubertal timing, parent–child conflict, and cohesion in families of young adolescents with spina bifida. *Journal of Pediatric Psychology, 27,* 461–473.

Dahlquist, L. M., & Switkin, M. C. (2003). Chronic and recurrent pain. In M. C. Roberts (Ed.), *Handbook of pediatric psychology* (3rd ed., pp. 198–215). New York: Guilford Press.

Davis, C., Delamater, A., Shaw, K., La Greca, A., Eidson, M., Perez-Rodriques, J., & Nemery, R. (2001). Brief Report: Parenting styles, regimen adherence and glycemic control in 4–10 year old children with diabetes. *Journal of Pediatric Psychology, 26,* 123–129.

DeVries, A. P. J., Kassam-Adams, N., & Cnaan, A. (1999). Looking beyond the physical injury: Post-traumatic stress disorder in children and parents after pediatric traffic injury. *Pediatrics, 104,* 1293–1299.

DuPaul, G. J., McGoey, K. E., & Mautone, J. A. (2003). Pediatric pharmacology and psychopharmacology. In M. C. Roberts (Ed.), *Handbook of pediatric psychology* (3rd ed., pp. 234–250). New York: Guilford Press.

Fiese, B., & Wamboldt, F. (2000). Family routines, rituals and asthma management: A proposal for family-based strategies to increase treatment adherence. *Families, Systems, and Health, 18*, 405–418.

Gettinger, M., & Seibert, J. K. (2002). Best practices in increasing academic learning time. In A. Thomas & J. Grimes (Eds.), *Best practices in school psychology IV*. Bethesda, MD: National Association of School Psychologists.

Hall, M. A., Camacho, F., Dugan, E., & Balkrishnan, R. (2002). Trust in the medical profession: Conceptual and measurement issues. *Health Services Research, 37*, 1419–1421.

Hall, M. A., Zheng, B., Dugan, E., Camacho, F., Kidd, K. E., Mishra, A., & Balkrishnan, R. (2002). Measuring patients' trust in their primary care providers. *Medical Care Research and Review, 59*, 293–318.

Holmbeck, G., Coakley, R., Hommeyer, J., Shapera, W., & Westhoven, V. (2002). Observed and perceived dyadic and systemic functioning in families of preadolescents with spina bifida. *Journal of Pediatric Psychology, 27*, 177–189.

Institute of Medicine. (1994). *Reducing risks for mental disorders: Frontiers for preventive intervention research*. Washington, DC: National Academy Press.

Johnson, B. (2000). Family-centered care: Four decades of progress. *Families, Systems, and Health, 18*, 137–156.

Kazak, A. (2001). Comprehensive care for children with cancer and their families: A social ecological framework guiding research, practice and policy. *Children's Services: Social Policy, Research and Practice, 4*, 217–233.

Kazak, A., Barakat, L., Meeske, K., Christakis, D., Meadows, A., Casey, R., et al. (1997). Posttraumatic stress, family functioning, and social support in survivors of childhood leukemia and their mothers and fathers. *Journal of Consulting and Clinical Psychology, 65*, 120–129.

Kazak, A. E., Rourke, M. T., & Crump, T. A. (2003). Families and other systems in pediatric psychology. *Handbook of pediatric psychology* (3rd ed., 159–175). New York: Guilford Press.

Kelleher, K. J., Childs, G. E., Wasserman, R. C., McInerney, T. K., Nutting, P. A., & Gardner, W. P. (1997). Insurance status and recognition of psychosocial problems: A report from PROS and ASPN. *Archives of Pediatrics and Adolescent Medicine, 151*, 1109–1115.

La Greca, A. M., & Bearman, K. J. (2003). Adherence to pediatric treatment regimens. In M. C. Roberts (Ed.), *Handbook of pediatric psychology* (3rd ed., pp. 119–140). New York: Guilford Press.

Leff, S. S., Costigan, T., & Power, T. J. (2004). Using participatory research to develop a playground-based prevention program. *Journal of School Psychology, 42*, 3–22.

Lemanek, K. (2001). Empirically supported treatments in pediatric psychology: Regimen adherence. *Journal of Pediatric Psychology, 26*, 253–275.

Madan-Swain, A., Katz, E. R., & LaGory, J. (2004). School and school reintegration after a serious illness or injury. *Handbook of pediatric psychology in school settings* (pp. 637–655). Mahwah, NJ: Erlbaum.

Nassau, J. H., & Drotar, D. (1995). Social competence in children with IDDM and asthma: Child, teacher, and parent reports of children's social adjustment, social performance, and social skills. *Journal of Pediatric Psychology, 20*, 187–204.

Noll, R. B., Garstein, M. A., Vannatta, K., Correll, J., Bukowski, W. M., & Davies, W. H. (1999). Social, emotional, and behavioral functioning of children with cancer. *Pediatrics, 103*, 71–78.

Noll, R. B., Kozlowski, M. A., Gerhardt, C. A., Vannatta, K., Taylor, J., & Russo, M. H. (2000). Social, emotional, and behavioral functioning of children with juvenile rheumatoid arthritis. *Arthritis and Rheumatism, 43*, 1387–1396.

Patterson, G. R., Reid, J. B., & Dishion, T. J. (1992). *Antisocial boys*. Eugene, OR: Castalia.

Phelps, L., Brown, R. T., & Power, T. J. (2002). *Pediatric psychopharmacology: Combining medical and psychosocial interventions*. Washington, DC: American Psychological Association.

Pianta, R. C. (1999). *Enhancing relationships between children and teachers*. Washington, DC: American Psychological Association.

Pianta, R. C., & Walsh, D. (1996). *High-risk children in the schools: Creating sustained relationships*. New York: Routledge.

Pope, A., & Ward, J. (1997). Factors associated with peer social competence in preadolescents with craniofacial anomalies. *Journal of Pediatric Psychology, 22*, 455–469.

Power, T. J., DuPaul, G. J., Shapiro, E. S., & Kazak, A. E. (2003). *Promoting children's health: Integrating school, family, and community*. New York: Guilford Press.

Power, T. J., DuPaul, G. J., Shapiro, E. S., & Parrish, J. M. (1995). Pediatric school psychology: The emergence of a subspecialty. *School Psychology Review, 24*, 244–257.

Power, T. J., Eiraldi, R. B., Clarke, A. T., Mazzuca, L. B., & Krain, A. L. (2005). Improving mental health service utilization for children and adolescents. *School Psychology Quarterly*, 206–221.

Power, T. J., Shapiro, E. S., & DuPaul, G. J. (2003). Preparing psychologists to link systems of care in managing and preventing children's health problems. *Journal of Pediatric Psychology, 28*, 147–156.

Reiter-Purtill, J., & Noll, R. B. (2003). Peer relationships of children with chronic illness. In M. C. Roberts (Ed.), *Handbook of pediatric psychology* (3rd ed., pp. 176–197). New York: Guilford Press.

Roberts, M. C., & Hurley, L. K. (1997). *Managing managed care*. New York: Plenum Press.

Rolland, J. (1994). *Families, illness and disability: An integrative treatment model*. New York: Basic Books.

Sameroff, A., Bartko, W., Baldwin, A., Baldwin, C., & Seifer, R. (1998). Family and social influences in the development of child competence. In M. Lewis & C. Feiring (Eds.), *Families, risk and competence* (pp. 165–185). Mahwah, NJ: Erlbaum.

Shapiro, E. S. (1996). *Academic skills problems: Direct assessment and intervention* (2nd ed.). New York: Guilford Press.

Sheridan, S. M., Eagle, J. W., Cowan, R. J., & Mickelson, W. (2001). The effects of conjoint behavioral consultation: Results of a 4-year investigation. *Journal of School Psychology, 39,* 361–385.

Sherry, D. D. (2000). An overview of amplified musculoskeletal pain syndromes. *The Journal of Rheumatology, 27,* 44–48.

Spirito, A., DeLawyer, D. D., & Stark, L. J. (1991). Peer relations and social adjustment of chronically ill children and adolescents. *Clinical Psychology Review, 11,* 539–564.

Tucker, C. M. (2002). Expanding pediatric psychology beyond hospital walls to meet the healthcare needs of ethnic minority children. *Journal of Pediatric Psychology, 27,* 315–324.

Wahler, R. G., & Dumas, J. E. (1989). Attentional problems in dysfunctional mother–child interactions: An interbehavioral model. *American Psychologist, 105,* 116–130.

Walker, L. S. (1999). The evolution of research on recurrent abdominal pain: History, assumptions, and a conceptual model. In P. J. McGrath (Ed.), *Chronic and recurrent pain in children and adolescents, progress in pain research and management* (pp. 141–172). Seattle, WA: IASP Press.

Walker, L. S., & Johnson, W. S. (2004). Recurrent abdominal pain and functional gastrointestinal disorders in the school setting. In R. T. Brown (Ed.), *Handbook of pediatric psychology in school settings* (pp. 299–312). Mahwah, NJ: Erlbaum.

Worchel-Prevatt, F. F., Heffer, R. W., Prevatt, B. C., Miner, J., Young-Saleme, T., Horgan, D., & Lopez, M. A. (1998). A school reentry program for chronically ill children. *Journal of School Psychology, 36,* 261–279.

2

PROVISION OF PSYCHOEDUCATIONAL SERVICES IN THE SCHOOLS: IDEA, SECTION 504, AND NCLB

STEVEN W. LEE AND MELISSA JANIK

The many systems of care that assist children with chronic health conditions to develop and adjust into adulthood must collaborate to ensure that all services and environments in which the child lives are taken into account (Shaw & Páez, 2002). If parents, educators, and medical caregivers cannot work together and speak a common language, it is unlikely that the best services will be provided to the child and the family. This chapter seeks to provide medical personnel, psychologists, and educators with information regarding how the Individuals With Disabilities Education Improvement Act of 2004 (IDEA) and Section 504 of the Rehabilitation Act of 1973 (Section 504) affords these children with the educational and medical services they need to grow, learn, and adjust to the challenging problems they face. The chapter begins with a brief description of the effects of chronic illness on school functioning and covers the procedures and services of IDEA, Section 504, and the No Child Left Behind Act of 2001 (NCLB) that may be made available to these children depending on the degree to which their illness affects their academic progress. The chapter also includes information on the rights of parents, procedural safeguards, and information on specific illnesses as they relate to these federal laws.

CHRONIC ILLNESS AND SCHOOL FUNCTIONING

Although there are many educational ramifications that are associated with a child experiencing chronic illness, the majority of such children are able to attend their regular classrooms without any program modifications; most will simply require brief tutorial help to "catch up" with their classmates (Sexson & Madan-Swain, 1993). Although school absence has been found to be related to academic difficulties, it is unclear which specific diagnosis increases a child's vulnerability for school absence (Shapiro & Manz, 2004). In their 1998 investigation into the results of the 1992–1994 National Health Interview Survey, Newacheck and Halfon (1998) found that "23% of those children with disabling chronic conditions were either unable to attend school or were limited in their ability to attend school on a long-term basis" (p. 613). Students may miss school because of chronic illness, complications from the illness (e.g., pneumonia), or the effects of treatments including medications.

School absence is obviously not the only factor associated with educational adjustment for children with chronic illness. In some cases, a chronic illness may have a direct effect on academic achievement. Conditions such as cerebral palsy, epilepsy, and other diseases resulting in diminished neuropsychological functioning, as well as autism, leukemia, and other cancers affecting the brain are examples of this direct effect. Achievement test scores were found to be significantly lower for chronically ill students compared with their healthy peers (Madan-Swain, Katz, & LaGory, 2004). For children who have prior histories of learning problems, illness may exacerbate their academic difficulties, possibly requiring some form of program modification or support service from the school. Special education services may also be needed for illnesses involving the central nervous system for the child to adjust back into the general school curriculum (Madan-Swain et al., 2004).

There is an obvious need for parents, caregivers, and educators to know and understand the provisions set forth in IDEA, NCLB, and Section 504. These federal policies help parents and professionals to understand the services that are available to children with chronic illnesses and the rationale for educational decisions made in schools. IDEA and Section 504 outline the procedures required to identify whether a child with chronic illness is eligible for services. Screening and assessment of these individuals then takes place through an evaluation process found in both IDEA and Section 504. If a child qualifies for services under IDEA, then he or she is provided with an Individualized Education Plan (IEP) or an Individual Family Service Plan (IFSP) that includes a detailed explanation of what services will be implemented to maximize the child's educational progress. In a similar way, Section 504 defines the accommodations that must be made to meet the needs of the child with a disability. IDEA also allows for related services, such as transportation and developmental, corrective, and support services, that may be implemented for such a child to benefit from the educational setting. Finally, procedural safeguards are in place under both IDEA and Section 504 to protect the rights of the parents and child at all stages of the process. The remainder of this chapter focuses on the provisions of IDEA, Section 504, and NCLB in an effort to help teachers and medical and mental health workers to understand how to work within the law to assist chronically ill children and their families.

IDEA AND CHILDREN WITH CHRONIC ILLNESS

We know that children with chronic health conditions are likely to face more psychosocial adjustment problems than healthy children (Wallander & Thompson, 1995). The concept of the severity of chronic illness in children may be viewed quite differently. Even in a well-documented case of asthma, parents and teachers may have different views on the degree to which they believe the illness interferes with the ability of the child to benefit maximally from his or her education. However, Theis (1999) stated that

> No legal mandate exists to serve children with chronic illness. Many children with asthma, diabetes, or cancer do not fit either the eligibility criteria for or philosophies of traditional special education programs created by IDEA. More to the point, eligibility for services under IDEA for children who are "health impaired" is based on "health problems" that "adversely affect a child's educational performance." Academic performance must be compromised before a child is deemed in need of educational services at school, and performance difficulties must be ascribed to the health impairment. Several problems exist with the current approach to identifying the educational needs of children with chronic illness. (p. 393)

Even if a teacher or parent believes that a chronic illness substantially influences a student's education, it may still be unclear whether the problem represents an identifiable educational disability under IDEA and what the school's responsibility is to respond. To attempt to answer these questions, we review the provisions of IDEA as they apply to children with chronic illnesses. Figure 2.1 shows the general processes that lead from general education through to special education under IDEA.

Evaluation, Eligibility, and Reevaluation

For parents and teachers, the ultimate goal of seeking a psychoeducational evaluation is to access the special services that may be afforded to

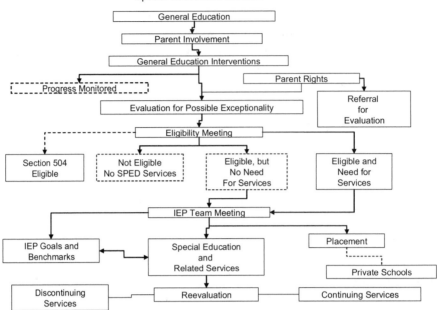

Special Education Flowchart

Figure 2.1. Special education flowchart. IEP = Individualized Education Plan.

the student. To best understand the treatment or interventions that can be provided to the student with chronic illness under IDEA, a brief discussion of the psychoeducational evaluation process is in order. In fact, the most mysterious aspect of disability determination for many is the process through which children become eligible for services under IDEA. By definition, a child with a disability

> means a child with mental retardation, hearing impairments (including deafness), speech or language impairments, visual impairments (including blindness), serious emotional disturbance (hereinafter referred to as emotional disturbance), orthopedic impairments, autism, traumatic brain injury, other health impairments or specific learning disabilities; and who by reason thereof, needs special education and related services. (IDEA, 20 U.S.C. § 1401 (3)(A)(i), 2004)

The definition for young children

> aged 3 through 9 may at the discretion of the State and the local education agency, include a child experiencing developmental delays as defined by the State and as measured by appropriate diagnostic instruments and procedures, in one or more of the following areas: physical development, cognitive development, communication development, social or emotional development, or adaptive development and who, by reason

thereof, needs special education and related services. (IDEA, 20 U.S.C. § 1401 (3)(B), 2004)

As these definitions show, IDEA covers both specific and nonspecific disorders. For young children, it is only sufficient to show that they are experiencing developmental delays. The reason for those delays may well be due or related to chronic or acute health conditions. Special attention should be drawn to the category Other Health Impaired (OHI). This category

> means having limited strength, vitality or alertness, including a heightened alertness to environmental stimuli, that results in limited alertness with respect to the educational environment, that (i) Is due to chronic or acute health problems such as asthma, attention deficit disorder or attention deficit hyperactivity disorder, diabetes, epilepsy, a heart condition, hemophilia, lead poisoning, leukemia, nephritis, rheumatic fever, and sickle cell anemia; and (ii) Adversely affects a child's educational performance. (IDEA, 34 U.S.C. § 300.7 (c)(9), 2004)

Another category under which a student with a chronic illness might be served is orthopedic impairment. This means

> a severe orthopedic impairment that adversely affects a child's educational performance. The term includes impairments caused by congenital anomaly (e.g., clubfoot, absence of some member), impairments caused by disease (e.g., poliomyelitis, bone tuberculosis, etc.) and impairments from other causes (e.g., cerebral palsy, amputations, and fractures and burns that cause contractures). (IDEA, 34 U.S.C. § 300.7 (c)(8), 2004)

Finally, students with chronic illness may be served under the category titled "traumatic brain injury." This category means

> an acquired injury to the brain caused by an external physical force, resulting in total or partial functional disability or psychosocial impairment, or both, that adversely affects a child's educational performance. The term applies to open or closed head injuries resulting in impairments in one or more areas, such as cognition; language; memory; attention; reasoning; abstract thinking; judgment; problem-solving; sensory, perceptual and motor abilities; psychosocial behavior; physical functions; information processing; and speech. The term does not apply to brain injuries that are congenital and degenerative, or to brain injuries induced by birth trauma. (IDEA, 34 U.S.C. § 300.7 (c)(12), 2004)

In these definitions, one can see the two critical elements required for an IDEA diagnosis. Unequivocal documentation of the chronic health condition by a physician or qualified health professional is required along with information to document the way in which the condition adversely affects the child's educational performance. Although it has been shown that chronic health conditions of sufficient severity may negatively affect educational performance (Madan-Swain et al., 2004), these effects vary significantly by the type and course of the disorder as well as the etiology and current method of treatment (Power, Heathfield, McGoey, & Blum, 1999). It is incumbent on the school staff and mental health workers to demonstrate carefully the student's educational delays using methods that are sensitive to the educational effects of the disorder.

When a student's chronic illness has adversely affected her or his educational performance there are many interested parties including the parents, teacher(s), and physician or other health care provider. Under IDEA only the parent or school staff may make a direct referral to request a comprehensive, multidisciplinary psychoeducational evaluation. Therefore, health care providers should work with the parents and the school when suggesting that the student be evaluated for possible special services.

When parents request a comprehensive evaluation and the school district agrees, the evaluation must be done within 60 days following the written request. In the case of parental referral, the parents should provide a release of information to allow the school to contact the physician to obtain the written documentation of the chronic health condition. Where possible, the school may request a physician's letter documenting that the child's illness or disability would have a significant impact on her or his educational performance (Shaw & Páez, 2002). The ensuing psychoeducational evaluation should use nondiscriminatory procedures, be multisourced (e.g., different instruments or respondents), and be completed by a multidisciplinary team of professionals, thus emphasizing a comprehensive approach and corroboration of findings through different psychometrically sound instruments and methods. The psychoeducational evaluation should identify the onset of the illness and its course by carefully interviewing the parents or guardians, the child's physician, or both. The child's educational progress may be evaluated through the examination of cumulative school records (e.g., grades, records of absences, standardized group achievement test scores), as well as broadband instruments and specific and informal tools to find both general areas of concern and specific areas of academic weakness. Power et al. (1999) recommended a functional analysis for selecting interventions that have the most promise for both medical and academic interventions.

The process for a teacher or school staff member making a referral for a comprehensive evaluation is somewhat different. As is evident in Figure 2.1, general education interventions must be developed, implemented, and evaluated prior to starting a comprehensive evaluation for a possible disability. These interventions usually emerge from a team meeting (sometimes multiple meetings) in which school personnel develop interventions for trial in the classroom through the use of a problem-solving, collaborative process with the referring teacher. These teams are generally referred to as student assistance teams (Lee & Jamison, 2003). These team meetings provide an excellent opportunity for the parents and health care providers of the chronically ill child to meet and discuss the most promising interventions that might be used in the classroom. As Shaw, Kelly, Joost, and Parker-Fisher (1995) pointed out, there are significant barriers to this type of collaboration including funding, time, and terminology differences. However, creative ways to involve health professionals (e.g., conference calls) need to be explored in an effort to increase the involvement of all of the important players in the child's life.

When a comprehensive evaluation is completed, parents and all involved professionals meet to discuss the results, draw conclusions, and promulgate recommendations to be forwarded to the team that will meet to create the IEP. If the parents disagree with the conclusions, they may request an independent educational evaluation to be done at public expense. This may be requested when a parent of a chronically ill child believes that an evaluation did not fully take into account their child's illness. Although the school may disagree with the parents and request a hearing to allow an independent hearing officer to assess the merit of the parents' request, any evaluation results that are obtained from an independent source (whether paid for by the parents or the school) must be considered when making final eligibility decisions.

Reevaluations are required for all students in special education at least every 3 years or if the parents or local education agency "determines that the educational or related services needs, including improved academic achievement and functional performance, of the child warrant a reevaluation" (IDEA, 20 U.S.C. § 1414 (a)(2)(A), 2004). The focus of the reevaluation includes the progress the student has made in the current special education placement. For children with chronic illness, their need for educational assistance may vary depending on changes in their health status. Therefore, parents and medical and teaching staff should be alert to changing medical status that might warrant a reevaluation of the child with chronic illness. Finally, for any comprehensive evaluation, the goals are twofold: (a) to assess eligibility for services and (b) to determine the type(s) and quantity of services the child needs. The final determination of school services to be provided to the child with chronic illness rests with the IEP team.

Provision of Services

The IEP is a plan of strategies and services designed to assist the child to make the largest academic improvement possible. The development of the IEP is akin to treatment planning that medical and mental health professionals do and should include a health service worker or medical liaison who is familiar with the child's health condition and planned medical treatments (Shaw & Páez, 2002).

Successful collaboration at the IEP meeting can result in well-integrated goals that take into account the child's medical condition as well as her or his academic needs. The development of the IEP should include measurable annual goals as well as clearly defined short-term objectives. The team is also charged with ensuring that

> to the maximum extent appropriate, children with disabilities, including children in public or private institutions or other care facilities, are educated with children who are not disabled, and special classes, separate schooling, or other removal of children with disabilities from the regular educational environment occurs only when the nature or severity of the disability of the child is such that education in regular classes with the use of supplementary aids and services cannot be achieved satisfactorily. (IDEA, 20 U.S.C. § 1412 (a)(5), 2004)

This principle is referred to as the least restrictive environment (LRE), and it focuses the attention of all caregivers on the notion that children may learn best and face the least social obstacles when maintained in the regular classroom environment (Hallahan & Kauffman, 2003).

When chronically ill children miss a significant amount of school during the year, there are provisions within IDEA that allow for extended school year services. To access these services, the child's IEP team must determine the need and recommend such service continuation. IDEA also has provisions to provide the chronically ill student that qualifies for special education with assistive technology devices or equipment that would "increase, maintain, or improve the functional capabilities of a child with a disability" (IDEA, 20 U.S.C. § 1401 (1), 2004).

Related and Supplementary Services

Supplementary services include aids, services, and supports (e.g., math manipulatives, tutoring) that help all children, including those with chronic illness, to benefit maximally from regular education classes (Wright & Wright, 2004). Additionally, chronically ill students who are eligible and require special education services may also receive related services such as speech, physical therapy, counseling, and school health services. Unlike supplementary services, related services are designed to help the child to benefit maximally from special education (Wright & Wright, 2004). The list of professionals and services available to the chronically ill child should be considered during program planning for the child. It should be noted that medical services from a licensed physician are available for diagnostic or evaluation purposes only. In contrast, a school nurse usually provides school health services; these include services (e.g., catheter insertion, ventilator maintenance) designed to help the child to benefit from special education and keep the child in school to the maximum extent possible. An additional related and critical service for chronically ill children is transportation.

Parents' Rights and Procedural Safeguards

The parents of a chronically ill child are under considerable stress. Studies have shown that the ability of the parents and family to cope with the illness and sequelae affects the adjustment and to some extent, the medical progress of the ill child (Wallander & Thompson, 1995). Parents are defined under IDEA as natural or adoptive parents, legal guardians, or educational advocates and should know their rights under IDEA. Parents have the right to (a) participate in meetings, including meetings with the student assistance, multidisciplinary (comprehensive evaluation), and IEP teams; (b) invite whomever they wish to the meeting, including the child's health care provider; (c) be informed of the child's progress in school; (d) give or revoke consent for evaluations, IEP goals or objectives, and any significant change in special education services for their child; (e) examine records or give consent for the release of records; (f) request an independent educational evaluation when the parent disagrees with the results or conclusions of an evaluation done at the school; and (g) receive a document that describes these rights.

Many of the interactions that parents of chronically ill children have under IDEA are meetings with school and or medical personnel. In meetings with parents, "the professional who fails to view the parent as a coequal agent in the care and treatment of the child may jeopardize the quality of care to the child and diminish the probability of an optimal treatment outcome" (Lee, 1991, p. 202). To welcome parental participation to the fullest extent, professionals should consider strategies for meetings with parents that would make them feel comfortable and encourage their involvement and participation (Lee & Guck, 2000, 2001). To encourage maximal parent participation, the following approaches are recommended:

- Reduce the number of participants at the meeting. Include only those that are absolutely necessary in the meeting.
- Create an informal atmosphere (e.g., talk to anyone, whenever you want).
- Provide information to the parents before the meeting. Although parents may hear information again at the meeting, they will have had time to consider it and its implications.
- Encourage parental participation. Include welcoming statements and include "door-opening" statements for involving parents.
- Communicate information to parents about available community services for which they may be eligible.
- Have regular meetings with parents, not just meetings that are required by law or when problems crop up.
- Provide the parents with a consistent contact person at the school, and call parents to remind them of meetings and what to bring.

- Reduce the use of jargon at meetings and check for parental understanding of the main points.

Procedural safeguards protect both the parents and the school, and these are designed to ensure that children obtain the best services that can be afforded to them under the law. If parents and the school district disagree on the educational diagnosis or plans for the child's education and cannot resolve the issue(s) on their own, three avenues may resolve such disputes. Either party may opt for mediation, which involves a disinterested third party who works to resolve the dispute. If successful, the parties reach a mutual agreement and sign a document affirming the agreement. If unsuccessful, the mediation is considered to be at an impasse. In this case, either party may request a due process hearing. The due process hearing has the appearance of a legal proceeding resulting in a binding ruling by an impartial hearing officer. Finally, parents may make a formal complaint in writing to the special education division of their state. Following an investigation, the complaint investigator will file a report that may contain corrective actions.

Parents have a right to limited confidentiality of educational records for their son or daughter under the Family Educational Rights and Privacy Act of 1976 (FERPA). Under this act, only parents or the student at age 18 may request the release of educational information and records to outside agencies with prior written consent. Within the school, personnel who have a "legitimate educational interest" in the student may view educational records. This would typically include the child's current teachers, the principal, and any related service personnel who work with the child at school. Under FERPA, parents and the student at age 18 may review their own records and may request to have their records amended if they choose.

SPECIFIC CHRONIC ILLNESSES AND IDEA

The specific service types and interventions used on behalf of children with chronic illnesses must take into account the specific needs of the child. It is clear that children with the same chronic health condition vary significantly in their ability to cope with the ramifications of the illness. Factors such as age, sex, socioeconomic status, ethnicity, coping strategies, family support, and social skills, to name a few, influence the specific educational, medical, mental health, and social needs of each child (Nabors & Lehmkuhl, 2004). As a result, even children with the same illness represent a heterogeneous group. The provisions of IDEA take this notion into account by requiring that assessment services and the development of interventions be tailored to the needs of the child through the use of multidisciplinary teams in the diagnostic and intervention planning process. In this way, children with the same educational diagnosis may have significantly different educational plans.

Nonetheless, there are some commonalities related to the specific nature of certain disease processes that affect many of the children afflicted. Theis (1999) pointed out that children with pulmonary conditions (e.g., asthma, cystic fibrosis) may have impaired memory, vision, or hearing, or feel anxious because of the long-term use of medications used to treat these disorders (e.g., steroids). Under IDEA, these children are eligible for special education services if it can be documented that the illness influences learning. The services such a child receives could include learning strategies delivered by the regular or special education teacher to enhance and improve memory and study skills (Gleason, Archer, & Colvin, 2002). Under IDEA, the child's special or regular education teacher may provide these and other needed services depending on the provisions of the student's IEP. For example, children with leukemia may experience impaired attention, short-term memory problems, or poor visuomotor coordination due to radiation treatments (Theis, 1999). Metacognitive or cuing strategies (Swanson, 2005) may be used to enhance short-term memory, and motor skills may be improved through exercises and regular practice of motor tasks under the supervision of a school-based occupational therapist (Semrud-Clikeman & Walkowiak, 2005). These examples illustrate how a school may tailor services on the basis of the specific needs of children with chronic illnesses.

SECTION 504 OF THE REHABILITATION ACT OF 1973

Section 504 is concerned with equal access and treatment for disabled persons for employment, education, and any public activity. State and local agencies that receive federal funds cannot discriminate against people with disabilities. Historically, Section 504 was primarily concerned with equal employment practices, but over the past 20 years, the Office of Civil Rights has become more active in enforcing Section 504 in education.

Under Section 504, a school discriminates against a chronically ill student when it denies the individual the right to participate in or benefit from school activities that are afforded to nonhandicapped students (e.g., clubs, sports, recognition). The school district must provide aids or services that are equivalent or afford the chronically ill student an equal opportunity to achieve in school as those afforded nonhandicapped children.

The definition of a disability under Section 504 includes people who have a mental or physical disability that limits major life activities (e.g., performing manual tasks, walking, seeing, hearing, breathing, learning, working). Chronic illnesses such as arthritis, asthma, and cancer are examples of conditions that would most likely fall under this broad definition. All students that carry an IDEA handicap are also qualified under Section 504, but not all students qualified under Section 504 qualify under IDEA. For example, a student with Crohn's disease featuring remitting and relapsing symptoms may require special accommodations such as special bathroom privileges, supervision while taking medications, or counseling services to treat the effects of stigmatization or low self-esteem (Proctor & Kranzler, 1998). Provided the student was able to maintain sufficient school progress with these accommodations, the child generally would not be eligible for special education services under IDEA.

To avoid discriminatory practices, schools must provide the chronically ill child with accommodations (e.g., aids, services, opportunities) that are effective in allowing the child to participate in the same education curriculum and school activities as their nondisabled counterparts. A school may evaluate children with a chronic illness to assess the degree to which the disability affects their education. The nature of the evaluation may vary depending on the nature of the disability, but key persons familiar with the student (parents, teachers, the child's physician) should be included in the process. The evaluation should focus on the educational impact of the disability on the child to determine the most appropriate educational services. The results of the evaluation should draw conclusions about the child's eligibility for accommodations under Section 504, the student's unmet needs, and services or accommodations that should be afforded the child.

The plan for accommodations or services for students should be evaluated periodically. Although all school staff should be aware of the provisions of Section 504 and the 504 plan for children in their charge, schools should have a Section 504 coordinator who can faciliatate training for staff and manage the process of evaluations, providing accommodations and scheduling periodic reviews for all disabled students in need within the building.

NO CHILD LEFT BEHIND ACT OF 2001

The goal of NCLB was to improve the quality of education in the United States and to narrow the gap between low-achieving and high-achieving students. To accomplish this, the law requires states to set challenging standards for students and to administer periodic assessments of academic progress against those standards. Schools are held accountable for the progress of all students. NCLB promotes school reform and the use of evidence-based approaches for instruction to help schools improve the academic performance of all students.

The reauthorized IDEA aligns itself with the NCLB. Students with disabilities are now able to receive appropriate accommodations on regular all-school assessments as dictated by the student's IEP team. In evaluating a student with a disability, IDEA states that the child's IEP must "include a statement of any individual modifications in the administration of State or district-wide assessments of student achievement that are needed in order for the child to participate in the assessment" (IDEA, 34 U.S.C. § 300.347 (a)(5), 2004). In addition, the IEP team is responsible for determining whether a student will participate in all or part of the State or district assessment. Under the 2005 proposed revisions to IDEA, states may adopt alternate achievement standards to measure the achievement of those children who have been identified as having a disability.

NCLB requires that schools maintain steady progress in achievement for all students in the core subjects of math, reading, and science. If annual yearly progress (AYP) is not met for 2 consecutive years, then the school must be designated as "in need of improvement." With this designation, the school is required to notify parents and offer the choice to all students to attend a different school that is meeting its AYP goals. Students with disabilities are also given this choice, although the school district has the right to place a student at a school that will still provide that student with a free appropriate public education, as mandated by IDEA.

If the school has not met AYP goals for 3 consecutive years, then the school must notify the parents of all students, including those with disabilities, of their failure to meet AYP. In addition, the school is required to provide additional supplemental educational services for all students to ensure that AYP may be met. Students with disabilities are also entitled to such supplemental educational services, provided by the school district.

CONCLUSION

The lack of a clear understanding of the laws that govern the educational services that are available to children with chronic illness represents a significant barrier to the academic progress of these children. This lack of knowledge reduces the quality of collaboration between children's health care providers and parents and the school personnel. Although this volume seeks to fill this void, it must be acknowledged that chronically ill children vary significantly in their need for remedial educational services. For those whose chronic illness can be shown to affect directly their educational progress, the schools provide an impressive array of services to assist the child to maximize his or her scholastic potential. Federal laws govern the processes for assessment, identification, and service provision, and parents and health care providers should be aware of and conform to these laws that mandate the procedural steps involved in accessing special services for chronically ill children. The processes and services provided to children through IDEA, NCLB, and Section 504, although not perfect, do attempt to provide adequate safeguards to protect parents and children with a goal of providing the best educational environment for learning.

REFERENCES

Family Educational Rights and Privacy Act. Implementing Regulations, 34 C.F.R. § 99.3 (1976).

Gleason, M. M., Archer, A. L., & Colvin, G. (2002). Interventions for improving study skills. In M. Shinn, H. Walker, & G. Stoner (Eds.), *Interventions for academic and behavioral problems II: Preventive and remedial approaches* (pp. 651–680). Bethesda, MD: National Association of School Psychologists.

Hallahan, D. P., & Kauffman, J. M. (2003). *Exceptional learners: Introduction to special education*. Boston: Allyn & Bacon.

Individuals With Disabilities Education Improvement Act of 2004, 20 U.S.C. § 1401 (2004).

Lee, S. W. (1991). The family with a chronically ill child. In M. J. Fine (Ed.), *Collaboration with parents of exceptional children* (pp. 201–218). Brandon, VT: Clinical Psychology.

Lee, S. W., & Guck, T. P. (2000). The family with a chronically ill child. In M. J. Fine & R. L. Simpson (Eds.), *Collaboration with parents and families of children and youth with exceptionalities* (2nd ed., pp. 257–276). Austin, TX: Pro-Ed.

Lee, S. W., & Guck, T. P. (2001). Parenting chronically ill children. In M. J. Fine & S. W. Lee (Eds.), *Handbook of diversity in parent education* (pp. 277–297). San Diego, CA: Academic Press.

Lee, S. W., & Jamison, T. R. (2003). Including the FBA process in student assistance teams: An exploratory study of team communications and intervention selection. *Journal of Educational and Psychological Consultation, 14*, 209–239.

Madan-Swain, A., Katz, E. R., & LaGory, J. (2004). School and social reintegration after a serious illness or injury. In R. T. Brown (Ed.), *Handbook of pediatric psychology in school settings* (pp. 637–655). Mahwah, NJ: Erlbaum.

Nabors, L. A., & Lehmkuhl, H. D. (2004). Children with chronic medical conditions: Recommendations for mental health clinicians. *Journal of Developmental and Physical Disabilities, 16*, 1–15.

Newacheck, P. W., & Halfon, N. (1998). Prevalence and impact of disabling chronic conditions in children. *American Journal of Public Health, 88*, 610–617.

No Child Left Behind Act of 2001, 20 U.S.C. § 6301 *et seq.* (2001).

Power, T. J., Heathfield, L. T., McGoey, K. E., & Blum, N. J. (1999). Managing and preventing chronic health problems in children and youth: School psychology's expanded mission. *School Psychology Review, 28*, 251–263.

Proctor, B. E., & Kranzler, J. H. (1998). Crohn's disease. In L. Phelps (Ed.), *A guide to understanding and educating health related disorders in children and adolescents* (pp. 197–203). Washington, DC: American Psychological Association.

Rehabilitation Act of 1973, 20 C.F.R. § Part 104 (1973).

Semrud-Clikeman, M., & Walkowiak, J. (2005). Motor assessment. In S. W. Lee & P. Lowe (Eds.), *Encyclopedia of school psychology*. Thousand Oaks, CA: Sage.

Sexson, S. B., & Madan-Swain, A. (1993). School reentry for the child with chronic illness. *Journal of Learning Disabilities, 26*, 115–125.

Shapiro, E. S., & Manz, P. H. (2004). Collaborating with schools in the provision of pediatric psychological services. In R. T. Brown (Ed.), *Handbook of pediatric psychology in school settings* (pp. 49–64). Mahwah, NJ: Erlbaum.

Shaw, S. R., Kelly, D. P., Joost, J. C., & Parker-Fisher, S. J. (1995). School-linked and school-based health services: A renewed call for collaboration between school psychologists and medical professionals. *Psychology in the Schools, 32,* 190–201.

Shaw, S. R., & Páez, D. (2002). Best practices in interdisciplinary service delivery to children with chronic medical issues. In A. Thomas & J. Grimes (Eds.), *Best practices in school psychology IV* (pp. 1473–1483). Bethesda, MD: National Association of School Psychologists.

Swanson, H. L. (2005). Memory. In S. W. Lee & P. Lowe (Eds.), *Encyclopedia of school psychology.* Thousand Oaks, CA: Sage.

Theis, K. M. (1999). Identifying the educational implications of chronic illness in school children. *Journal of School Health, 69,* 392–397.

Wallander, J. L., & Thompson, R. J., Jr. (1995). Psychosocial adjustment of children with chronic physical conditions. In M. C. Roberts (Ed.), *Handbook of pediatric psychology* (2nd ed., pp 124–141). New York: Guilford Press.

Wright, P. W., & Wright, P. D. (2004). *Wrightslaw: Special education law.* Harfield, VA: Harbor House Law Press.

3

CHILDREN WITH CANCER

MICHAEL K. CRUCE AND TERRY A. STINNETT

Cancer is a major public health burden in the United States accounting for one in four deaths (Jemal et al., 2004). Cancer typically refers to a group of related diseases that are distinguished by uncontrolled cell growth and the resulting spread of abnormal cells. These cells are considered to be malformed but may outlive normal cells and continue to reproduce additional deviant cells, resulting in a breakdown of organ functioning in the body. Many cancers take the form of tumors; however, other cancers, such as leukemia, affect the blood, resulting in complications across numerous organs. Cancer is believed to be caused by both genetic and environmental factors with at least 5% to 10% of cancers being hereditary in nature (American Cancer Society, 2003). Cancer may also be a result of contacts with chemicals, infectious diseases, or radiation exposure. Additionally, there appears to be a strong behavioral component to the acquisition of several cancer types, resulting in medical professionals actively discouraging in recent decades potentially dangerous contributing activities such as smoking and sunbathing.

Medical advances have greatly increased longevity and quality of life in both children and adolescents with cancer. Consequently, it has been reconceptualized from an inevitably fatal illness to a life-threatening chronic difficulty, resulting in a paradigm shift from preparing families for end-of-life scenarios to a focus on issues related to quality of life. Survivors of childhood and adolescent cancer are a high-risk population for experiencing chronic and late-occurring health problems as well as diminished quality of life associated with previous cancer therapy (Oeffinger & Hudson, 2004). The emergence of survivorship of cancer in children and adolescents has prompted psychologists to examine the psychosocial, cognitive, behavioral, and quality-of-life difficulties that these young people experience. There is increasing interest in empirically supported psychosocial and behavioral treatments for these youth. Furthermore, siblings of children with cancer may also experience adjustment difficulties, particularly social and academic functioning (Labay & Walco, 2004). Finally, educational systems have been presented with the challenging task of providing effective services to children with these potentially life threatening health impairments.

This chapter provides an overview of pediatric cancer; its related medical, psychosocial, and educational sequelae; treatment options; and outcomes. Prevalence rates, staging of the disease, and different types of cancer in children are given attention. Potential emotional and behavioral difficulties related to childhood cancer, chronic pain, and traumatizing treatments and the idea of cancer as a lifelong illness are discussed. The chapter ends with a brief conclusion.

OVERVIEW

Prevalence estimates of childhood cancer indicate that approximately 9,000 new cases of cancer occurred in 2003, resulting in about 1,500 deaths. The American Cancer Society (2003) reported that cancer is currently the chief cause of death by disease in children and is the third leading cause of death overall in children, behind unintentional injuries and homicides (American Cancer Society, 2003). Currently, the 5-year survival rate of children with cancer is at 75%, the 10-year survival rate is approaching 70%, and the cure rate is greater than 60%. The incidence rates of cancer are higher in boys than in girls; highest in Caucasians, followed by Hispanics, Asian/Pacific Islanders, and African Americans; and are lowest in American Indians/Alaska Natives (American Cancer Society, 2003). Although data on childhood cancer prevalence were not kept before the 1970s, trends over time suggest that cancer rates in children increased until the start of the 1990s when they leveled off and began to decline. There have been slight increases in several of the classes of cancer in children since the mid-1990s, but these increases have been attributed to newer diagnostic techniques that enable doctors to identify and treat cancer at younger ages than were previously detected by medical science (American Cancer Society, 2003). Still, childhood cancer is considered rare, comprising less than 1% of all malignancies diagnosed each year in developed countries.

Although cancer in adults is typically categorized by its location within the body (e.g., breast or lung cancer), cancers in children are classified into 12 major categories under the International Classification of Childhood Cancers (ICCC). Additionally, cancer is categorized, or staged, based on the extent of spread from the site of origin. Cancer is studied by the extent of the primary tumor (T), whether there is lymph node involvement (N), and whether the cancer has spread or metastasized (M; spread through the body). Each of the TNM categories is then given a stage of I, II, III, or IV, with stage I considered early and stage IV considered advanced. This staging procedure assists oncologists in determining the most appropriate treatment protocol. Although this broad classification system exists, the largest percentage of young people with cancer have one of a small handful of diagnoses, with the largest percentage of young people being diagnosed with leukemia, central nervous system tumors, or lymphoma.

The most prevalent type of cancer found in children is leukemia, which accounts for about one third of all oncology cases in children under 15 and affects approximately 2,600 children in the United States each year (American Cancer Society, 2003). Prior to the early 1970s, leukemia was considered to be a fatal diagnosis, but with the advent of central nervous system prophylaxis such as cranial radiation therapy (CRT), the survival rate has approached 70%. Leukemia is known to be a malignant disorder of the blood-forming tissues, specifically the bone marrow, lymph nodes, and spleen. The blood-forming tissues flood the bloodstream and lymph system with abnormal and immature white blood cells, and these immature cells cannot carry out the normal cells' function of fighting infections in the body. They also reduce production of normal red blood cells (which prevent anemia), as well as tiny discs called platelets (which regulate coagulation and bleeding). If left uncontrolled, leukemia will cause (a) infections because of the lack of normal infection-fighting white blood cells; (b) severe anemia, because of the lack of oxygen-carrying red blood cells; and (c) bruising and hemorrhaging, because of the lack of platelets. Leukemia is further classified into two broad categories: acute and chronic. Acute leukemia affects immature white blood cells, progresses rapidly, and is the type most often seen in children. Chronic leukemia occurs most frequently in adults and progresses slowly, often over a period of many years (Leukemia Society of America, 2000). Additionally, leukemia can be either lymphocytic/lymphoblastic, which involves cells that are formed in the lymph nodes and spleen, or myelocytic/myelogenous, which affects cells directly in the bone marrow (Leukemia Society of America, 2000). Acute lymphoblastic leukemia is more prevalent than acute myeloblastic leukemia (Lightfoot & Roman, 2004).

Central nervous system tumors are the second most common type of cancer in children, making up approximately 20% of cases of childhood cancer and occurring most frequently in people less than 10 years of age. This translates to about 1,500 children per year in the United States. This category of childhood cancer consists of tumors in the brain or spinal column. A tumor may create pressure in an afflicted area, resulting in damage regardless of whether the tumor is benign or malignant. More than half of central nervous system tumors are a specific subtype called *astrocytomas* (brain tumors that develop from a star-shaped cell called an astrocyte), which have incidence rates highest in children from birth to age 7 and survival rates that are better the later the onset of the disease. Pediatric brain tumors have a much better prognosis than adult brain tumors do, but clinicians face associated problems for children. First, pediatric brain tumors are often misdiagnosed or diagnosed late because of their rarity. Additionally, current treatments may damage the developing brain, and, because there are several tumor types, there are only a small number of patients with specific tumor types to enroll in therapy trials.

Lymphomas are the third most common form of childhood cancer and make up approximately 10% to 15% of the cases of childhood cancer. Lymphomas directly affect the lymphatic system, the part of the body that fights disease and infections. Lymphatic vessels carry lymph, a colorless, watery fluid containing infection-fighting cells known as lymphocytes to areas known as lymph nodes (American Cancer Society, 2003). Lymphomas in children are classified as Hodgkin's disease or non-Hodgkin's lymphomas. Hodgkin's disease is a specific lymphoma subtype that contains an abnormal cell known as the Reed–Sternberg cell, which is not found in other lymphomas. In Hodgkin's disease, lymphoma cells spread from their original site to affect other sites as well as other organs through the bloodstream. The incidence rates of Hodgkin's disease have steadily declined between 1975 and 1995, and the 5-year survival rate for Hodgkin's patients has increased to 91% (American Cancer Society, 2003). Non-Hodgkin's lymphomas, by contrast, consist of abnormal cells in the lymphatic system that can occur in one or more parts of the body simultaneously. Non-Hodgkin's lymphoma rates typically increase throughout childhood with incidence rates remaining stable in recent years and with a 5-year survival rate of 73% among those diagnosed from 1989 to 1995 (American Cancer Society, 2003).

Additionally, a variety of diverse and more unique cancer diagnoses may be seen in children and adolescents, but these subtypes occur infrequently in young people and are certainly rarer than the previously mentioned types of cancers. These additional cancers include (a) osteosarcomas, a bone cancer comprising 2.4% of all childhood cancers; (b) Ewing's sarcoma, another cancer of the bone, making up 1.7% of the cases; (c) neuroblastomas, occurring in the abdomen in 7.5% of cancer cases; (d) rhabdomyosarcomas, a soft-tissue sarcoma typically occurring in the head or neck in 3.4% of the cases; (e) retinoblastomas, which comprise 3.1% of the cases and consist of an often curable cancer of the eye; and (f) Wilm's tumor, a kidney cancer that makes up approximately 6% of childhood cancers (American Cancer Society, 2003).

OUTCOMES

Children with cancer are likely to turn to family and friends for social support (Manne & Miller, 1998). This support may be difficult for the child to seek out at school for fear of social ostracism, however. For a child with cancer, school may prove to be an uncomfortable environment requiring interventions to facilitate the child's overall adjustment and well-being (Prevatt, Heffer, & Lowe, 2000). Children with cancer have been rated by their peers as more socially withdrawn and less likely to be thought of as a best friend by their classmates (Vannatta, Zeller, Noll, & Koontz, 1998). This may be due to decreased social functioning on the part of the child with cancer or a lack of empathy and understanding on the part of his or her classmates (Manne & Miller, 1998). The average size of peer groups of children with cancer is smaller than the peer groups of their healthy counterparts (Nichols, 1995). This may be in part explained by the young person displaying low self-confidence because of a perceived lack of social support from others, possibly coupled with noticeable signs of health impairment, for example, visible hair loss, nausea and vomiting, or use of assisted walking devices (Novakovic et al., 1996).

High rates of conflict are likely to be present for both mothers and fathers of children with cancer when compared to parents of children with no chronic health impairments (Manne & Miller, 1998). This has been attributed to the young person's desire for some degree of autonomy while facing the reality of needing increased assistance from parents due to illness. Also, as many as 25% to 35% of parents may eventually develop some level of psychological difficulty as a result of their child's diagnosis. Having a child diagnosed with a serious medical condition can provoke a variety of stressors in parents, including watching the child's condition deteriorate, helping the child deal with painful medical treatments and side effects in the hospital, and battling with health care bills. Some research, however, suggests that receiving information about a family member's cancer may be related to positive psychological adjustment in children and may be a protective factor for siblings of children with the disease (Eiser & Havermans, 1994; Labay & Walco, 2004; Lobato & Kao, 2002).

Children diagnosed with cancer may display a variety of behavioral and emotional difficulties. Little empirical evidence consistently supports that young people with cancer have higher rates of psychopathology than their healthy counterparts, however. Unfortunately, many young cancer patients are not routinely screened for difficulties such as depression, and few cancer patients are prescribed any type of antidepressant medication. An obstacle to obtaining reliable prevalence rates of depression in children with cancer is that the symptoms of cancer and side effects of treatments (e.g., sleep disturbances, weight loss, lack of energy, and loss of interest in previous activities) are the same vegetative symptoms and criteria used for diagnosis of a major depressive disorder. Additionally, fatigue and insomnia have been shown to occur in at least 40% to 50% of adult cancer patients and may be even higher in younger patients (Walsh, Donnelly, & Rybicki, 2000). Fatigue is the most distressing treatment-related symptom in children and adolescents. Children undergoing cancer treatments described fatigue as a profound sense of being physically tired or having difficulty moving their arms or legs, whereas adolescents discussed it as a changing state of mental exhaustion that could include physical, mental, and emotional tiredness. Pediatric oncology staff members have reported it as emotional or mental withdrawal, mood changes such as irritability and decreased cooperation, and a physical desire to rest or lie down (Hockenberry et al., 2003). Engstrom, Strohl, and Rose (1999) found chronic sleep problems in 44% of a sample of 150 participants who had cancer. To complicate diagnosis further, symptoms of depression are often seen as a developmentally appropriate response to having been diagnosed with a chronic medical condition, and, as a result, some physicians may pay inadequate attention to the depressive symptoms of cancer patients.

Children diagnosed with cancer may also display symptoms associated with various anxiety disorders. The child diagnosed with cancer has the potential to experience fear and avoidance of the topic of cancer. Children may or may not grasp the meaning of the diagnosis or its ramifications on their lives. These children also deal with a course of treatment that may be unusual and painful. For example, children with acute lymphoblastic leukemia must endure a series of invasive procedures including lumbar punctures, which are associated with intense pain and anxiety. This may be especially unnerving if the child also senses dread on the part of his or her parents. Children who are more pain sensitive and receive intervention may show greater decreases in distress over time than do pain-sensitive children who do not receive intervention. Consequently, those children who are most vulnerable to distress and anxiety during medical procedures should be identified prior to undergoing invasive procedures and provided psychological intervention (Chen, Craske, Katz, Schwartz, & Zeltzer, 2000). Finally, it is difficult to calculate the prevalence of anxiety disorders in pediatric cancer patients, and there are no reliable estimates of the percentage of children who experience serious anxiety symptoms.

Posttraumatic stress symptoms in children with cancer or their parents were reported in approximately 20 studies between 1991 and 2005. Prevalence estimates for posttraumatic stress disorder (PTSD) symptomology across these studies have been estimated between 2% and 20% in children and between 10% and 30% in their parents, even years after the end of cancer treatment (Taieb, Moro, Baubet, Revah-Levy, & Flament, 2003). Although results across studies varied, in general, adults who had survived childhood cancer had fairly good long-term adaptation with relatively low levels of psychiatric sequelae (Eiser, Hill, & Vance, 2000; Mackie, Hill, Kondryn, & McNally, 2000). Interestingly, Kazak et al. (1997) examined anxiety and posttraumatic stress sequelae in 130 former childhood leukemia patients and their families, and there were significantly more posttraumatic stress symptoms in both mothers and fathers of childhood leukemia survivors and few reports of the symptoms by the children. Kazak et al. also found no long-term anxiety or avoidance behaviors in cancer survivors. Stuber, Kazak, Meeske, and Barakat (1998) speculated that considering cancer as an extreme stressor and applying a trauma model to the disease has shifted clinicians away from considering the psychological effects as part of an adjustment disorder. Reluctance of parents or of the childhood survivors to participate in long-term studies may be understood as avoidance, a symptom of PTSD. These individuals may also minimize their difficulties to avoid reminders of the cancer and its treatment (Taieb et al., 2003). Nonetheless, identifying PTSD in children who have survived cancer may be problematic because there is a lack of adequate instrumentation for assessing it in children and an overreliance on parental report (American Academy of Child and Adolescent Psychiatry Official Action, 1998; Perrin, Smith, & Yule, 2000). Nonetheless, children with cancer should receive routine screenings for internalizing problems as they may experience anxiety and depressive symptomology on initial diagnosis, when faced with treatment procedures, and when discussing future life events related to their cancer experience.

The treatments for cancer (e.g., radiation therapies and chemotherapies) may also result in adverse cognitive effects on the child, and the young person may experience deficits in cognitive and academic areas where he or she previously displayed no difficulties. The long-term cognitive effects of various cancer treatments are not well documented. There may, however, be modest negative effects on cognitive functioning following central nervous system prophylactic chemotherapy in children. It has also been suggested that other diseases of the blood (i.e., sickle cell anemia), may negatively affect cognitive functioning, suggesting that hematological diseases in general may yield similar results.

A comprehensive understanding of cancer pain is necessary because it is often one of the presenting symptoms in the initial cancer diagnosis. Management of cancer pain in children is critical to minimize psychological distress and physiologic responses to the illness and its treatment (Anghelescu & Oakes, 2000). Prior to the widespread use of conscious sedation in childhood cancer patients, these children endured bone marrow aspirations, lumbar punctures, and intravenous injections as highly painful treatments. Even with sedation, however, all three procedures continue to elicit symptoms of anxiety and fear before, during, and after their implementation. Children may become nauseated, vomit, and develop skin rashes or insomnia in anticipation of the procedures; cry, scream, and resist during the procedures; and become withdrawn, angry, or embarrassed afterward (Kazak et al., 1997). In some cases, the procedures and related pain are so traumatic that long-lasting fear of hospitals, medical staff, and medical paraphernalia can occur.

Assessment of pain is critical to manage it successfully. Sources of pain related to childhood cancer vary; however, pain precursors can be categorized into three broad classes: (a) disease-related, (b) procedure-related, and (c) treatment-related pain. Disease-related pain occurs prior to diagnosis and usually disappears upon initial treatment efforts. Disease-related pain occurs as a result of cells having been invaded by cancer material. This may result in a variety of symptoms, including headache, joint and bone pain, and neuropathic pain. Procedure-related pains usually result from the diagnostic measures that accompany cancer treatment. Such invasive procedures include lumbar punctures, venipunctures, and bone marrow aspirations. Finally, treatment-related pain is associated with cancer management. Treatments such as radiation therapy and chemotherapy can result in nausea, infections, and abdominal pain. Both anticipatory and post-chemotherapy symptoms are noted to occur in children and youth, with greater percentages of adolescents being affected than children, probably because the chemotherapy protocols for adolescents use agents with more potential to cause nausea and vomiting (McQuaid & Nassau, 1999).

MEDICAL AND PSYCHOEDUCATIONAL IMPLICATIONS

The American Cancer Society (2003) posits two challenges related to pediatric oncology: to continue progress in effectively destroying the cancer and to minimize the impact of treatments on the child's long-term quality of life. It would be erroneous to conclude that a child will return to normal functioning simply because of an absence of disease at the end of therapy. Survivors of childhood cancer are a high-risk population because the curative therapies administered for it affect growing and developing tissues, and late-occurring health problems may not become clinically apparent until decades after treatment. Also, although the causes of childhood cancer may be unknown or difficult to determine, parents and children often make attributions as to the origin of the disease. As would be expected, children and parents who make external causal attributions about the cancer and related difficulties display a significantly better quality of life than those who make internal attributions about the source. Furthermore, children often report that addressing psychosocial difficulties is a top priority after diagnosis and treatment. Adults who are active participants in the life of the child are able to play a significant role in relieving the associated difficulties that these children exhibit. Behavioral training for families and teachers may help adults assist children with chronic illnesses to behave more confidently, thereby reducing the risk of further emotional and behavioral problems (Cleave & Charlton, 1997).

Recent effective medical treatments for children with cancer have resulted in the new paradigm of cancer as a lifelong chronic illness. As a result, there are a variety of pharmacological options available for children living with pain. Treatments prescribed by physicians for these youth typically consist of local anesthetics, general anesthetics, sedative hypnotics, and opioids. Modern medical regimens to combat cancer in children typically consist of chemotherapy, surgery, radiation therapy, immunotherapy, or a combination of these treatments based on the initial diagnosis and staging of the cancer. Chemotherapy consists of an individually designed care protocol in which a child is given medications either orally or through injections for the purposes of treating cancer that has metastasized. This treatment procedure often occurs over a period lasting approximately 6 months and may prevent the cancer from returning if it is completely destroyed. Although chemotherapy is an effective treatment or an adjunct treatment for a variety of cancers, it often yields side effects that are unpleasant for the child. Many children report fatigue, nausea, and vomiting after treatment sessions, and children may have an increased chance of infections or temporary hair loss after treatment (American Cancer Society, 2003).

In radiation therapy, the site of the child's cancer is exposed to radioactive materials, which prevents the cancerous cells from continually dividing, resulting in the death of malignant cells. Healthy cells may also be affected during radiation treatments, so oncologists attempt to localize the radiation treatments to affect only the specific site of the tumor. Side effects are typically relegated to the area affected by radiation and most frequently consist of a sunburn-type skin condition at the site of exposure, fatigue, and nausea (American Cancer Society, 2003). Depending on the type of tumor, its site, and its growth, another potential medical treatment option is surgery, whereby the cancerous material and the surrounding tissue are removed. Sometimes lymph nodes near the site of the tumor will also be removed. Radiation therapy and chemotherapy may initially be used in conjunction with surgery to shrink the tumor or to make sure that all of the cancerous material is destroyed (American Cancer Society, 2003).

Oncologists may also use biologic therapy, also known as immunotherapy, a treatment option in which the body's immune system is used to fight cancerous cells and promote the continued growth of healthy cells. In immunotherapy, chemicals called biological response modifiers are given to the child to repair damaged cells and directly interfere with malignant cell growth. Side effects of biologic therapies include nausea, chills, fever, rash, loss of appetite, and diarrhea (American Cancer Society, 2003). Finally, some children with leukemia, lymphoma, or brain tumors may undergo a bone marrow transplant (BMT), a procedure whereby the damaged spongy tissue inside of bones is replaced with healthy stem cells to grow new, healthy cells (American Cancer Society, 2003). The healthy bone marrow may be harvested from the child (done previously while he or she was in remission), a family member, or a donor whom the child does not know. Children who receive BMTs are frequently in the hospital for a period of several months and require a high degree of supervision and monitoring.

After conducting a meta-analysis on pharmacological and cognitive–behavioral interventions, Kuppenheimer and Brown (2002) indicated that cognitive–behavioral treatment protocols are effective for relieving procedural distress and that pharmacological therapies are relatively safe and effective when administered and monitored by medical personnel. Common effective cognitive–behavioral strategies for children with cancer include reframing, active coping, distraction, imagery, making a pain plan, motivation and messages, and breathing exercises (Woznick & Goodheart, 2002). Other specific techniques designed to reduce anxiety and distress include progressive muscle relaxation, positive self-talk, filmed modeling, behavioral rehearsal and precoaching, reinforcement schedules, and the simultaneous practices of ignoring pain and replacing negative thoughts with positive coping self-statements. Distraction has also been used to divert the child's attention from noxious stimuli by either redirecting the child's attention or actively involving the child in the performance of a diversionary task (Kleiber & Haper, 1999). It should be noted that even when coping strategies are taught to children, not all improvements are maintained over time without receiving a booster session or verbal prompts for the continued use of learned skills (Gil et al., 1996). Some longitudinal studies have suggested that the capacity for coping with pain may be stable over time even if intervention does not continue, however (Gil, Wilson, & Edens, 1997).

Another psychosocial treatment option for children with cancer is stress inoculation and education. Stress inoculation procedures emphasize reducing the amount of anxiety experienced by the child, which will, in turn, decrease perceived levels of pain and increase relaxation. By adding an educational component, the child may feel more secure and in control of his or her cancer related experiences. Stress inoculation typically starts with a preparation phase in which the child is included in the discussion about stress, pain, and medical procedures. The child may be given a tour of the treatment room, allowed to handle the equipment, and encouraged to talk to others who have undergone treatment. Parental involvement is highly encouraged in both stress inoculation and education because research supports that parental involvement may reduce anxiety stressors.

Controversial and untested methods are also in use for treating children with cancer. Kelly (2004) reports that 31% to 84% of children with cancer also use complementary and alternative medicine (CAM) therapies to alleviate pain and symptoms of cancer, especially to reduce the side effects of cancer treatments. These are used mostly as adjuncts to support conventional medical treatment and include alternative medical systems (e.g., homeopathy, traditional Chinese medicine), mind–body medicine (e.g., meditation, prayer, art, music), biologically based therapy (e.g., dietary supplements, herbal products), manipulative and body-based methods (e.g., chiropractic or osteopathic manipulation), energy and biofield therapies (e.g., qiqong, reiki, therapeutic touch), and bioelectromagnetic-based techniques (e.g., pulsed fields, magnetic fields, alternating or direct current fields; Kelly, 2004). These fall outside the mainstream, are generally unregulated, and most have been subjected to little, if any, scientific scrutiny. Therefore, they cannot be endorsed as potentially promising interventions. Even more alarming, less than half of parents who use CAM notify the child's physician (Kelly et al., 2000; McCurdy, Spangler, Wofford, Chauvenet, & McClean, 2003). Parents may resort to CAM because of the desire to do everything possible for their child. Other factors related to the use of CAM include poor prognosis, prior CAM use, older age, and religiosity (Gagnon & Recklitis, 2003; Kelly et al., 2000). Other techniques are also available and widely publicized—for example, hypnosis or traditional counseling—but are used less frequently because there is some question as to the efficacy of the outcome for the child when comparing the treatments to ones that emphasize a pharmacological or behavioral component (Smith, Barabasz, & Barabasz, 1996).

The role of the psychologist in preparing the child and the school for the child's return after the student's diagnosis or treatment has received an increased focus in the scientific literature over the course of the last decade. This is important considering that children often report that the most difficult part of their cancer experience is the return to school. Off-task behavior, truancy, and work refusal are frequently seen difficulties for these young people, and they may have continued absences because of medical appointments, hospitalizations for treatment, or school avoidance. Although the child's environment and life circumstances may have changed drastically over the course of cancer treatment, life at the school has probably changed little during this time, resulting in an environment that may not suit the particular needs of the child with cancer. Because school is the environment where children practice socialization, young people with newly diagnosed cancer are encouraged to return to school and their premorbid social experiences as soon as possible. Research has shown, however, that lower perceived social support from classmates may increase the risk for psychopathology in the child with cancer and may result in avoidance behavior on the part of the child (Varni, Katz, Colegrove, & Dolgin, 1994).

A variety of school-reintegration programs are available to families and academic personnel, and many large medical centers offer school reintegration as a part of their related services. If the child's hospital does not offer this, a reintegration program may be undertaken by a school social worker or psychologist, focusing on topics such as listening skills, identifying behavioral difficulties, educating school staff, and intervention planning at home and at school. Most reintegration programs contain similar components consisting of an educational protocol for teachers and students along with written materials for the school explaining cancer terminology and research. Prevatt et al. (2000) reviewed available reintegration programs and found that they primarily fit into three categories: school personnel education programs, peer education programs, or combined programs. Educating both school personnel and peers on information related to cancer is considered a promising strategy for assisting children with the transition back to school. Nonetheless, none of the reintegration programs reviewed follow a strict theoretical foundation, the teacher and peer interventions have not been followed longitudinally, and many of the combined programs rely heavily on qualitative reports of effectiveness. Educating school staff and peers on cancer should assist in social acceptance, which is a developmental factor in the positive adjustment of the child with cancer.

CONCLUSION

Cancer has been identified as a major public health problem in the United States and has been indicated to be the third leading cause of death in children. Medical advances have, however, increased the life span and number of survivors of childhood and adolescent cancer. These children and youth have been recognized as a high-risk population for developing further health, social, educational, and psychological difficulties that can have a negative impact on quality of life. Children and adolescents with cancer may be more socially withdrawn in school settings, and may display various behavioral, social, educational, and emotional difficulties, although there is little evidence that they have higher rates of psychopathology than their healthy counterparts. These difficulties include depressive, anxious, and post-traumatic stress symptoms; school adjustment problems; and fears and avoidance behavior related to treatment. Treatments for the cancers found in these youth include radiation therapies, chemotherapy, immunotherapy, and surgery, or some combination of these. Some complementary and alternative medical therapies are also used in children with cancer, but these have generally not been systematically studied and are not widely accepted. Additionally, various cognitive–behavioral, pharmacological, and stress inoculation interventions have been used to reduce anxiety in childhood cancer patients, and school reintegration programs have been developed to assist them with educational adjustment problems. Psychologists will continue to have an important role in providing treatment to these children and families. Furthermore, research focused on the psychological, social, and educational difficulties of these youth is needed to add to the understanding of the challenges they face in response to the disease and its psychological, educational, and social effects. Thus, through treatment and research, psychologists may help ensure that these children can function to their best potential as they progress through life as survivors of cancer.

REFERENCES

American Academy of Child and Adolescent Psychiatry Official Action. (1998). Practice parameters for the assessment and treatment of children and adolescents with posttraumatic stress disorder. *Journal of the American Academy of Child and Adolescent Psychiatry, 37*(Suppl. 10), 4–26.

American Cancer Society. (2003). *2000 facts and figures special section: Childhood cancer* [Brochure]. Atlanta, GA: Author.

Anghelescu, D., & Oakes, L. (2000). Working toward better cancer pain management for children. *Cancer Practice, 10*(Suppl. 1), S52–S57.

Chen, E., Craske, M. G., Katz, E. R., Schwartz, E., & Zeltzer, L. K. (2000). Pain-sensitive temperament: Does it predict procedural distress and response to psychological treatment among children with cancer? *Journal of Pediatric Psychology, 25*, 269–278.

Cleave, H., & Charlton, A. (1997). Evaluation of a cancer-based coping and caring course used in three different settings. *Child: Care, Health and Development, 23*, 399–413.

Eiser, C., & Havermans, T. (1994). Long term social adjustment after treatment for childhood cancer. *Archives of Disease in Childhood, 70*, 66–70.

Eiser, C., Hill, J. J., & Vance, Y. H. (2000). Examining the psychological consequences of surviving childhood cancer: Systematic review as a research method in pediatric psychology. *Journal of Pediatric Psychology, 25*, 449–469.

Engstrom, C. A., Strohl, R. A., & Rose, L. (1999). Sleep alterations in cancer patients. *Cancer Nursing, 22*, 143–148.

Gagnon, E. M., & Recklitis, C. J. (2003). Parents' decision-making preferences in pediatric oncology: The relationship to health care involvement and complementary therapy use. *Psychooncology, 12*, 442–452.

Gil, K. M., Wilson, J. J., & Edens, J. L. (1997). The stability of pain coping strategies in young children, adolescents, and adults with sickle cell disease over an 18-month period. *Clinical Journal of Pain, 13*, 110–115.

Gil, K. M., Wilson, J. J., Edens, J. L., Webster, D. A., Abrams, M. A., Orringer, E., et al. (1996). The effects of cognitive coping skills training on coping strategies and experimental pain sensitivity in African American adults with sickle cell disease. *Health Psychology, 15*, 3–10.

Hockenberry, M. J., Hinds, P. S., Barrera, P., Bryant, R., Adams-McNeill, J., Hooke, C., et al. (2003). Three instruments to assess fatigue in children with cancer: The child, parent, and staff perspectives. *Journal of Pain and Symptom Management, 25*, 319–328.

Jemal, A., Tiwari, R. C., Murray, T., Ghafoor, A., Samuels, A., Ward, E., et al. (2004). Cancer statistics, 2004. *CA: A Cancer Journal for Clinicians, 54*, 8–29.

Kazak, A. E., Barakat, L. P., Meeske, K., Christakis, D., Meadows, A., Casey, R., et al. (1997). Posttraumatic stress, family functioning, and social support in survivors of childhood leukemia and their mothers and fathers. *Journal of Consulting and Clinical Psychology, 65*, 120–129.

Kelly, K. M. (2004). Complementary and alternative medical therapies for children with cancer. *European Journal of Cancer, 40*, 2041–2046.

Kelly, K. M., Jacobson, J. S., Kennedy, D. D., Braudt, S. M., Mallick, M., & Weiner, M. A. (2000). Use of unconventional therapies by children with cancer at an urban medical center. *Journal of Pediatric Hematology/Oncology, 22*, 412–416.

Kleiber, C., & Haper, D. (1999). Effects of distraction on children's pain and distress during medical procedures: A meta-analysis. *Nursing Research, 48,* 44–49.

Kuppenheimer, W. G., & Brown, R. T. (2002). Painful procedures in pediatric cancer: A comparison of interventions. *Clinical Psychology Review, 22,* 753–786.

Labay, L. E., & Walco, G. A. (2004). Brief report: Empathy and psychological adjustment in siblings of children with cancer. *Journal of Pediatric Psychology, 29,* 309–314.

Leukemia Society of America. (2000). *Leukemia. Long-term survival rates are rising: Cures are now possible* [Brochure]. New York: Author.

Lightfoot, T. J., & Roman, E. (2004). Causes of childhood leukaemia and lymphoma. *Toxicology and Applied Pharmacology, 199,* 104–117.

Lobato, D., & Kao, T. (2002). Integrated sibling–parent group intervention to improve sibling knowledge and adjustment to chronic illness and disability. *Journal of Pediatric Psychology, 27,* 711–716.

Mackie, E., Hill, J., Kondryn, H., & McNally, R. (2000). Adult psychosocial outcomes in long-term survivors of acute lymphoblastic leukaemia and Wilm's tumour: A controlled study. *Lancet, 355,* 1310–1314.

Manne, S., & Miller, D. (1998). Social support, social conflict, and adjustment among adolescents with cancer. *Journal of Pediatric Psychology, 23,* 121–130.

McCurdy, E. A., Spangler, J. G., Wofford, M. M., Chauvenet, A. R., & McClean, T. W. (2003). Religiosity is associated with the use of complementary medical therapies by pediatric oncology patients. *Journal of Pediatric Hematology/Oncology, 25,* 125–129.

McQuaid, E. L., & Nassau, J. H. (1999). Empirically supported treatments of disease-related symptoms in pediatric psychology: Asthma, diabetes, and cancer. *Journal of Pediatric Psychology, 24,* 305–328.

Nichols, M. L. (1995). Social support and coping in young adolescents with cancer. *Pediatric Nursing, 21,* 235–240.

Novakovic, B., Fears, T. R., Wexler, L. H., McClure, L. L., Wilson, D. L., & McCalla, J. L. (1996). Experiences of cancer in children and adolescents. *Cancer Nursing, 19,* 54–59.

Oeffinger, K. C., & Hudson, M. M. (2004). Long-term complications following childhood and adolescent cancer: Foundations for providing risk-based health care for survivors. *CA: A Cancer Journal for Clinicians, 54,* 208–236.

Perrin, S., Smith, P., & Yule, W. (2000). Practitioner review: The assessment and treatment of post-traumatic stress disorder in children and adolescents. *Child Psychology and Psychiatry, 41,* 277–289.

Prevatt, F. F., Heffer, R. W., & Lowe, P. A. (2000). A review of school reintegration programs for children with cancer. *Journal of School Psychology, 38,* 447–467.

Smith, J. T., Barabasz, A., & Barabasz, M. (1996). Comparison of hypnosis and distraction in severely ill children undergoing painful medical procedures. *Journal of Counseling Psychology, 43,* 187–195.

Stuber, M. L., Kazak, A. E., Meeske, K., & Barakat, L. (1998). Is posttraumatic stress a viable model for understanding responses to childhood cancer? *Child and Adolescent Psychiatric Clinics of North America, 7*, 169–182.

Taieb, O., Moro, M. R., Baubet, T., Revah-Levy, A., & Flament, M. F. (2003). Posttraumatic stress symptoms after childhood cancer. *European Child and Adolescent Psychiatry, 12*, 255–264.

Vannatta, K., Zeller, M., Noll, R. B., & Koontz, K. (1998). Social functioning of children surviving bone marrow transplantation. *Journal of Pediatric Psychology, 23*, 169–178.

Varni, J. W., Katz, E. R., Colegrove, R., & Dolgin, M. (1994). Perceived social support and adjustment of children with newly diagnosed cancer. *Developmental and Behavioral Pediatrics, 15*, 20–26.

Walsh, D., Donnelly, S., & Rybicki, L. (2000). The symptoms of advanced cancer: relationship to age, gender and performance status in 1000 patients. *Supplemental Cancer Care, 8*, 175–179.

Woznick, L., & Goodheart, C. (Eds.). (2002). *Living with childhood cancer: A practical guide to help families cope*. Washington, DC: American Psychological Association.

4

CRANIOFACIAL ANOMALIES

KRISTAL EHRHARDT, MICHAEL HIXSON, AND ALAN POLING

Craniofacial anomalies (CFAs) are congenital abnormalities in the bone or soft tissue of the face or head (Richards, 1994; World Health Organization [WHO], 2002). CFAs comprise a wide range of heterogeneous conditions with many associated syndromes. Some CFAs and their associated syndromes are relatively common, such as cleft lip with or without cleft palate, with an estimated prevalence of 1 in 600 newborn babies (WHO, 2002). Others are more rare, such as Crouzon syndrome, which results in flattening of the back and top of the head, shallow eye sockets, retrusion (concavity) of the middle face, and protrusion of the lower jaw and has an estimated prevalence of 0.2 per 10,000 births (WHO, 2002). This chapter provides a synopsis of the probable causes of craniofacial anomalies, the related psychoeducational and medical outcomes, and the various treatment options.

In some cases, labeled syndromes are defined by and consist of CFAs; in others, syndromes comprise signs and symptoms in addition to CFAs. A given CFA typically is associated with at least several, and sometimes many, syndromes. As a case in point, about 350 different syndromes are associated with facial clefts (Shpritzen & Goldberg, 1995).

OVERVIEW

Chromosomal disorders, teratogens, and prenatal mechanical stresses can produce CFAs and the syndromes associated with them, although the etiology of a specific CFA often is speculative or unknown (Fiorello, Wright, & Mason, 1998). The past 2 decades have been marked by dramatic progress in understanding human genetics and the association between genotypes and CFAs (Nuckolls, Shum, & Slavkin, 1999). Researchers have established, for example, that CFAs can result from autosomal recessive inheritance (e.g., Meckel–Gruber syndrome, Smith–Lemli–Opitz syndrome), autosomal dominant inheritance (e.g., Apert syndrome, Treacher–Collins syndrome), X-linked recessive inheritance (Chitayat syndrome, Lowe syndrome), and X-linked dominant inheritance (e.g., Aarskog syndrome, Rett syndrome; Hopkin, 2001).

Gene–environment interactions resulting from exposure to teratogens have been shown to contribute to CFAs. For example, smoking appears to interact with an uncommon form of the TCF-alpha gene to increase the risk of cleft palates; infants having this allele were 6 times as likely to develop clefts if their mothers smoked tobacco than if they did not (Shaw et al., 1996). Although much more research is needed to determine the range of environmental variables that contribute to CFAs (WHO, 2002), in utero exposure to ethanol (beverage alcohol), retinoic acid, and phenytoin (an antiepilepsy drug) appear to increase the risks of CFAs (Nuckolls et al., 1999). According to WHO (2002), "The pathogenesis of the most common forms of CFA—non-syndromic clefts of lip and/or palate—is especially challenging because they appear to arise from complex polygenic interactions with environmental factors" (p. 2). Further understanding of these interactions might well provide a basis for developing strategies to reduce the prevalence of such clefts.

As noted previously, CFAs often occur in conjunction with other structural or functional abnormalities, which must be considered to provide appropriate services for patients and their families. For example, both Goldenhar syndrome (also known as oculo–auriculo–vertebral anomalad) and trisomy 18 are associated with CFAs involving the first and second branchial arches. Trisomy 18 leads to early death (typically within 1 year of birth) and severe mental impairment. Because they inevitably die at an early age, patients with trisomy 18 are not exposed to surgical interventions intended to ameliorate CFAs, and care in general is supportive.

OUTCOMES

Because CFAs differ dramatically in form and degree and because CFAs are often accompanied by other congenital anomalies, probable outcomes must be described in a very general way. For instance, children with a CFA who have a hearing impairment as the result of the malformation of the external or internal ear may experience delayed speech and receptive language skills. They are also at a greater risk for otitis media (i.e., middle ear infections) because of problems with eustachian tube functioning. During the infection period, hearing is impaired because of fluid buildup in the inner ear. Untreated otitis media can result in permanent hearing loss. Moreover, repeated bouts of otitis media can slow language development even if hearing is retained (refer to chap. 9, this volume, on language-related disorders).

A CFA that involves the vocal tract may affect the development of speech. Many infants and toddlers with a cleft palate show a delay in the onset and development of speech sounds. Before a cleft palate is surgically repaired, there is no separation between the mouth and nasal cavity, making it difficult or impossible to make certain sounds. This problem results in hypernasality, a resonance disorder that produces nasal-sounding speech. Velopharyngeal dysfunction is an anatomical defect that prevents adequate velopharyngeal valve closure, which can also result in hypernasality.

A malformation in the pharynx or larynx in an infant may cause feeding problems with an associated delay in weight gain. Children with a cleft palate may have problems such as choking, nasal regurgitation, excessive air intake, and poor oral suction. Breast-feeding may be difficult or impossible for children with a cleft palate. A cleft palate can also result in improper development in the number, size, and shape of the teeth, which may affect eating and speech.

Some CFAs are not predictive of intellectual or academic performance, as illustrated by Speltz, Endriga, and Mouradian (1997), who found that 19 infants with nonsyndromic sagittal synostosis (absence of connective tissue between the parietal bones of the skull) did not differ in any developmental aspect from matched control children without CFAs. Overall, however, children with CFAs appear to be at a somewhat elevated risk for cognitive impairment, poor academic performance, and learning disabilities, particularly in the area of reading (Delameter & Grus, 2002; Endriga & Kapp-Simon, 1999). For example, in a study of school children with clefts, 47% were functioning below grade level, and 46% were diagnosed with a learning disability (Broder, Richman, & Matheson, 1998). It is important to realize that CFAs may accompany, but not cause, intellectual and educational difficulties. That is, CFAs may be part of a syndrome that includes cognitive impairment. For instance, Down syndrome and CHARGE (an acronym describing a constellation of defects) syndrome are both associated with CFAs and cognitive impairment (Hartshorne & Hartshorne, 1998; Ramirez & Morgan, 1998).

As a group, children with a CFA demonstrate more emotional and behavioral difficulties than same-age peers without a CFA. These difficulties may be the result of teasing, social rejection, and poor social skills (Broder, Smith, & Strauss, 2001; Kapp-Simon & McGuire, 1997). Avoiding social interactions may develop as a method of coping with social difficulties. Likewise, adolescents with a CFA tend to be more withdrawn, and they more frequently report being unhappy with their facial appearance and social relationships (Broder, 2001; Kapp-Simon & McGuire, 1997).

MEDICAL AND PSYCHOEDUCATIONAL IMPLICATIONS

As Fiorello et al. (1998) related, "specific problems and treatments may be different for different syndromes, suggesting that diagnosis should be as specific as possible. Examination by a dysmorphologist (an expert in genetic diseases) is extremely important" (p. 168). Interestingly, diagnosis based on clinical signs and symptoms frequently disagrees with diagnosis based on genetic testing, in part because different genes can produce similar CFAs and the same gene can produce CFAs that differ in form and degree (Nuckolls et al., 1999).

Patients with CFAs are remarkably heterogeneous, even within diagnostic categories, and best-practice treatments are individualized. Unfortunately, in many cases, the research basis for making clinical decisions is relatively weak (WHO, 2000). Consider the surgical treatment of clefts, which is widely accepted. According to the WHO (2002), even for the longest established CFA intervention (i.e., management of cleft lip and palate), the scientific basis of the discipline is weak. Virtually no elements of treatment have been subjected to the rigors of contemporary clinical trial design (Roberts, Semb, & Shaw, 1991), and there is a bewildering diversity in practices. A recent survey of European cleft services revealed that in 201 teams, 194 different surgical protocols were followed for unilateral clefts alone (Shaw et al., 2001). Generally speaking, choices in surgical technique, timing and sequencing, and choices in ancillary procedures such as orthopedics, orthodontics, and speech therapy are determined after disappointment in the results of former practices rather than on the basis of firm evidence that the new protocol has succeeded elsewhere.

Given the foregoing, it appears impossible to specify empirically supported best practices for the surgical treatment of clefts, which are abnormal openings in an anatomical area, usually the palate or lip; cleft lips and palates can occur either alone or together. The same is true with respect to best practices for meeting the psychoeducational needs of children with CFAs. Relatively little research that is directly relevant to the needs of these children has appeared and the few published studies have typically involved small, nonrandom samples. Most of the relevant research is summarized elsewhere (Bennett, 1995; Broder, 1997, 2001; Endriga & Kapp-Simon, 1999; Hughes, 1998), and we recommend those overviews for more detailed coverage than is provided here.

Children born with a CFA may undergo multiple surgeries, often starting in infancy, for both functional and cosmetic purposes. For example, a cleft lip is usually repaired at 6 to 12 weeks of age and a cleft palate at 6 to 18 months (American Cleft Palate-Craniofacial Association, 2002). The repair of a cleft palate may ameliorate feeding problems and hypernasality. Ear tubes are often inserted between 2 and 6 months of age to release fluid buildup in the ears and to reduce the possibility of infection (American Cleft Palate-

Craniofacial Association, 2002). Repeated surgeries, continuing into adolescence or even adulthood, are needed to treat some CFAs; scheduling these surgeries during summer breaks may lessen their educational impact.

Early dental care is important for children with CFAs (Campbell & Dock, 2001). As the primary (baby) teeth erupt, a number of problems may be evident, such as a missing or an extra tooth in the area of the cleft. Dentists, orthodontists, and oral surgeons are all usually necessary for proper care of the teeth and jaws. The relationship between the maxillary (upper) teeth and mandibular (lower) teeth needs to be monitored to ensure proper occlusion (closing of the teeth). For children with a repaired cleft palate, bone grafting (i.e., the surgical introduction of bone-forming material into the cleft) usually takes place prior to the eruption of the permanent teeth. This helps to stabilize the maxillary arch and provide support for unerupted teeth and teeth next to the cleft. The maxillary arch is often underdeveloped in relation to the mandibular arch (lower jaw), which causes misalignment. This may be evident early in a child's life or not until adolescence and is corrected using a maxillary expansion device.

Other surgeries may be necessary to improve breathing, speech, mastication, swallowing, or aesthetics. An otolaryngologist (head and neck surgeon) may be needed for surgeries to improve breathing or feeding. The otolaryngologist may recommend nonsurgical procedures for some breathing and feeding problems. Coordination among the various professionals is necessary to ensure proper timing of surgeries and to combine treatments, when possible. Improvements in surgical procedures have reduced the need for prosthetic devices, but they may be needed in some cases for dental, speech, or aesthetic reasons (Kummer, 2001).

Velopharyngeal dysfunction refers to speech and resonance disorders attributable to an inability of the velopharyngeal valve to open and close properly. Velopharyngeal dysfunction is not diagnosed until the child can cooperate with a speech pathologist and emit multiword utterances (Billmire, 2001). Surgery to repair the anatomical structures usually takes place around 4 years. The diagnosis of velopharyngeal dysfunction is based on the perception of speech by a speech pathologist, so early evaluation is important.

A speech pathologist who is experienced in providing services to children with CFAs is a critical member of the CFA treatment team. Speech problems related to anatomical anomalies will require surgical or prosthetic intervention, not speech therapy. After velopharyngeal dysfunction surgery, however, intervention by a speech pathologist is often necessary to teach appropriate articulation and airflow (Kummer, 2001). Mild or inconsistent hypernasality may also be treated by a speech pathologist. Therapy is usually begun once the child is speaking in frequent multiword utterances, which typically occurs between 3 and 5 years of age, although a speech evaluation and some forms of intervention may occur earlier. Intervention with infants and very young children may prevent the development of some compensatory strategies that may be difficult to unlearn (Kummer, 2001; Sussman, Holt, Stone, & Ritter-Schmidt, 1992).

Auditory discrimination training is effective in treating hypernasality, as are other methods that provide some form of feedback to the child as to how closely they are approximating correct articulation (Kummer, 2001). One example involves a "listening tube," one end of which the child places at a nostril and the other end near an ear. When air leaves the nostril during speech, the child can easily hear the sound and is instructed to make adjustments in articulation to reduce it. The speech therapist, in some cases, can improve articulation problems that are due to dental problems or misalignment of the jaws, but greater success may occur after these structures have been surgically repaired. A speech pathologist should work closely with the dentist and oral surgeon to ensure appropriate treatment plans and to monitor the effectiveness of the various forms of treatment. Speech services provided before adolescence are generally more effective than those provided later in life because of the difficulty in changing habitual articulation practices (Kummer, 2001).

Many children with CFA have difficulty feeding. Certain structural problems, such as an opening between the trachea and esophagus, may preclude oral feeding until the problem can be surgically repaired. Children with a cleft lip or palate may be able to feed normally or with minor alterations to normal feeding procedures (Miller & Kummer, 2001). Breast-feeding may be possible, or a variety of modified nipples designed for children with cleft lips and palates may be used. Positioning the infant in an upright position reduces the chance of nasal regurgitation and permits gravity to assist in swallowing. The positioning of the nipple is also critical for successful feeding. A person specializing in feeding children with CFAs should consult with those who will feed the infant. This should occur before birth when CFAs are recognized prenatally, or shortly after birth when they are not. In all cases, the weight of the infant should be carefully monitored to ensure appropriate weight gain.

The hearing of a child with a CFA should be monitored on a regular basis. Hearing aids may be necessary. Preferential seating in classrooms may benefit a child with a mild hearing loss. Because these children are at a greater risk for language and reading problems, which is often because of a hearing or speech problem, these skills should be monitored and early intervention provided if necessary (Endriga & Kapp-Simon, 1999).

Teaching children with CFAs how to describe their condition to other children and to adults is an effective way for them to handle questions and may lessen a child's anxiety in new social situations (Cleft Palate Foundation, n.d.). Children may be taught various methods to deal with teasing, such as responding assertively or ignoring. Teasing will also be reduced if adults, particularly teachers, make it clear that teasing is not tolerated.

Although some of them will not have serious difficulties, the behavioral and emotional functioning of elementary and secondary students with CFAs should be monitored carefully and psychological services provided, if necessary (Endriga & Kapp-Simon, 1999; Schultz, 2001). The psychological challenges that young people with CFAs face are not fundamentally different from those faced by children and adolescents who are visibly different because of scars, burns, blemishes from dermatological diseases, or other factors. Being visibly different increases the likelihood of anxiety, depression, and low self-esteem; early detection and rapid intervention with proven techniques are essential to reduce their severity.

Social skills training and cognitive–behavioral techniques may be taught to adolescents to improve interpersonal skills and reduce anxiety associated with social situations (Thompson & Kent, 2001). Children with CFAs may also be extremely fearful of the surgical procedures they will need to undergo. In such cases, stress inoculation training, which involves educational, problem-solving, and coping skills components may be an effective intervention (Nash & Zevon, 1992). Cognitive–behavioral interventions are effective in countering depression and in improving self-image and should be provided when appropriate. People who are visibly different face two essential challenges: developing a satisfactory body image and dealing with other people's reactions to their appearance. A combination of cognitive–behavioral therapy and social skills training may be especially useful in meeting their psychological needs (Thompson & Kent, 2001).

Meeting the needs of children with CFAs requires the integrated services of a wide range of specialists. In 1995, Shpritzen described an idealized treatment team for patients with clefts that comprised more than two dozen specialists, and extant teams at many treatment centers approach this size, although not all specialties are involved in treating each child. Ensuring that communication is open and service provision is integrated among a large number of busy men and women is a difficult task but essential to ensuring the well-being of children with CFAs. Equally so is viewing those children as individuals, individuals who are homogeneous only insofar as they have one or more of a wide range of diverse congenital abnormalities known collectively as CFAs. Their CFAs may well influence the needs of these children, and therefore the special psychological and educational services they should receive, but a wide range of other factors also come into play. Hence, it is recommended that caregivers view children with CFAs in their totality, as complex individuals who function in dynamic educational, community, and family settings. Families of children with CFAs, as well as the children themselves, may well have special needs. Needs of the family are important in their own right and must be met to maximize the well-being of children with CFAs.

CONCLUSION

Craniofacial anomalies are heterogeneous and may result in a wide array of medical and psychoeducational outcomes. Various surgical procedures are usually necessary to provide essential structural alterations. Speech, language, and auditory discrimination services are generally required. Likewise, counseling and social skills training are frequently necessary to assist children diagnosed with a craniofacial anomaly to deal effectively with the related emotional and psychological effects of the disorder.

REFERENCES

American Cleft Palate-Craniofacial Association. (2002). *Core curriculum for cleft lip/palate and other craniofacial anomalies: A guide for educators.* Retrieved September 12, 2004, from http://www.acpa-pf.org/EducMeetings/Core%20Curriculum%202002.pdf

Bennett, M. E. (1995). Psychological and social consequences of craniofacial disfigurement of children. *Facial Plastic Surgery, 11,* 76–81.

Billmire, D. A. (2001). Surgical management of clefts and velopharyngeal dysfunction. In A. W. Kummer (Ed.), *Cleft palate and craniofacial anomalies: Effects on speech and resonance* (pp. 103–127). San Diego, CA: Singular.

Broder, H. L. (1997). Psychological research on children with craniofacial anomalies: Review, critique, and implications for the future. *Cleft Palate-Craniofacial Journal, 34,* 402–404.

Broder, H. L. (2001). Using psychological assessment and therapeutic strategies to enhance well-being. *Cleft Palate-Craniofacial Journal, 38,* 248–254.

Broder, H. L., Richman, L. C., & Matheson, P. B. (1998). Learning disability, school achievement, and grade retention among children with cleft: A two-center study. *Cleft Palate-Craniofacial Journal, 35,* 127–131.

Broder, H. L., Smith, F. B., & Strauss, R. P. (2001). Developing a behavior rating scale for comparing teachers' ratings of children with and without craniofacial anomalies. *Cleft Palate-Craniofacial Journal, 36,* 560–565.

Campbell, R., & Dock, M. (2001). Dental anomalies associated with cleft palate. In A. W. Kummer (Ed.), *Cleft palate and craniofacial anomalies: Effects on speech and resonance* (pp. 103–127). San Diego, CA: Singular.

Cleft Palate Foundation. (n.d.). *Preparing your child for social situations.* Retrieved September 12, 2004, from http://www.cleftline.org/publications/social.htm

Delameter, A. M., & Grus, C. L. (2002). Congenital abnormalities. In S. B. Johnson, N. W. Perry, Jr., & R. H. Rozensky (Eds.), *Handbook of clinical health psychology* (Vol. 1, pp. 443–481). Washington, DC: American Psychological Association.

Endriga, M. C., & Kapp-Simon, K. A. (1999). Psychological issues in craniofacial care: State of the art. *Cleft Palate-Craniofacial Journal, 36,* 3–11.

Fiorello, C. A., Wright, L. B., & Mason, E. J. (1998). Cleft lip and palate. In L. Phelps (Ed.), *Health-related disorders in children and adolescents* (pp. 167–178). Washington, DC: American Psychological Association.

Hartshorne, T. S., & Hartshorne, N. S. (1998). CHARGE Syndrome or Association. In L. Phelps (Ed.), *Health-related disorders in children and adolescents* (pp. 154–160). Washington, DC: American Psychological Association.

Hopkin, R. J. (2001). Genetics and patterns of inheritance. In A. W. Kummer (Ed.), *Cleft palate and craniofacial anomalies: Effects on speech and resonance* (pp. 33–71). San Diego, CA: Singular.

Hughes, M. J. (1998). *The social consequences of disfigurement.* Brookfield, VT: Ashgate.

Kapp-Simon, K. A., & McGuire, D. E. (1997). Observed social interaction patterns in adolescents with and without craniofacial conditions. *Cleft Palate-Craniofacial Journal, 34,* 380–384.

Kummer, A. W. (2001). *Cleft palate and craniofacial anomalies: Effects on speech and resonance.* San Diego, CA: Singular.

Miller, C. K., & Kummer, A. W. (2001). Feeding problems of infants with cleft lip/palate or craniofacial anomalies. In A. W. Kummer (Ed.), *Cleft palate and craniofacial anomalies: Effects on speech and resonance* (pp. 103–127). San Diego, CA: Singular.

Nash, L. B., & Zevon, M. A. (1992). Psychosocial aspects: Family, patient, and treatment issues. In L. Brodsky, L. Holt, & D. H. Ritter-Schmidt (Eds.), *Craniofacial anomalies: An integrated approach* (pp. 27–39). St. Louis, MO: Mosby.

Nuckolls, G. H., Shum, L., & Slavkin, H. C. (1999). Progress toward understanding craniofacial malformations. *Cleft Palate-Craniofacial Journal, 36,* 12–26.

Ramirez, S. Z., & Morgan, V. (1998). Down syndrome. In L. Phelps (Ed.), *Health-related disorders in children and adolescents* (pp. 254–265). Washington, DC: American Psychological Association.

Richards, M. E. (1994). Common pediatric craniofacial reconstructions. *Nursing Clinics of North America, 29,* 791–799.

Roberts, C. T., Semb, G., & Shaw, W. C. (1991). Strategies for the advancement of surgical methods in cleft lip and palate. *Cleft Palate-Craniofacial Journal, 28,* 141–149.

Schultz, J. R. (2001). Psychosocial aspects of cleft lip/palate and craniofacial anomalies. In A.W. Kummer (Ed.), *Cleft palate and craniofacial anomalies: Effects on speech and resonance* (pp. 103–127). San Diego, CA: Singular.

Shaw, W. C., Semb, G., Nelson, P., Brattstrom, V., Prahl-Andersen, B., & Gundlach, K. K. H. (2001). The Eurocleft Project 1996–2000: Overview. *Journal of Cranio Maxillo-Facial Surgery, 29,* 131–140.

Shaw, G. M., Wasserman, C. R., Lammer, E. J., O'Malley, C. D., Murray, J. C., Bassart, A. M., & Tolarova, M. M. (1996). Orofacial clefts, parental cigarette smoking and transforming growth factor-alpha gene variants. *American Journal of Human Genetics, 58,* 551–561.

Shpritzen, R. J. (1995). A new perspective on clefting. In R. J. Shpritzen & J. Bardach (Eds.), *Cleft palate and speech management* (pp. 1–15). St. Louis, MO: Mosby.

Shpritzen, R. J., & Goldberg, R. (1995). The genetics of clefting and associated syndromes. In R. J. Shpritzen & R. Bardach (Eds.), *Cleft palate and speech management* (pp. 16–43). St. Louis, MO: Mosby.

Speltz, M. L., Endriga, M. C., & Mouradian, W. E. (1997). Presurgical and postsurgical mental and psychomotor development of infants with sagittal synostosis. *Cleft Palate-Craniofacial Journal, 34,* 374–379.

Sussman, J. E., Holt, L., Stone, R., & Ritter-Schmidt, D. H. (1992). Speech and language treatment issues. In L. Brodsky, L. Holt, & D. H. Ritter-Schmidt (Eds.), *Craniofacial anomalies: An integrated approach* (pp. 27–39). St. Louis, MO: Mosby.

Thompson, A., & Kent, G. (2001). Adjusting to disfigurement: Processes involved in dealing with being visibly different. *Clinical Psychology Review, 21,* 663–682.

World Health Organization. (2002). *Global strategies to reduce the health-care burden of craniofacial anomalies.* Geneva, Switzerland: Author.

5

ENDOCRINE DISORDERS

DAVID E. SANDBERG AND LAUREN ZURENDA

The endocrine system comprises a collection of glands (pineal, pituitary, thyroid, parathyroid, thymus, adrenal, pancreas, testis, and ovary) and the hormones they produce. Hormones are chemical messengers that are secreted into the bloodstream and transported to organs and tissues throughout the body to regulate metabolism, growth, and development.

The clinical presentation of an endocrine disorder varies not only in terms of the manifestations of the particular condition but also with respect to the individual's adaptation to it. Although certain psychosocial or behavioral characteristics may be associated with a syndrome, they are not necessarily intrinsic to it. Instead, psychosocial problems may develop as a reaction of the child or family to the stress associated with the condition and its treatment. Likewise, physical or cognitive features related to the condition may elicit negative reactions from others. It is imperative that clinicians do not underestimate the role of such environmental factors.

This chapter summarizes information on the following conditions: growth hormone deficiency (and other indications for growth hormone therapy), diabetes mellitus (Types 1 and 2), thyroid disorders (congenital and acquired *hypothyroidism*, and acquired *hyperthyroidism*), disorders of puberty (precocious and delayed), and congenital adrenal hyperplasia (as an example of a disorder affecting sexual differentiation). The review is necessarily selective in terms of the conditions selected and the studies summarized.

GROWTH HORMONE DEFICIENCY

Overview

Growth is a complex process involving diverse factors. The pituitary gland is central to the endocrine component of the process insofar as it promotes growth through the release of growth hormone (GH). When stimulated by GH-releasing hormone from the hypothalamus, the anterior pituitary releases GH. In addition to promoting growth in youths, GH also exerts important metabolic and body composition effects in adulthood (Carroll et al., 1998; Rosen, Johannsson, Johansson, & Bengtsson, 1995).

GH deficiency (GHD) may result from a disruption of the GH axis in the higher brain, hypothalamus, or pituitary gland (Reiter & Rosenfeld, 2003). In cases where the deficiency is *congenital*, the cause may be a pituitary gland that is too small, deformed, or absent altogether. When GHD is *acquired*, the cause may be trauma to the head or neck, a tumor of the central nervous system (CNS), or radiation treatment. Disease factors in the etiology of GHD may also be responsible for deficits of other pituitary hormones. An additional cause of GHD is physical or psychological abuse or neglect (e.g., psychosocial short stature; Blizzard & Bulatovic, 1996). Although most instances of isolated GHD are idiopathic (i.e., of unknown cause), specific disease states are typically responsible when GHD is associated with multiple pituitary hormone deficiencies (MPHD). It is thus understandable that psychological adaptation will vary according to the etiology of the pituitary insufficiency.

Children with GHD are characterized by a progressive slowing of growth, delayed skeletal maturation, and delayed puberty. GHD occurs in 1 in 3,500 children, and although it is seen twice as often in boys as in girls, this discrepancy may reflect referral bias rather than a difference in disease manifestation (Lindsay, Feldkamp, Harris, Robertson, & Rallison, 1994). GHD was the first Food and Drug Administration–approved indication for human GH (rhGH) therapy, but by 2005 there were five additional indications: Turner syndrome, Prader–Willi syndrome, chronic renal insufficiency, growth failure in children born small for gestational age (SGA), and, most recently, idiopathic short stature. Only GHD is associated with a deficiency in GH. Despite the diversity of the conditions for which rhGH is an approved treatment, all share the feature of growth failure and "short stature" (SS; defined as height = 2 SD below age- and gender-adjusted populations norms).[1] An implicit rationale for rhGH treatment is the reduction of the perceived physical or psychosocial disabilities associated with marked SS (Sandberg, Colsman, & Voss, 2004).

---

[1]The height cutoff for the idiopathic short stature indication for rhGH is −2.25 SD (i.e., the shortest 1.2% of children).

Children presenting at a routine medical exam with SS and a pattern of growth failure consistent with GHD should be referred to a pediatric endocrinologist for a growth evaluation. This process includes lab testing for IGF-I (insulin-like growth factor 1) and IGFBP-3 (IGF-binding protein) levels, as well as thyroid function tests. When GHD is suspected, two GH-stimulation tests are required to confirm the diagnosis. Because these tests are imperfect in differentiating between a normal and abnormal GH axis, the endocrinologist must integrate all available data (clinical, growth history, radiological, and biochemical) when making a diagnosis (Reiter & Rosenfeld, 2003).

Outcomes

The psychosocial adaptation of youths with GHD has been the focus of many studies (for reviews, see Sandberg, 1996; Sandberg, Colsmann, & Voss, 2004; Sandberg & Voss, 2002). It has frequently been reported that youths with SS are treated according to height age (HA) rather than chronological age (CA). Because this misperception is associated with lower expectations, affected youths are at risk for decreased social maturity and functional independence (Meyer-Bahlburg, 1990). The discrepancy between physical appearance and CA may also lead to stigmatization or teasing by peers, which may contribute to an unhealthy body image or poor global self-concept. In an effort to make their SS less obvious, some children will seek younger peers as friends. One drawback of this strategy is that it may potentiate socialization according to HA (Meyer-Bahlburg, 1990), thereby making integration with the CA group even less likely.

Although numerous clinical and anecdotal reports validate the stereotype that SS is associated with problems of psychosocial adaptation, recent epidemiologically oriented research serves to challenge this assumption. For example, self-reported self-esteem scale scores for youths referred for evaluation of SS were higher (i.e., more positive) than questionnaire norms, despite reports that the majority of these individuals experienced teasing and juvenilization (Sandberg, Brook, & Campos, 1994; Sandberg & Michael, 1998). With regard to behavioral disturbances, patients reported significantly fewer problems than questionnaire norms. Likewise, parental reports indicated that patients were comparable to norms in terms of behavioral and emotional functioning (Sandberg et al., 1994; Zimet et al., 1995).

Additionally, in a recent community-based study using a novel research design, the reports of classmates were used to study the influence of height on students' psychosocial adaptation (Sandberg, Bukowski, Fung, & Noll, 2004). Statistically significant relationships were not detected between height, and measures of friendship, popularity, or most aspects of reputation among peers (despite substantial statistical power). Findings did not vary by participant gender, peer- or self-report, whether data from the entire sample were used or when subgroups of very short (= 2.25 height SD; 1st percentile) or very tall students (= 2.25 height SD; 99th percentile) were contrasted with average height (25th to 75th percentile for norms) classmates. In the lower grades, classmates perceived shorter students as younger than their CA. This perception was not meaningfully related to measures of social acceptance or other aspects of reputation among peers, however.

As with psychosocial adaptation, a consideration of academic achievement demands a clear distinction between isolated GHD and GHD secondary to a complex medical condition. Although increased rates of grade retention and academic underachievement have been reported among children with GHD, studies of those with isolated GHD demonstrate intellectual functioning within the average range (Sandberg, 1996). Although GHD may be associated with specific cognitive deficits, this remains in question (Abbott, Rotnem, Genel, & Cohen, 1982; Siegel, 1990). In one study of children receiving rhGH, 18% to 29% were performing poorly in at least one of four academic domains, and 26% had been classified as educationally "handicapped" (Sandberg et al., 1998). Those children with GHD as one feature of more complex medical states (e.g., MPHD) displayed greater academic failure than did those with isolate GHD or idiopathic SS, however (Sandberg et al., 1998). Because there was no association between academic performance and height, psychosocial stressors related to SS do not appear to be responsible for school difficulties.

Medical and Psychoeducational Implications

Medical treatment of GHD (and all other approved indications for rhGH) entails daily subcutaneous injections. Early initiation of treatment and appropriate dosing can allow youths to achieve full growth potential (August, Julius, & Blethen, 1998; Mauras, Attie, Reiter, Saenger, Baptista, & the Genentech Inc. Cooperative Study Group, 2000). The first year of treatment is associated with catch-up growth (MacGillivray, Baptista, & Johanson, 1996), after which growth velocity gradually decreases. Treatment generally continues for several years and is terminated when maximum growth potential is achieved. Although some individuals will remain GH-deficient throughout adulthood, others will not; for this reason, lab studies should be performed toward the end of the teen years to determine whether continuing therapy is necessary. The justification for lifelong GH replacement stems from its beneficial effects on body composition, bone density, lipid metabolism, cardiovascular function, and physical performance (Carroll et al., 1998).

Treatment for rhGH is not reliably associated with any changes in psychosocial or educational adaptation. Instead, if positive psychosocial or educational changes are observed at treatment onset, they are more likely due to the initiation of an intervention that promises increased growth velocity. Likewise, negative changes may result from the burdens associated with a chronic and invasive therapy.

Some children with GHD will also experience a delay (or absence of) pubertal development. For some of this group, this lag in sexual development will be experienced as a challenging personal problem. In cases in which delayed or absent puberty is a consequence of MPHD (or another medical condition), sex hormone replacement therapy is a treatment option. In determining the appropriate timing of treatment, clinicians should consider the importance of on-time puberty in terms of healthy psychosocial adaptation (even if treatment may result in attenuated adult height).

In the psychosocial domain, anticipation of predictable experiences related to SS can be helpful. The belief that SS is strongly associated with negative experiences can result in the attribution of problems to the child's stature, even when other factors are more directly responsible. If significant problems of psychosocial or educational adjustment are encountered, a referral to a pediatric psychologist should be considered. Individual or group counseling may benefit children who are experiencing teasing related to SS (Eminson, Powell, & Hollis, 1994). Because teasing may, in extreme cases, be associated with social isolation and a negative self-image, psychological intervention can serve a preventative function in the promotion of effective coping strategies.

Psychologists can also be helpful to children and families by promoting realistic expectations for treatment. This consideration is particularly important because unrealistic expectations may result in disappointment for children and parents when they are not realized. Accordingly, clinicians should emphasize that treatment will not result in an adult height beyond that which would be expected on the basis of genetic growth potential (and often will fall significantly below that; Grew, Stabler, Williams, & Underwood, 1983; Hunt, Hazen, & Sandberg, 2000).

Because of the tendency to treat children according to their HA rather than CA, adults should be encouraged to promote age-appropriate independence and self-help skills in children with SS. Any aspect of the physical environment that serves as a barrier to this goal should be targeted for modification. Additionally, teachers and coaches should be encouraged to maintain age-appropriate expectations and to encourage the child to remain in the mainstream of academic and extracurricular activities (Meyer-Bahlburg, 1990). Although SS is sometimes used as a reason to postpone school entry or repeat kindergarten, these options should be considered only if academic achievement and psychometric testing indicate marked developmental delays (and remediation is not an option). "Immaturity" of social behavior is best addressed by an alteration of adult expectations and the establishment of clear behavioral goals (Rieser & Meyer-Bahlburg, 1991).

DIABETES MELLITUS

Overview

Produced by the pancreas, insulin functions to regulate the level of glucose in the blood by allowing glucose to pass from the bloodstream into cells where it can be broken down and used for energy. In people with diabetes mellitus, the pancreas is unable to produce sufficient amounts of insulin; consequently, affected individuals have elevated levels of blood glucose. The ideal range for blood glucose is between 80 and 120 mg of glucose per 100 mL of blood (mg/dL). After eating, levels can rise to 180 mg/dL. *Hyperglycemia* occurs when glucose levels are elevated beyond 180 mg/dL, and is marked by excessive thirst or hunger (or both), frequent urination, weight loss, fatigue, irritability, and sweet-smelling breath. *Hypoglycemia* occurs when glucose levels drop below 70 mg/dL. Pronounced hypoglycemia can be associated with seizures and coma. If left untreated, it may result in death, because brain function cannot be supported without adequate glucose concentration.

The two major forms of diabetes mellitus affecting children are Type 1 (insulin-dependent diabetes mellitus) and Type 2 diabetes (non-insulin-dependent diabetes mellitus). Complete failure of the pancreas is characteristic of Type 1 diabetes; as a result, affected individuals require daily injections of insulin for survival. In Type 2 diabetes, the pancreas continues to produce insulin, although it cannot produce amounts that are sufficient to maintain normal glucose levels. Type 1 diabetes affects 1 in 600 children in the United States. It occurs 1.5 times more often in White male than in non-White male individuals but occurs equally in male and female individuals. Peak incidence is during puberty. The incidence of Type 2 diabetes has risen dramatically in recent years, and it is currently estimated that 1 to 50 in 1,000 children are affected (depending on the ethnic group surveyed; Eisenbarth, Polonsky, & Buse, 2003). The high prevalence of pediatric obesity is thought to account for the increasing incidence of this condition (Buse, Polonsky, & Burant, 2003). Type 2 diabetes does not result from a single cause, however, and genetic, physiologic, and lifestyle factors are all believed to be important contributions to disease onset.

Type 2 diabetes begins with insulin resistance, in which cells resist the action of insulin at the receptor level. Although the pancreas initially responds by producing higher levels of insulin (hyperinsulinemia), insulin secretion declines over time. As a result, hyperglycemia occurs. In contrast, Type 1 diabetes is thought to be caused by an autoimmune process whereby the insulin-producing beta cells of the pancreas are destroyed. There may also be a viral component to the disease, resulting in injury to the pancreas. Additionally, there is likely to be a genetic component of the disease, as both forms run in families. However, a specific mode of inheritance has not been identified (Buse et al., 2003; Eisenbarth et al., 2003).

Outcomes

Medical outcomes of diabetes depend on the amount of glycemic control achieved through treatment. Long-term complications of diabetes can include eye problems (e.g., cataracts and blindness), kidney disease, heart attack, stroke, numbness and pain in legs, and increased infections (especially of skin, upper and lower extremities, legs, and feet). Not surprisingly, these types of complications are associated with depression (typically in adulthood). Although the risk of negative outcomes is heightened by prolonged poor glycemic control that may be affected by treatment adherence, adherence does not guarantee their prevention (Eisenbarth et al., 2003).

Although depression is more prevalent in adults with diabetes, it may also occur in children upon diagnosis. When depression does occur in children, it typically fades within a 6-month period. Children may also experience anxiety related to the condition. The risk of hypoglycemic episodes (which can involve shaking, sweating, and loss of consciousness) can be one source of anxiety because these episodes are likely to be embarrassing. For this reason, some children consciously maintain glucose levels above the normal range to prevent their occurrence. Prolonged hyperglycemia can be detrimental to long-term health, and thus psychoeducational intervention is necessary for youths who engage in this behavior (Jacobson, 1996).

As with all chronic health conditions, the period of adolescence can be particularly challenging for youths with diabetes, and decisions that may be stressful for all adolescents may be especially consequential for this population. For instance, alcohol can cause a prolonged episode of hypoglycemia lasting 8 to 12 hours. The symptoms of excess alcohol and hypoglycemia can be similar—sleepiness, dizziness, and disorientation. For this reason, it is important that individuals with diabetes always wear an ID bracelet to inform others of their health status (e.g., "I have diabetes").

Issues related to body image may also manifest differently in affected adolescents. Those with Type 2 diabetes stemming from obesity are at risk for stigmatization (Strauss & Pollack, 2003). Youths, especially girls, with Type 1 diabetes are at an increased risk for eating disorders, with studies demonstrating that 30% to 40% of female adolescents with Type 1 diabetes use insulin manipulation as a means of losing weight (Jacobson, 1996). Individuals concerned with weight gain may reduce the insulin dose (or skip injections) to promote weight loss.

Autonomy issues may also be particularly challenging for adolescents with diabetes because activities of day-to-day life may be restricted for safety reasons related to hypoglycemic episodes. Specifically, the risk of such an episode may have implications for certain types of employment and other activities (e.g., driving). Finally, the stressors related to adolescence common to all individuals may hinder treatment adherence. The inadequate glycemic control that results is likely to exacerbate medical and psychosocial challenges.

Type 1 diabetes is associated with increased risk of learning disabilities (Desrocher & Rovet, 2004). When onset occurs prior to age 5, children are at risk for lower Performance and Full Scale IQ scores. Academic achievement is also associated with earlier disease onset, with arithmetic being affected less than spelling or reading. In contrast, lower Verbal IQ scores are associated with later onset Type 1 diabetes. Specific neurocognitive deficits associated with Type 1 diabetes include verbal ability, memory, attention, visuomotor skill, and visuospatial processing. Deficits in this latter domain are also associated with repeated hypoglycemic seizures during childhood. Although there is no pattern of cognitive deficits associated with Type 2 diabetes, poor glycemic control may adversely affect academic performance.

Medical and Psychoeducational Implications

Two types of insulin, short acting and intermediate acting, are typically used (in combination) to regulate glucose levels. Injections are administered once or twice daily, usually before breakfast and dinner. Glucose levels are measured multiple times daily and recorded by computerized glucose meters. Because diet is important in terms of glucose regulation, meals and snacks must be coordinated with the timing and amount of insulin injections. As an alternative to injections, the insulin pump can be used to regulate blood glucose levels. The pump delivers small amounts of insulin continuously into the bloodstream to maintain a "basal" level. When food is consumed, the pump can be programmed to release more insulin (bolus). Basal and bolus rates are established by patients and health care providers in the initial stages of treatment and can be adjusted to meet the body's changing needs. This method of treatment allows patients to lead a more relaxed lifestyle without strictly regimented meal planning. Some adolescents may feel self-consciousness about carrying a device that may be visible to others, however.

Although weight management is an integral treatment component for individuals with Type 2 diabetes, pharmacological treatment is also necessary for most. Medications such as metformin (e.g., Glucophage) are typically prescribed to improve glycemic control, as well as to preserve beta-cell function and reduce insulin resistance (Buse et al., 2003). Few controlled studies of the efficacy of these medications have been conducted, however. The American Diabetes Association has recommended that all children with Type 2 diabetes receive self-management education that includes instruction with regard to the monitoring of blood glucose, as well as behavior modification (Mensing et al., 2005). Because lifestyle factors play a significant role in the development of Type 2 diabetes, family involvement is particularly important for this population.

Lifestyle factors play an important role in Type 1 diabetes as well. For instance, because physical exercise lowers blood glucose by enhancing the use of insulin, it can be a particularly important intervention strategy. An added benefit of exercise derives from its capacity to moderate psychological stress. This relationship is important because psychological stress can impede insulin action and lead to hyperglycemia. Relaxation training is another common intervention that may help stress-prone children cope adaptively. Other useful interventions include psychotherapy groups, self-help consumer support groups, and "diabetes camps." Goals of these groups include the enhancement of social and coping skills (e.g., assertiveness) particularly with regard to diabetes-specific challenges (American Diabetes Association, 2005; Mensing et al., 2005).

Mental health professionals should be alert to many issues when working with children who have diabetes. For example, accurate diagnoses may be challenging within this population because some symptoms of diabetes overlap with those of psychological disorders. For instance, the physical symptoms of anxiety can mimic symptoms of poor glycemic control, making anxiety disorders particularly difficult to diagnose in children with diabetes (Perrin, Stein, & Drotar, 1991). Typically, a diagnosis is made when psychological symptoms (e.g., obsessions, compulsions, persistent fears) outweigh physical symptoms and occur during periods of adequate glycemic control. An eating disorder diagnosis may be similarly difficult to diagnose in children with Type 1 diabetes because symptoms of eating disorders and diabetes may overlap (Jacobson, 1996). Additionally, mental health professionals should take care when prescribing psychotropics because some of these medications (e.g., selective serotonin reuptake inhibitors) can adversely affect blood sugar concentrations (Jacobson, 1996).

THYROID DISORDERS

Overview

Located in the front of the neck below the larynx, the thyroid gland produces hormones that influence many states and functions of the body (e.g., energy, temperature, metabolism, growth, and intelligence). A thyroid disorder occurs when a deficiency or excess of thyroxine (T4) and triiodothyronine (T3) results from under- or overproduction by the thyroid gland or when the hormones are unable to carry out their functions for other reasons. Congenital hypothyroidism (CH) is marked by a deficiency of thyroid hormone (Dallas & Foley, 1996a). When the site of the defect is the thyroid gland itself (i.e., primary hypothyroidism), the condition may take one of several forms: the gland may be absent (*athyreosis*), it may function inadequately (*dyshormonogenesis*), or it may be abnormally positioned (*ectopic*). There is an association between the etiology of the disorder and its severity; unsurprisingly, athyreosis is associated with the most severe symptoms (Dallas & Foley, 1996a).

Abnormalities along the hypothalamic–pituitary–thyroid axis during fetal life can result in damage to organ systems, including the CNS and skeleton. If left untreated, CH results in a host of problems, the most grave of which is *cretinism*, a reduction in brain size associated with severe mental retardation. Without early intervention, CH can also lead to impaired bodily growth, feeding problems, constipation, hypotonia, excessive sleeping, protruding tongue, and hoarse voice. Since 1974, all newborns in developed countries have been screened for this disease, allowing for early detection and treatment. As a result, severe mental retardation related to CH has essentially been eliminated. The primary screening test for CH involves the measurement of thyroid-stimulating hormone (TSH) from blood collected by a heel stick the day after birth. CH affects 1 in 4,000 births and affects the sexes equally (Fisher & Foley, 1989).

Acquired hypothyroidism also results from a deficiency in thyroid hormones. The most common cause is Hashimoto's thyroiditis, a condition in which the immune system's antibodies attack thyroid tissue and impair glandular function. Hypothyroidism occurs with increased frequency in other conditions associated with autoimmune processes (e.g., Type 1 diabetes and Down, Klinefelter, and Turner syndromes). Although acquired hypothyroidism appears to run in families, a specific mode of inheritance has not been identified (Larsen & Davies, 2003).

Children with hypothyroidism typically have an enlarged thyroid gland, or goiter. In many cases, this is the only sign that the individual may be hypothyroid. Some children, however, may experience nonspecific symptoms including physical weakness, lethargy, decreased appetite (but with mild obesity), cold intolerance, constipation, and dry skin. Most children will demonstrate growth deceleration with delayed skeletal maturation and puberty, and girls may feature *galactorrhea* (i.e., milk flow at times other than nursing). The clinical assessment for hypothyroidism comprises a physical exam and family history, along with lab tests of thyroid function (including levels of TSH, thyroxine, and thyroid antibodies). Acquired hypothyroidism is estimated at 1 in 500 to 1,000 school-age children and is observed more often in girls than boys (Cooper, 2001; Dallas & Foley, 1996b).

Acquired hyperthyroidism is a condition characterized by the excessive production of thyroid hormone in an individual born with a normally functioning thyroid gland. Although acquired hyperthyroidism might arise for several reasons, in at least 95% of childhood cases, the overproduction of thyroid hormone is caused by an autoimmune condition known as Grave's disease (Larsen & Davies, 2003). In approximately 60% of patients with hyperthyroidism, a family history of autoimmune thyroid disease is present. Physical symptoms may include goiter, a sudden growth spurt, heat intolerance, rapid fingernail growth, and protruding eyes (referred to as exophthalmos), and irritated eyes. The diagnostic procedure is similar to that for hypothyroidism, with low levels of TSH and elevated thyroxine levels confirming the diagnosis. Hyperthyroidism affects 1 in 500 to 1,000 children. Although onset can occur any time after birth, symptoms emerge between 10 and 15 years in more than two thirds of childhood cases (Dallas & Foley, 1996b).

Outcomes

Newborn screening for CH, along with early intervention, can serve to prevent the debilitating effects of this hormone deficiency. Findings from the longitudinal studies reveal global IQs falling within the average range. Although some research indicates the presence of selective neurocognitive deficits in children with CH, there is little agreement concerning the specific type or extent of the impairment (Rovet & Daneman, 2003; Rovet & Ehrlich, 2000). Suggested problems include speech and language delays, poor motor function (especially balance), and weak perceptuomotor abilities. It has also been suggested that children with CH exhibit a cognitive profile resembling that of children with nonverbal learning disabilities (Rovet, Ehrlich, & Sorbara, 1992). Additionally, there is an association between CH and hearing loss, which is an especially important consideration when language delays are observed (Debruyne, Vanderschueren-Lodeweyckx, & Bastijns, 1983; Vanderschueren-Lodeweyckx, Debruyne, Dooms, Eggermont, & Eeckels, 1983).

Some studies have indicated that a subgroup of children with CH— those with athyreosis—exhibit deficits in intellectual potential compared with unaffected children (Oerbeck, Sundet, Kase, & Heyerdahl, 2003; Tillotson, Fuggle, Smith, Ades, & Grant, 1994). In response to such findings, the recommended starting dose of thyroxine has been increased (Fisher & Foley, 1989). Although the higher dose regimen is associated with higher IQs and better school performance, there have also been reports of increased temperamental difficulty and attention problems (Rovet, 2000; Rovet, Ehrlich, & Sorbara, 1987). It has been suggested that although a higher starting dose may be beneficial for those with severe CH, children with mild forms of the condition may be at an increased risk for hormone excess (Rovet, 2004; Simoneau-Roy et al., 2004).

The risk to intellectual functioning is a major factor distinguishing acquired hypothyroidism from CH. Whereas children with CH, if left untreated, will experience impaired intellectual functioning, children who acquire hypothyroidism before age 3 years are less at risk when the child receives prompt and adequate treatment. When onset occurs later in life, affected children are not at risk for related CNS damage (Foley, 2000).

Children with acquired hypothyroidism may demonstrate deterioration in school performance prior to treatment. This phenomenon is attributable to decreased energy and resolves after treatment. Although most other features of the disorder reverse on treatment as well, final adult height is compromised in some cases. This depends on the age of onset, severity of the deficiency, and timing of treatment. Most prepubertal children with severe hypothyroidism and SS will experience a period of catch-up growth in response to treatment, however (Foley, 2000).

Children with acquired hyperthyroidism may demonstrate a number of behavioral and emotional changes as a result of their condition, and most will experience a change in sleeping patterns. The heightened metabolic state (associated with sleeplessness and insomnia) can result in extreme mental and physical exhaustion and accompanying mood changes. As with children with acquired hypothyroidism, school performance may deteriorate (Dallas & Foley, 1996b).

Medical and Psychoeducational Implications

Medical treatment for infants diagnosed with congenital hypothyroidism begins within the first few weeks after birth. The regimen involves thyroxine replacement (levothyroxine, taken orally) and is necessary throughout life. The initial 3 to 4 weeks of treatment are critical in terms of growth and development; for this reason, tight adherence is essential during this period. As noted earlier, the recommended starting dose for thyroxine has increased (Fisher & Foley, 1989). Although there are long-term benefits to more aggressive dosing for children with severe hypothyroidism, these may be less apparent among those showing less severe hormonal deficiency in whom the higher doses may be associated with restlessness and distractibility (Rovet, 2000; Rovet et al., 1987). Because children within the athyreotic subgroup may be at heightened risk for cognitive and learning deficits, they are good candidates for educational assessment and remedial services.

The treatment of acquired hypothyroidism is the same as that for children with the congenital form: daily doses of levothyroxine (Synthroid) taken orally. When symptoms appear before age 3, prompt treatment is crucial to prevent damage to the CNS. Regardless of age of onset, treatment should begin as early as possible to allow the achievement of full growth potential. When normal thyroid levels are attained too quickly, side effects (e.g., distractibility, sleep disturbances) may be observed. Dosing must be monitored closely for this reason (Dallas & Foley, 1996a).

For children with acquired hyperthyroidism, medical treatment entails antithyroid medication. Hormone levels are typically brought within the normal range within weeks. Unfortunately, not all children tolerate the medication, and some exhibit allergic reactions (e.g., fever, hives, rash). Other children (approximately 1 in 300) develop *agranulocytosis,* a condition in which white blood cell count drops significantly, thereby inhibiting the body's ability to fight off disease (Dallas & Foley, 1996b). Symptoms of agranulocytosis include fever, sore throat, and mouth sores. If these symptoms are observed, treatment should be discontinued immediately and the pediatrician should be contacted. For children who cannot tolerate the medication, radioactive iodine treatment is another option. This treatment typically results in hypothyroidism, which is then treated with levothyroxine. Although it has been suggested that radioiodine may cause leukemia or other cancers, there is currently no evidence to support this claim (Ron et al., 1998).

Because the maintenance of adequate thyroid hormone levels is necessary to support optimal cognitive functioning, the importance of adherence extends beyond childhood. This applies to all three thyroid conditions described here. The period of adolescence presents particular challenges in this regard, and psychoeducational intervention may be beneficial for adolescents who encounter difficulties adhering to the regimen.

DISORDERS OF PUBERTY

Overview

Puberty is the transitional period between the onset and completion of sexual maturation during which sexual organs develop, secondary sex characteristics emerge, and a "growth spurt" occurs. Descriptive standards for the assessment of pubertal advancement have been developed to aid in the objective recording of sexual characteristics. This system of assessment uses "Tanner stages" to distinguish among sequential stages of development (Tanner, 1962), where Tanner Stage 1 refers to prepubescence, and Tanner Stage 5 refers to a fully sexually mature state. Although normal healthy individuals vary greatly with regard to the age of pubertal onset, age cutoffs derived from cross-sectional and longitudinal studies of healthy children are used to distinguish between normal puberty and puberty that is considered aberrant (precocious or delayed).

The initial sign of normal puberty in girls (breast budding) commences as early as 7 years among White girls, and 6 years among Black girls (Herman-Giddens et al., 1997). For boys, the initial sign of normal puberty is increased testicular size; this may begin as early as 9 years. Girls who begin puberty before age 6 and boys who begin before age 9 are said to have precocious puberty (PPUB). Because PPUB is associated with the normal physical signs of puberty, affected children tend to be taller than their classmates. An assessment of PPUB includes a family history and a medical examination, as well as lab tests to measure sex hormones and gonadotropins (pituitary-derived gonad stimulating factors). A radiograph of the hand and wrist is often ordered to determine bone age, and imaging studies of the brain (e.g., magnetic resonance imaging) may also be ordered to detect abnormalities (Lee, 1996).

PPUB can be caused by several factors, although most cases are idiopathic. Girls exhibit PPUB 5 times more often than boys, and the idiopathic form 8 times more often than boys. In contrast, neurologic abnormalities occur at least as frequently as idiopathic PPUB in boys. Among girls, neurologically based PPUB is only one fifth as common as the idiopathic form (Grumbach & Styne, 2003).

Like PPUB, delayed puberty (DPUB) is diagnosed according to descriptive standards of healthy children. A girl is considered to have DPUB if (a) the pubertal process has not begun by age 13, (b) the process is not complete over the course of 4 years, or (c) *menarche* (first menses) has not occurred by age 16. Boys are considered to have DPUB if they have not commenced puberty by age 14 (Grumbach, Hughes, & Conte, 2003). As with PPUB, children presenting with DPUB should be referred to a pediatric endocrinologist to rule out pathological causes of the delay. The majority of children who are considered to have DPUB are physically healthy, and most cases can be attributed to constitutional growth delay (CGD), a variant of normal development characterized by slow but consistent growth throughout infancy and childhood. Ultimately, children with CGD achieve a height commensurate with their genetic growth potential.

For a minority of children, DPUB has an underlying pathological cause. *Hypogonadism* (i.e., a state of inadequate production of sex hormones) can stem from insufficient stimulation of the gonads by pituitary-derived stimulating factors (*hypogonadotropic hypogonadism*), such as that commonly associated with brain tumors and Kallmann syndrome. Hypogonadism can also arise as a consequence of a problem with the ovary or testis itself (*hypergonadotropic hypogonadism*), as in that observed as a feature of Klinefelter syndrome, Turner syndrome, or other instances of primary testicular or ovarian failure.

Outcomes

Studies show that children with PPUB or DPUB are not at an increased risk for clinically significant psychological disturbances. Both groups, however, may face stresses related to the incongruence between physical appearance and CA (similar to those discussed for children with SS; Mazur & Clopper, 1991). As a result of this discrepancy, adults may hold expectations that are inconsistent with the child's capacities. For children with PPUB, adults' expectations may be unrealistically high, resulting in misperceptions of the child as socially immature or intellectually slow. Conversely, adults may have lower than appropriate expectations of children with DPUB. This tendency can result in the child being inadequately challenged—academically or socially—in ways that interfere with the realization of his or her potential.

Additionally, children may be embarrassed by premature or delayed physical development and may avoid activities where secondary sex characteristics are more salient (e.g., swimming, dating). Parents may be particularly concerned about premature physical development, especially as it relates to psychosexual development. Although parents can be assured that children with PPUB do not seek out sexual experiences at an age earlier than children with on-time puberty, these children may be vulnerable to the advances of others because of their physical maturity. Research findings indicate that children with PPUB achieve psychosexual milestones at an age that falls in line with norms for their CA, and not their physical appearance. Affected children may engage in masturbation at a younger age, however (Mazur & Clopper, 1991).

For children with DPUB, there is some evidence to suggest that psychosexual milestones are achieved at a slightly later age. The psychosocial effects of this do not seem to be far-reaching, however, because adults with a history of CGD are indistinguishable from adults who experienced on-time puberty. The psychosocial prognosis for children with DPUB attributable to other causes (e.g., Klinefelter or Turner syndrome) may be less optimistic (refer to chap. 15, "Sex Chromosome Anomalies"). The specific influence of DPUB on quality of life in these individuals is confounded by syndrome-specific features associated with such conditions, however.

A similar caveat applies to intellectual functioning: Whereas DPUB associated with CGD is not associated with a particular cognitive profile, the more complex conditions listed earlier are associated with specific cognitive strengths and weaknesses. For children with PPUB, intellectual functioning falls within the average to high average range. The slight increase in functioning is likely due to the higher academic expectations placed on them.

Medical and Psychoeducational Implications

When PPUB is the consequence of premature activation of the hypothalamic–pituitary–gonadal axis, treatment consists of a gonadotropin-releasing hormone (GnRH) agonist (Lupron). Early intervention is important in terms of the achievement of final adult height because the hormones responsible for early puberty also cause the growth plates at the ends of the bones (epiphyses) to fuse. Because this fusion marks the end of linear growth, final adult height will be compromised if treatment begins too late. On discontinuation, treatment has not been shown to have negative side effects on later pubertal development or subsequent fertility. In addition to psychoeducational counseling, academic acceleration (i.e., skipping a grade) may be helpful for children with PPUB who socialize better with older children. This option is only feasible in cases in which the child's intellectual capacity supports such an option.

Because most cases of DPUB are variations of normal growth, medical treatment is typically not necessary. For children who experience emotional distress that would be relieved by the acceleration of pubertal onset, however, short-term therapy with sex hormones is an option. This treatment does not compromise final adult height. Psychoeducational counseling may be useful as a supplement, or alternative, to medical treatment.

DISORDERS OF SEXUAL DIFFERENTIATION

Overview

Disorders of sexual differentiation (intersexuality) encompass diverse and complex conditions characterized by discordance among sex chromosomes, gonads, sex hormones, and phenotypic sex (internal reproductive structure and external genital appearance; Grumbach et al., 2003). These conditions include (a) true hermaphroditism (in which both ovarian and testicular tissue are present in the same or opposite gonads); (b) genetic females (i.e., 46, XX) with congenital adrenal hyperplasia, (c) genetic males (46, XY) with partial androgen insensitivity; (d) 46, XY individuals with 5-alpha-reductase deficiency; (e) 46, XY individuals with very small but normally formed penis (micropenis) or malformed penis (microphallus); and (f) 46, XY individuals with cloacal exstrophy (a severe birth defect wherein many of the abdominal organs, particularly the bladder and intestines, are exposed). The prevalence rate for these conditions combined may be as high as 1 in 3,000 (Melton, 2001). Because congenital adrenal hyperplasia (CAH) is the most frequently occurring condition associated with ambiguous genitalia (in girls), it is the focus of the section that follows.

Overview

In the United States, CAH affects approximately 1 in 15,000 live births, although there is considerable variation among ethnic–racial populations (Grumbach et al., 2003). CAH is a genetically inherited disorder that is associated with errors in the synthesis of hormones, resulting from a deficiency in any one of several enzymes. Ninety-five percent of all cases are characterized by a deficiency in the enzyme 21-hydroxylase. There are two major subgroups of "classic" 21-hydroxylase CAH: salt-wasting CAH, in which affected individuals experience varying degrees of salt loss secondary to a deficiency in the production of the hormone aldosterone, and simple-virilizing CAH, in which excess androgen production is not accompanied by salt loss. Salt-wasting CAH, experienced by the majority (75%) of those affected, is potentially life threatening (particularly during the first few weeks of life prior to diagnosis). Because of the serious implications of late treatment, the majority of states have established a newborn screening test.

Transmitted as an autosomal recessive trait (i.e., both parents must carry the mutation to have an affected child), CAH results in an impaired ability of the adrenal cortex to produce cortisol. As a consequence, adrenocorticotropic hormone (ACTH) secretion from the pituitary gland is stimulated, leading to the enlargement of the adrenal cortex. The enlarged adrenal cortex, along with the blocked metabolic pathway, results in excessive androgen production. Because this excess production begins in early fetal development, female newborns may exhibit ambiguous genitalia with labial fusion and clitoral enlargement. In severe cases, this may result in an announcement of male sex at birth. Late diagnosis (or inadequate hormone replacement) can result in accelerated growth during childhood and precocious puberty, but SS in adulthood.

Some expecting couples may know that both partners carry a classical gene mutation (either because they have had a child with CAH or through DNA testing). These couples may consider prenatal therapy, whereby the pregnant mother takes dexamethasone (a glucocorticoid) as soon as pregnancy is confirmed. Prenatal testing by chorionic villus sampling is then performed. If the fetus is unaffected, therapy is discontinued. If the fetus is female and is affected with classical CAH, treatment is continued until term. By working to suppress excess androgen production by the fetal adrenal glands, dexamethasone serves to minimize genital anomalies of affected female fetuses. Very early treatment (within 9 weeks of last menstrual period) substantially diminishes or eliminates genital virilization in girls.

Outcomes

Since the introduction of newborn screening, the incidence of salt-loss related deaths has been greatly reduced, particularly among affected boys. Although adequate hormone replacement prevents postnatal virilization in female infants, genital surgery is an option for those with masculinized genitalia. Inadequate metabolic control, whether due to late diagnosis or poor adherence to the hormone replacement medical regimen, may lead to PPUB.

In addition to the challenges associated with any chronic and potentially life-threatening illness, children with CAH (and their parents) may face stresses associated with PPUB, as well as SS. Although cognitive impairment is not characteristic of CAH, salt-wasting crises during infancy can potentially place children at risk for deficits (Berenbaum, 2001).

Androgen-Related Effects in Girls

Extensive animal research has demonstrated that the brains and behavior of males and females are sexually dimorphic and that these differences are influenced by exposure to prenatal androgens during sensitive periods of brain development. These differences, then, do not stem directly from the genetic sex of the animal (Collaer & Hines, 1995; Goy & McEwen, 1980). In humans, overlap in the gender distributions for most behaviors or traits are the rule rather than the exception and are influenced by an interaction of genetic, hormonal, and environmental factors (Ruble & Martin, 1998).

Gender dimorphisms are usually expressed as differences in the quantity of the behavior exhibited under specific conditions. For instance, social play is gender dimorphic in many mammalian species, with males consistently exhibiting higher levels of what can be described as rough-and-tumble play. Because girls with CAH are exposed to abnormally high levels of prenatal androgens, many researchers have examined the behavioral development of these individuals.

Although the gender identity of females with CAH is (with few exceptions) unequivocally female (Meyer-Bahlburg et al., 1996), girls with CAH exhibit a masculine shift in behavioral pattern (Zucker, 1999). Interestingly, it is girls with the salt-wasting form of CAH that show the most pronounced behavioral effects, possibly reflecting the greater severity of this form compared with simple virilizing CAH (Hall et al., 2004; Nordenstrom, Servin, Bohlin, Larsson, & Wedell, 2002).

In addition to the behavioral sequelae in childhood, data also suggest that the sexual behavior of adolescents and adults with CAH differs significantly from that of comparison groups. For instance, during adolescence, girls with CAH tend to achieve psychosexual milestones later than unaffected control subjects. Furthermore, women with CAH report less heterosexual activity than unaffected control subjects. These women are more likely to develop a bisexual or homosexual orientation, as indicated by sexual imagery (erotic or romantic fantasies and dreams), sexual attractions, and, to a lesser extent, overt homosexual activity (e.g., Zucker et al., 1996). Because the majority of women with CAH are heterosexual, however, it is clear that factors other than prenatal androgen exposure contribute to sexual orientation in women with CAH.

Androgen-Related Effects in Boys

Relatively little research has been directed toward the examination of psychosocial effects of increased androgen exposure in boys. Generally, affected boys are difficult to distinguish from unaffected siblings in ways that would translate to significant problems of psychosocial adjustment (Berenbaum, Korman, Duck, & Resnick, 2004).

Medical and Psychoeducational Implications

The primary aims of the treatment are to replace deficient hormones, suppress excess androgen formation, and promote normal growth and development. After the period of infancy ends and the condition has been stabilized, glucocorticoid replacement (Cortef) is the most common treatment. Dosage must be carefully monitored, because excessive amounts of cortisol may result in growth retardation and other side effects. By replacing the deficient cortisol and suppressing ACTH production, overstimulation of the adrenal cortex ceases. This results in the suppression of excessive adrenal androgen production, which, in turn, averts further virilization in girls, slows accelerated growth, and allows for the normal onset of puberty.

Mineralocorticoid replacement treatment is also essential to maintain salt and water homeostasis for patients with the salt-wasting forms of CAH. This is accomplished with the oral administration of fludrocortisone acetate (Florinef) and sometimes the addition of dietary salt. Because excessive amounts of mineralocorticoid and salt can result in severe hypertension, blood pressure must be monitored carefully. It is not uncommon for youngsters to "outgrow" the need for daily mineralocorticoid treatment. In some cases, they may cease to require treatment except on very hot days or when they are extremely active.

In rare cases where a CAH diagnosis is overlooked and a salt-wasting crisis occurs, emergency care is required. Infants must be treated immediately with intravenous hydration with saline, supplementation with hydrocortisone (Solu-Cortef), and correction of electrolyte abnormalities.

For girls born with masculinized genitalia, surgical management is an additional aspect of treatment. This typically occurs within the first year of life. Because infants do not have the ability to give informed consent and surgery may damage the sensitivity of genital tissue, the issues surrounding genital reconstruction are entangled in heated controversy (Beh & Diamond, 2000). Psychoeducational counseling with a professional who is informed of the different viewpoints surrounding the controversy may be useful in providing families with unbiased information that will help them arrive at a decision.

Whether genital surgery is under consideration or not, psychoeducational counseling is recommended upon diagnosis for the families of boys and girls with CAH. As the child gets older, family and individual counseling should correspond with the occurrence of major developmental milestones. For both sexes, challenges related to PPUB or learning disabilities may arise. Girls may benefit from assistance in dealing with issues related to atypical genital appearance, the discomfort associated with repeated genital examinations, and the possibility of surgery in later life. Mental health professionals should expect parents of daughters to have concerns regarding gender-atypical behavior and questions about later psychosexual development.

CONCLUSION

The endocrine disorders reviewed in this chapter have varied etiologies, as well as varied psychosocial and educational sequelae. Despite this heterogeneity, each of these conditions presents challenges to a positive quality of life. In many (perhaps even the majority) of cases, this "risk" does not advance to "disorder." Thus, one may encounter a child with congenital adrenal hyperplasia or growth hormone deficiency who does not exhibit all (or any) of the intellectual or behavioral–emotional features summarized in this review. This is likely due to the variable clinical presentation of all of these conditions, or because additional factors in the affected individual's environment mitigate the detrimental effects associated with the condition.

The task of the parent, clinician, teacher, and other adults who participate in the care and education of the child is to be aware of and to anticipate predictable sequelae—educational, behavioral, and emotional—associated with a particular condition. Early identification of syndrome-characteristic cognitive and behavioral deficits, together with the development of remedial strategies tapered to the individual, can greatly facilitate educational and psychosocial development. A note of caution is warranted: Common features associated with a condition will appear variably across affected individuals. The assumption of limitations based on studies of groups may result in a disservice to individuals. Unwarranted assumptions may prompt a "self-fulfilling prophecy," resulting in a foreclosure—rather than a broadening—of life options for the child or adolescent.

REFERENCES

Abbott, D., Rotnem, D., Genel, M., & Cohen, D. J. (1982). Cognitive and emotional functioning in hypopituitary short-statured children. *Schizophrenia Bulletin, 8*, 310–319.

American Diabetes Association. (2005). Standards of medical care in diabetes. *Diabetes Care, 28*(Suppl. 1), S4–S36.

August, G. P., Julius, J. R., & Blethen, S. L. (1998). Adult height in children with growth hormone deficiency who are treated with biosynthetic growth hormone: The National Cooperative Growth Study experience. *Pediatrics, 102*, 512–516.

Beh, H. G., & Diamond, M. (2000). An emerging ethical and medical dilemma: Should physicians perform sex assignment surgery on infants with ambiguous genitalia? *Michigan Journal of Gender & Law, 7*, 1–63.

Berenbaum, S. A. (2001). Cognitive function in congenital adrenal hyperplasia. *Endocrinology & Metabolism Clinics of North America, 30*, 173–192.

Berenbaum, S. A., Korman, B. K., Duck, S. C., & Resnick, S. M. (2004). Psychological adjustment in children and adults with congenital adrenal hyperplasia. *Journal of Pediatrics, 144*, 741–746.

Blizzard, R. M., & Bulatovic, A. (1996). Syndromes of psychosocial short stature. In F. Lifshitz (Ed.), *Pediatric endocrinology* (3rd ed., pp. 83–93). New York: Marcel Dekker.

Buse, J. B., Polonsky, K. S., & Burant, C. F. (2003). Type 2 diabetes mellitus. In P. R. Larsen, H. M. Kronenberg, S. Melmed, & K. S. Polonsky (Eds.), *Williams textbook of endocrinology* (10th ed., pp. 1427–1483). Philadelphia: W. B. Saunders.

Carroll, P. V., Christ, E. R., & the members of Growth Hormone Research Society Scientific Committee. (1998). Growth hormone deficiency in adulthood and the effects of growth hormone replacement: A review. *Journal of Clinical Endocrinology Metabolism, 83*, 382–395.

Collaer, M. L., & Hines, M. (1995). Human behavioral sex differences: A role for gonadal hormones during early development? *Psychological Bulletin, 118*, 55–107.

Cooper, D. S. (2001). *Medical management of thyroid disease.* New York: Marcel Dekker.

Dallas, J. S., & Foley, T. P. (1996a). Hypothyroidism. In F. Lifshitz (Ed.), *Pediatric endocrinology* (3rd ed., pp. 391–399). New York: Marcel Dekker.

Dallas, J. S., & Foley, T. P. (1996b). Hyperthyroidism. In F. Lifshitz (Ed.), *Pediatric endocrinology* (3rd ed., pp. 401–414). New York: Marcel Dekker.

Debruyne, F., Vanderschueren-Lodeweyckx, M., & Bastijns, P. (1983). Hearing in congenital hypothyroidism. *Audiology, 22*, 404–409.

Desrocher, M., & Rovet, J. (2004). Neurocognitive correlates of Type 1 diabetes mellitus in childhood. *Child Neuropsychology, 10*, 36–52.

Eisenbarth, G. S., Polonsky, K. S., & Buse, J. B. (2003). Type 1 diabetes mellitus. In P. R. Larsen, H. M. Kronenberg, S. Melmed, & K. S. Polonsky (Eds.), *Williams textbook of endocrinology* (10th ed., pp. 1485–1508). Philadelphia: W. B. Saunders.

Eminson, D. M., Powell, R. P., & Hollis, S. (1994). Cognitive behavioral interventions with short statured boys: A pilot study. In B. Stabler & L. E. Underwood (Eds.), *Growth, stature, and adaptation* (pp. 135–150). Chapel Hill: University of North Carolina.

Fisher, D. A., & Foley, B. L. (1989). Early treatment of congenital hypothyroidism. *Pediatrics, 83*, 785–789.

Foley, T. P., Jr. (2000). Acquired hypothyroidism in infants, children and adolescents. In L. E. Braverman & R. D. Utiger (Eds.), *Werner and Ingbar's the thyroid* (8th ed., pp. 983–988). Philadelphia: Lippincott-Raven.

Goy, R. W., & McEwen, B. S. (1980). *Sexual differentiation of the brain.* London: Oxford University Press.

Grew, R. S., Stabler, B., Williams, R. W., & Underwood, L. E. (1983). Facilitating patient understanding in the treatment of growth delay. *Clinical Pediatrics, 22*, 685–690.

Grumbach, M. M., Hughes, I. A., & Conte, F. A. (2003). Disorders of sexual differentiation. In P. R. Larsen, H. M. Kronenberg, S. Melmed, & K. S. Polonsky (Eds.), *Williams textbook of endocrinology* (10th ed., pp. 842–1002). Philadelphia: W. B. Saunders.

Grumbach, M. M., & Styne, D. M. (2003). Puberty: Ontogeny, neuroendocrinology, physiology, and disorders. In P. R. Larsen, H. M. Kronenberg, S. Melmed, & K. S. Polonsky (Eds.), *Williams textbook of endocrinology* (10th ed., pp. 1117–1286). Philadelphia: W. B. Saunders.

Hall, C. M., Jones, J. A., Meyer-Bahlburg, H. F. L., Dolezal, C., Coleman, M., Foster, P., et al. (2004). Behavioral and physical masculinization are related to genotype in girls with congenital adrenal hyperplasia. *Journal of Clinical Endocrinology Metabolism, 89*, 419–424.

Herman-Giddens, M. E., Slora, E. J., Wasserman, R. C., Bourdony, C. J., Bhapkar, M. V., Koch, G. G., et al. (1997). Secondary sexual characteristics and menses in young girls seen in office practice: A study from the Pediatric Research in Office Settings network. *Pediatrics, 99*, 505–512.

Hunt, L., Hazen, R. A., & Sandberg, D. E. (2000). Perceived versus measured height. Which is the stronger predictor of psychosocial functioning? *Hormone Research, 53*, 129–138.

Jacobson, A. M. (1996). The psychological care of patients with insulin-dependent diabetes mellitus. *New England Journal of Medicine, 334*, 1249–1253.

Larsen, P. R., & Davies, T. F. (2003). Hypothroidism and thyroiditis. In P. R. Larsen, H. M. Kronenberg, S. Melmed, & K. S. Polonsky (Eds.), *Williams textbook of endocrinology* (10th ed., pp. 423–455). Philadelphia: W. B. Saunders.

Lee, P. A. (1996). Disorders of puberty. In F. Lifshitz (Ed.), *Pediatric endocrinology* (3rd ed., pp. 175–193). New York: Marcel Dekker.

Lindsay, R., Feldkamp, M., Harris, D., Robertson, J., & Rallison, M. (1994). Utah Growth Study: Growth standards and the prevalence of growth hormone deficiency. *Journal of Pediatrics, 125*, 29–35.

MacGillivray, M. H., Baptista, J., & Johanson, A. (1996). Outcome of a four-year randomized study of daily versus three times weekly somatropin treatment in prepubertal naive growth hormone-deficient children. Genentech Study Group. *Journal of Clinical Endocrinology Metabolism, 81*, 1806–1809.

Mauras, N., Attie, K. M., Reiter, E. O., Saenger, P., Baptista, J., & the Genentech Inc. Cooperative Study Group. (2000). High dose recombinant human growth hormone (GH) treatment of GH-deficient patients in puberty increases near-final height: A randomized, multicenter trial. *Journal of Clinical Endocrinology Metabolism, 85*, 3653–3660.

Mazur, T., & Clopper, R. R. (1991). Pubertal disorders. Psychology and clinical management. *Endocrinology & Metabolism Clinics of North America, 20*, 211–230.

Melton, L. (2001). New perspectives on the management of intersex. *Lancet, 357*, 2110.

Mensing, C., Boucher, J., Cypress, M., Weinger, K., Mulcahy, K., Barta, P., et al. (2005). National standards for diabetes self-management education. *Diabetes Care, 28*, S72–S79.

Meyer-Bahlburg, H. F. L. (1990). Short stature: Psychological issues. In F. Lifshitz (Ed.), *Pediatric endocrinology* (2nd ed., pp. 173–196). New York: Marcel Dekker.

Meyer-Bahlburg, H. F. L., Gruen, R. S., New, M. I., Bell, J. J., Morishima, A., Shimshi, M., et al. (1996). Gender change from female to male in classical congenital adrenal hyperplasia. *Hormones and Behavior, 30*, 319–332.

Nordenstrom, A., Servin, A., Bohlin, G., Larsson, A., & Wedell, A. (2002). Sex-typed toy play behavior correlates with the degree of prenatal androgen exposure assessed by CYP21 genotype in girls with congenital adrenal hyperplasia. *Journal of Clinical Endocrinology & Metabolism, 87*, 5119–5124.

Oerbeck, B., Sundet, K., Kase, B. F., & Heyerdahl, S. (2003). Congenital hypothyroidism: Influence of disease severity and L-thyroxine treatment on intellectual, motor, and school-associated outcomes in young adults. *Pediatrics, 112,* 923–930.

Perrin, E. C., Stein, R. E., & Drotar, D. (1991). Cautions in using the Child Behavior Checklist: Observations based on research about children with a chronic illness. *Journal of Pediatric Psychology, 16,* 411–421.

Reiter, E. O., & Rosenfeld, R. G. (2003). Normal and aberrant growth. In P. R. Larsen, H. M. Kronenberg, S. Melmed, & K. S. Polonsky (Eds.), *Williams textbook of endocrinology* (10th ed., pp. 1003–1114). Philadelphia: W. B. Saunders.

Rieser, P. A., & Meyer-Bahlburg, H. F. L. (1991). *Short & OK.* Glen Head, NY: Human Growth Foundation.

Ron, E., Doody, M. M., Becker, D. V., Brill, A. B., Curtis, R. E., Goldman, M. B., et al. (1998). Cancer mortality following treatment for adult hyperthyroidism. Cooperative Thyrotoxicosis Therapy Follow-up Study Group. *Journal of the American Medical Association, 280,* 347–355.

Rosen, T., Johannsson, G., Johansson, J. O., & Bengtsson, B. A. (1995). Consequences of growth hormone deficiency in adults and the benefits and risks of recombinant human growth hormone treatment. A review paper. *Hormone Research, 43,* 93–99.

Rovet, J. F. (2000). Neurobehavioral consequences of congenital hypothyroidism identified by newborn screening. In B. Stabler & B. B. Bercu (Eds.), *Therapeutic outcome of endocrine disorders. Efficacy, innovation, and quality of life* (pp. 235–254). New York: Springer-Verlag.

Rovet, J. F. (2004). In search of the optimal therapy for congenital hypothyroidism. *Journal of Pediatrics, 144,* 698–700.

Rovet, J., & Daneman, D. (2003). Congenital hypothyroidism: A review of current diagnostic and treatment practices in relation to neuropsychologic outcome. *Paediatric Drugs, 5,* 141–149.

Rovet, J. F., & Ehrlich, R. (2000). Psychoeducational outcome in children with early-treated congenital hypothyroidism. *Pediatrics, 105,* 515–522.

Rovet, J., Ehrlich, R., & Sorbara, D. (1987). Intellectual outcome in children with fetal hypothyroidism. *Journal of Pediatrics, 110,* 700–704.

Rovet, J. F., Ehrlich, R. M., & Sorbara, D. L. (1992). Neurodevelopment in infants and preschool children with congenital hypothyroidism: Etiological and treatment factors affecting outcome. *Journal of Pediatric Psychology, 17,* 187–213.

Ruble, D. N., & Martin, C. L. (1998). Gender development. In N. Eisenberg (Vol. Ed.), *Handbook of child psychology: Vol. 3. Social, emotional, and personality development* (5th ed., pp. 933–1016). New York: Wiley.

Sandberg, D. E. (1996). Short stature: Intellectual and behavioral aspects. In F. Lifshitz (Ed.), *Pediatric endocrinology* (3rd ed., pp. 149–162). New York: Marcel Dekker.

Sandberg, D. E., Brook, A. E., & Campos, S. P. (1994). Short stature: A psychosocial burden requiring growth hormone therapy? *Pediatrics, 94,* 832–840.

Sandberg, D. E., Bukowski, W. M., Fung, C. M., & Noll, R. B. (2004). Height and social adjustment: Are extremes a cause for concern and action? *Pediatrics, 114,* 744–750.

Sandberg, D. E., Colsman, M., & Voss, L. D. (2004). Short stature and quality of life: A review of assumptions and evidence. In O. H. Pescovitz & E. Eugster (Eds.), *Pediatric endocrinology: Mechanisms, manifestations, and management* (pp. 191–202). Philadelphia: Lippincourt, Williams & Wilkins.

Sandberg, D. E., & Michael, P. (1998). Psychosocial stresses related to short stature: Does their presence imply psychiatric dysfunction? In D. Drotar (Ed.), *Assessing pediatric health-related quality of life and functional status: Implications for research* (pp. 287–312). Mahwah, NJ: Erlbaum.

Sandberg, D. E., Ognibene, T. C., Brook, A. E., Barrick, C., Shine, B., & Grundner, W. (1998). Academic outcomes among children and adolescents receiving growth hormone therapy. *Children's Health Care, 27,* 265–282.

Sandberg, D. E., & Voss, L. D. (2002). The psychosocial consequences of short stature: A review of the evidence. *Best Practice & Research. Clinical Endocrinology & Metabolism, 16,* 449–463.

Siegel, P. T. (1990). Intellectual functioning and academic functioning in children with growth delay. In C. S. Holmes (Ed.), *Psychoneuroendocrinology: Brain, behavior, and hormonal interactions* (pp. 17–39). New York: Springer-Verlag Telos.

Simoneau-Roy, J., Marti, S., Deal, C., Huot, C., Robaey, P., & Van Vliet, G. (2004). Cognition and behavior at school entry in children with congenital hypothyroidism treated early with high-dose levothyroxine. *Journal of Pediatrics, 144,* 747–752.

Strauss, R. S., & Pollack, H. A. (2003). Social marginalization of overweight children. *Archives of Pediatrics & Adolescent Medicine, 157,* 746–752.

Tanner, J. M. (1962). *Growth at adolescence.* Springfield, IL: Charles C Thomas.

Tillotson, S. L., Fuggle, P. W., Smith, I., Ades, A. E., & Grant, D. B. (1994). Relation between biochemical severity and intelligence in early treated congenital hypothyroidism: A threshold effect. *British Medical Journal, 309,* 440–445.

Vanderschueren-Lodeweyckx, M., Debruyne, F., Dooms, L., Eggermont, E., & Eeckels, R. (1983). Sensorineural hearing loss in sporadic congenital hypothyroidism. *Archives of Disease in Childhood, 58,* 419–422.

Zimet, G. D., Cutler, M., Litvene, M., Dahms, W., Owens, R., & Cuttler, L. (1995). Psychological adjustment of children evaluated for short stature: A preliminary report. *Journal of Developmental & Behavioral Pediatrics, 16,* 264–270.

Zucker, K. J. (1999). Intersexuality and gender identity differentiation. *Annual Review of Sex Research, 10,* 1–69.

Zucker, K. J., Bradley, S. J., Oliver, G., Blake, J., Fleming, S., & Hood, J. (1996). Psychosexual development of women with congenital adrenal hyperplasia. *Hormones & Behavior, 30,* 300–318.

6

EPILEPSY AND SEIZURES

ROWLAND P. BARRETT AND HENRY T. SACHS III

OVERVIEW

This chapter provides an overview of seizure disorders; the related medical, psychosocial, and educational outcomes; and the treatment options. The term *epilepsy* is derived from the Greek word *epilambabein* meaning "to attack" or "to seize upon." It is defined by paroxysmal or sudden and dramatic changes in cerebral neuron firing with or without disturbance of consciousness or alterations in perceptual motor functioning. The term *seizure* is derived from the Latin word *sacire*, which means "to take possession of." A seizure is defined by paroxysmal or sudden and dramatic changes in cerebral functioning associated with abnormal cerebral neuron firing. Seizures are always linked with a disturbance of consciousness, alterations of perceptual motor functioning, or both. Depending on the distribution of the abnormal neuronal discharges, the disturbance of consciousness and alterations of perception may vary widely and range from spectacular convulsive activity to a personal experiential occurrence not readily discerned by the naïve observer.

It is important to distinguish epilepsy from seizures. Although the terms are commonly (and wrongly) used synonymously, they are quite different. A seizure is an event that may be initiated by either a central nervous system process, such as head injury or lead poisoning, or a process external to the central nervous system, such as fever, drug withdrawal, and electroconvulsive therapy. Epilepsy is a disorder in which seizures recur because of a chronic underlying pathology that invariably is initiated by the central nervous system. Consequently, a person who presents with a single seizure (or recurrent seizures) because of a temporary or correctable condition, such as a high fever or drug withdrawal, does not necessarily have epilepsy. A person who presents with recurrent seizures due to a chronic underlying pathology that affects the central nervous system, such as vascular and metabolic abnormalities or head trauma, is correctly diagnosed with epilepsy.

Epidemiology

Ten percent of Americans will experience a seizure in their lifetime, and by age 75, 3% will have developed epilepsy (Epilepsy Foundation of America, 1999). The disparity between these rates is largely due to the potential among infants and young children to experience a so-called "single-episode febrile seizure," a rare occurrence in older children and adults. Febrile seizures occur when body temperature rises rapidly during an illness. Infants and young children are more prone than adults to febrile illness, such as otitis media and respiratory infection, and more likely to experience high fever during bouts of ill health. The vast majority (60%) of infants and young children who experience a febrile seizure do not experience more than one febrile seizure event.

Epidemiologic studies have found the average annual incidence of epilepsy to approximate 85 cases per 100,000 (Annegers, 1997). Thirty percent of epilepsies occur between birth and 5 years of age, and 75% of epilepsies present by age 20 (Cowan, Bodensteiner, Leviton, & Doherty, 1989). The remaining 25% of epilepsies are distributed throughout adulthood with a disproportionate number of adult-onset epilepsies affecting the geriatric (65+ years) population (Epilepsy Foundation of America, 2003).

Prevalence rates of epilepsy in children vary widely with study results being highly dependent on methodological issues. When stringent research diagnostic criteria have been applied, a prevalence rate of 10 cases per 1,000 individuals has been commonly accepted. Cowan et al. (1989) reported prevalence rates of 5.2 cases per 1,000 in children aged birth to 4 years and 4.6 cases per 1,000 in children and adolescents aged 5 to 19. A conservative estimate is that 500,000 children and adolescents experience nonfebrile, recurrent seizures each year due to epilepsy and that approximately 180,000 new cases of epilepsy are identified annually for all age groups including adulthood (Epilepsy Foundation of America, 2003).

Classification

There have been many attempts to classify seizures, and with good reason. Accurate delineation of seizure type is critical to determining etiology and prognosis and selecting the appropriate treatment protocol. The most commonly used and widely accepted classification system remains the *International Classification of Epileptic Seizures* (Dreifuss, 1981). Seizures in this classification system are divided into two broad categories: (a) partial seizures, which begin focally at a single site within the brain and usually affect only one sensory or motor system, and (b) generalized seizures, which affect both hemispheres of the brain and the body, bilaterally (and symmetrically), at onset. Partial seizures are further subclassified as those that do not impair consciousness (simple) and those in which consciousness is impaired (complex). Within each of these subclassifications are numerous additional subcategories differentiated by symptom presentation or how the seizure event progresses within the brain.

Partial Seizures

Partial seizures are those in which the first clinical or behaviorally observable (including electroencephalogram [EEG]) changes indicate activation of a system of neurons limited to one part of the cerebral hemisphere (Dreifuss, 1981). Simple partial seizures (SPS) may present either with motor, sensory, autonomic, or psychic symptoms. Motor symptoms are the classic form of presentation, often beginning as uncontrollable bending (flexion), alternating with extending (extension) around a joint of a distal extremity, such as a finger or wrist, creating a tapping or flailing appearance. Although this may be the observable extent of the seizure, it also may expand to involve the entire extremity (arm), unilateral extremities (arm and leg), an entire side of the body, or eventually the entire body, at which time it is reclassified as a partial seizure that has evolved secondarily into a generalized seizure. This progression is rarely observed in children, but not in adults, where it is usually indicative of a cortical lesion. Motor seizures also may affect body posture and vocalizations, including arresting speech. A subclass of motor seizures called *versive* seizures characteristically consist of eye and (often) head turning in a stereotypic manner opposite the site of the cortical damage.

Complex partial seizures (CPS) may begin as simple partial seizures or as a complex partial seizure from the outset. These seizures are among the most controversial in the interface among psychiatry, psychology, and neurology. CPS may present in a variety of fashions with the single requirement that consciousness is altered. The alteration in consciousness may be subtle or dramatic and may affect mood, cognition, memory, personality traits, and well-established behavior patterns. Although 20% to 30% of patients with all types of epilepsy also have psychiatric diagnoses, several studies indicate a much greater likelihood of behavioral disturbance (50%–70%) in patients having CPS with temporal lobe involvement (Tucker, 1998).

Complex partial seizures (CPS) may be accompanied by *automatisms*. Often described as stereotypic, repetitive activities ranging from simple lip smacking to complex motor tasks such as marching or even undressing. Attempts to interrupt these activities often lead to agitation and undirected aggression by the individual who is experiencing them, of which they are later unaware. Observers may wrongly attribute this behavior to oppositional or acting-out behavior. Directed aggression is rarely observed in individuals with CPS.

Prodromal symptoms or *auras* associated with CPS often are described as senses of deja vu, abdominal discomfort, or olfactory hallucinations such as burning rubber, hot tar, or other unpleasant odors, possibly representing a simple partial seizure (SPS) progressing to become a CPS. Once the episode is concluded, the individual will often be disoriented, tired, and unable to recall the event(s). Common sources of abnormal neuronal firing in CPS are the deep structures of the brain's limbic system, especially the amygdala. Because standard EEG studies only record relatively superficial cortical activity, these abnormal discharges may not be detected. Therefore, up to three normal EEG studies should be conducted before a seriously considered diagnosis of CPS is ruled out.

Primary Generalized Seizures

Both simple and complex partial seizures can evolve secondarily into generalized seizures. Primary generalized seizures, however, are those in which the first clinical changes indicate initial involvement of both cerebral hemispheres. Impairment of consciousness may be the presenting symptom, and any motor manifestations will affect the body bilaterally. Generalized seizures (Dreifuss, 1989) are a heterogeneous group of seizures including absence seizures (formerly known as petit mal seizures) and tonic–clonic seizures (formerly known as grand mal seizures).

Tonic–clonic seizures may present without warning or following an aura, which is most commonly a period of abdominal discomfort, dizziness, or occasionally an irritable mood but may take many forms. Following the aura, the individual's eyes may roll up into the head accompanying a loss of consciousness, and the individual may emit a grunt or piercing cry, caused by the constriction of the thoracic muscles and subsequent forced exhalation through constricted vocal chords. Classically, the individual will then become rigid, extending the extremities and arching the back (tonic phase) for a few seconds, followed by rhythmic contractions of the extremities (clonic phase), more so than the trunk. The primary safety concerns during a tonic–clonic seizure are physical injury secondary to a fall following the alteration of consciousness and injury to the extremities as they flail during the seizure event. *Hypoxia* also is a concern if the individual is unable to breathe spontaneously because of constant forceful contraction of the thoracic muscles and tight closing of the jaw. *Cyanosis*, in the form of a bluish tinge around the lips, mouth, and tongue, is the clearest sign of inadequate oxygenation and indicative of the need for supplemental oxygen. In all cases of tonic–clonic seizure activity, individuals should be placed on their side to prevent aspiration of vomit or sinus mucous and moved away from furniture, walls, and other objects to prevent trauma to their extremities during flailing. Seizures or *ictal* events are usually self-limiting, lasting from a few seconds to 20 to 30 minutes. Typically, they are followed by a period of confusion and a semiconscious state known as the *postictal* period. Individuals may lose bladder control during the course of seizure activity and usually will sleep for an hour or more after the event has concluded, often complaining of headache.

Absence seizures (Mirsky, 1989) are classically described as brief periods of loss of consciousness without accompanying motor activity. They appear as momentary lapses in attention characterized by staring. Practically speaking, however, upward of two thirds of individuals with absence seizures will have some accompanying motor movements, typically eyelid fluttering at a rate of 3 per second, lip smacking, head drooping with decreased muscle tone, or motor activities resembling the automatisms seen in complex partial seizures. Absence seizures may be as brief as 1 second in duration but typically last 5 to 10 seconds. Onset is without warning. There is no aura, and the individual has no awareness that the episode has occurred. The typical EEG pattern for absence seizures is specific, making identification of the disorder relatively straightforward, if the diagnosis is being considered.

Within the category of primary generalized seizures there are numerous subgroups (Dreifuss, 1989), including tonic, clonic, atonic, and myoclonic seizures. *Tonic seizures* are characterized by violent muscle contractions of the extremity or axial muscles in a strained position with eye deviation and, occasionally, complete rotation of the entire body. Respirations are inhibited by the contractions of the respiratory muscles and face, which is contorted with a tight jaw. Cyanosis is not unusual in tonic seizures. *Clonic seizures* are primary generalized seizures in which the tonic phase does not precede the rhythmic clonic phase and repetitive clonic jerks. *Atonic seizures* are differentiated by the sudden decrease or loss of muscle tone involving either a limb, the head, neck, or entire body. This phenomenon also is known as a "drop attack." However, atonic seizures are not the only cause of drop attacks, which appear to occur most frequently in the morning hours. Atonic seizures comprising drop attacks are potentially dangerous and increase the risk of injury, especially involving the face and head. Children with intractable atonic seizures are usually required to wear protective headgear to protect against injury from sudden falls. Myoclonic jerks—sudden brief contractions of single muscle groups that may be repetitive—are the observable or clinical representation of *myoclonic seizures* as well as other benign and significant physiologic processes, including falling asleep in healthy individuals. An EEG study may be required to differentiate potential etiologies of myoclonic jerks, including differentiating them from chronic motor tics.

OUTCOMES

OUTCOMES

Mortality and Morbidity

Mortality rates from childhood through early adulthood are significantly higher for individuals with epilepsy than in the general population. The risk of death is 2 to 3 times greater for individuals with epilepsy compared with cohorts across the life span (Tomson, 2000). A 30-year follow-up study in Finland by Sillanpaa (1992) reported a mortality rate that was clearly higher for patients with epilepsy than patients without epilepsy. The annual mortality risk for male patients with epilepsy was 7.5 per 1,000 patient years compared with an expected value of 1.9 per 1,000 patient years for male patients without epilepsy. Female patients with epilepsy also had a higher mortality rate (4.8 per 1,000 patient years) compared with female patients without epilepsy (0.7 per 1,000 patient years). These findings represented a four- and sevenfold increase in the mortality rates of male and female patients, respectively, because of epilepsy. Accidents (drowning), respiratory infection (pneumonia), *status epilepticus* (a condition defined by the onset of second and subsequent attacks of seizure activity without full recovery from the previous seizure episode), suicide, and cerebrovascular disease are among the most common causes of death in people with epilepsy (Morgan & Kerr, 2002).

The morbidity of epilepsy related to physical injury is not well established. The relative risk of physical injury for patients with epilepsy compared with the general population is thought to be substantially higher but remains understudied. Research assessing injury in the epilepsy population has more closely examined the types of injuries sustained and the relationship with seizure type and seizure frequency. Buck, Baker, Jacoby, Smith, and Chadwick (1997) reported that 35% of patients who had experienced at least one seizure within the past year experienced a physical injury related to the seizure. Head injury, burns and scalds, dental injury, and fractures were the most frequently reported injuries. Injuries generally doubled for patients presenting with more than one seizure per month, with the greatest risk associated with primary generalized seizures (Beghi & Cornaggia, 2002).

The costs of epilepsy are considerable. The total annual cost of epilepsy in the United States is $12.5 billion, with $10.8 billion primarily associated with employment (Begley, Famulari, & Annegers, 2000). Personal, intellectual, and social disabilities associated with epilepsy not measured in dollars are also costly, however. Results of a survey by Beran (1999) indicated that 53% of individuals with epilepsy reported restrictions in activities of daily living, 46% reported difficulties in memory and concentration, 39% indicated concern about having children, 36% reported an impaired ability to drive a car, 28% reported difficulties in interpersonal relationships with spouses or partners, and 21% reported sexual difficulties. Similarly, results of a Roper poll (Roper Organization, 2000) indicated that 61% of those surveyed cited limitations to thinking clearly, 51% cited driving limitations, 44% cited work-related limitations, and 38% cited limitations to participating in sports as affecting their daily living.

In the United States, 25% of working-age people with epilepsy are unemployed. Of these, 64% stated that they were not working as a direct result of their epilepsy (Epilepsy Foundation of America, 1999). It is difficult to establish the precise burden of epilepsy in unemployment and underemployment. Many occupations prohibit the hiring of individuals with epilepsy for valid safety reasons. Concomitant psychological morbidity in terms of the cognitive and behavioral changes associated with epilepsy, social prejudice, the side effects of antiepileptic drugs, as well as psychiatric aspects of living with a chronic illness (Aldenkamp, DeKrom, & Reijs, 2003; Jokeit, Daamen, Zang, Janszky, & Ebner, 2001; Meador, 2002) all may come to bear on gaining and maintaining employment, however. A number of studies (cf. Epilepsy Foundation of America, 1999) have confirmed academic underachievement and specific reading difficulties, as well as higher rates of psychiatric disorder in patients with epilepsy compared with patients who have other types of chronic medical illnesses. It may be argued that low rates of performance and behavioral problems are characteristics most employers are opposed to seeing in their employees. Consequently, it is difficult to separate the relative contribution of the medical disorder of epilepsy from its comorbid psychological features in determining the occupational hardship associated with the disorder.

Psychological and Social Sequelae

Generally speaking, children with epilepsy do not achieve academically as well as expected and require a high rate of special education services (Seidenberg, Beck, & Geisser, 1986). The relationship between seizure activity and cognitive functioning is complicated and not yet fully understood. Seizures can be divided into two categories, those with known associated structural damage to the central nervous system and those that are *idiopathic* (i.e., of unknown etiology). For those individuals having epilepsies associated with neuroanatomical and neurophysiological abnormalities, it is difficult to differentially attribute cognitive dysfunction to the seizure disorder itself, the structural damage to the brain, or a combination of both. What is clear, however, is that individuals with known etiologies for their seizures have less favorable outcomes on neuropsychological testing than those with idiopathic seizures (Dodrill, 1992). In all individuals with epilepsy, the confounding influence of various antiepileptic drug treatments on cognitive functioning must be taken into consideration.

The role of antiepileptic drugs in the cognitive impairment experienced by individuals with epilepsy is controversial (Trimble & Cull, 1988). What appear to be less controversial are the effects of *polypharmacy*. Multiple antiepileptic drugs are more likely to have adverse effects on attention, memory, and general intellectual functioning (Bourgeois, 1988). There is, however, the confounding fact that individuals who require multiple antiepileptic drug treatment to maintain adequate management of their seizure disorder are most likely to have more serious underlying observable neuroanatomical or neurophysiological abnormalities, a known risk for cognitive deficit.

Even when allowances for attention, memory, and learning difficulties, as well as seizure control are taken into consideration, most children with epilepsy still fail to meet academic expectation (Suurmeijer, 1991). Parents of children with epilepsy traditionally have reported lower academic expectations of their children, as well as attitudes of disapproval of participation in extracurricular activities. School systems also show a willingness to view the student with epilepsy differently. It is much more likely that a child with epilepsy who makes poor progress academically will be placed in a special education classroom than an underachieving or poorly performing child without epilepsy (Zelnik, Saado, Silman-Stolar, & Goikhman, 2001). Lower expectations of parents and teachers and accommodations to the traditional academic curriculum conspire to motivate most students with epilepsy to seek vocational training and develop vocational careers (Kokkonen, Kokkonen, Saukkonen, & Pennanen, 1997).

Numerous behavioral problems have been attributed to epilepsy and seizures (cf. Kim, 1991; Sackellares & Berent, 1997). Surveys of schoolteachers have indicated that 20% to 30% of students with epilepsy have problematic personal and social behavior, including aggression. Similar findings established the rule of thumb that one third of children, adolescents, and adults with epilepsy will experience comorbid psychiatric disorder. More recent studies (Tucker, 1998) have indicated that this may be an underestimate. Depression alone is observed in 20% to 55% of individuals with epilepsy and suicide rates are 3 to 5 times higher than in the general population (Epilepsy Foundation of America, 2003). The new rule of thumb is to expect one half of individuals with epilepsy to encounter comorbid behavioral health issues at some point in their lifetimes.

Epilepsy is a chronic illness that carries with it numerous psychosocial stressors (Shackleton, Kasteleijn-Nolst Trenite, De Craen, Vandenbrouke, & Westendorp, 2003). Prejudice against individuals with epilepsy is longstanding and may lead to ostracism. The role as outcast may evolve around peers, parents, family, teachers, or coworkers, regardless of age of onset. Generalized convulsive seizure activity is frightening to observe and some of the behaviors associated with complex partial seizures are odd and difficult for the naïve observer to reconcile. Children may quickly distance themselves from classmates with epilepsy who, during seizure episodes, may urinate, defecate, vomit, fall and damage their face, or display some inappropriate behavior (self-biting, scratching, or pinching) accompanied by an exaggerated emotional response. The child's own embarrassment when told of the events and the sense of lacking control may lead to increasing and voluntary social isolation, as well as the development of a powerful negative self-image.

The same holds true for adolescents, made worse by additional restrictions on critical activities such as driving an automobile, participation in sports and recreational activities, and work performance. These restrictions typically lead to less satisfying interactions with peers, parents, family members, and coworkers and result in an increased dependency on others at a time when personal autonomy, social initiative, independence, and personal and social accomplishments are used as the milestones of success and happiness (Bishop & Allen, 2003). Adolescence is a time of many significant changes, and the frequency and severity of seizure activity may be among those changes. Absence seizures diminish, generalized seizures may increase, and complex partial seizures may remain unchanged. Medication compliance is a huge issue in adolescence, especially if weight gain, hirsutism (i.e., excessive hair growth), and gum hyperplasia are untoward effects of antiepileptic drug treatment. The adverse effects of medication are contrasted with the requirement to be seizure free for a substantial period to be issued a driver's license. Few things represent the normal developmental assertions of independence and identity in a more compelling manner than driving an automobile (Gilliam et al., 1997), especially for an adolescent. Since the first traffic accident attributed to epilepsy was reported in 1906, all 50 states in the United States impose restrictions on driving for individuals diagnosed with epilepsy. Restrictions vary from state to state but typically require 3 months to 1 year of seizure-free status before issuing a driver's license. In addition to the obstacles involved in obtaining a driver's license, actuarial data support the need for increased insurance premiums. Individuals with epilepsy are found to be involved in twice as many automobile accidents compared with the general population (Epilepsy Foundation of America, 1999). The increased expense of auto insurance may be prohibitive and unfavorably affect already limited employment opportunities for both adolescents and young adults with epilepsy.

MEDICAL AND PSYCHOEDUCATIONAL IMPLICATIONS

Antiepileptic Drug (AED) Treatments

Antiepileptic drug therapy is the typical treatment for the vast majority of patients with epilepsy. Approximately two thirds of patients with epilepsy can obtain control of their seizure disorder through the use of a single antiepileptic drug. An additional 10% to 15% of patients will obtain control by using a second and, in some cases, a third drug. The goal of antiepileptic drug therapy is twofold: (a) no seizures and (b) no side effects (Engel, 2004).

Accurate diagnosis of seizure type is important to the selection of the most appropriate medication. Certain antiepileptic drugs control certain seizure types better than others. There is, however, considerable overlap in the general effectiveness of most antiepileptic drugs. Individual patient needs and the drug side effect profile are considered equally important to the history of drug effectiveness with a particular class of seizure.

Barbiturate compounds, such as *phenobarbital*, have been the most studied of the antiepileptic drugs. There is a long history of their use as an effective first-line antiepileptic drug. There is an equally long-standing concern, however, that barbiturates produce sedation in adults and irritability, aggressiveness, and hyperactivity in children (Forsythe & Sills, 1984), as well as adverse cognitive effects. Decreases in intellectual performance, as well as attention and short-term memory have been reported in patients with epilepsy who were being treated with phenobarbital, as well as volunteer control subjects without epilepsy who received phenobarbital (Smith, 1991).

Phenytoin (Dilantin) is another antiepileptic drug that has been well studied and has a long history of successful employment as a first-line therapeutic agent for the treatment of partial seizures. Phenytoin has a relatively long half-life, making it amenable to an easy, twice daily, dosing schedule. Side effects, such as hirsutism, coarsening of facial features, and gingival hyperplasia are common and usually poorly tolerated, often leading to discontinuation of the drug. Studies conducted across the past 20 years have reached a consensus that phenytoin is safe and effective but requires careful monitoring to prevent a wide range of untoward effects, such as memory impairment (Herranz, Armijo, & Arteaga, 1988) and cerebellar atrophy (Ney, Lantos, Barr, & Schaul, 1994), which may occur secondary to toxicity (Pellock, 2002).

Ethosuximide (Zarontin) is used as the treatment of choice for absence seizures. It appears to be safe and effective, resulting in significant reduction or total elimination of absence seizure activity for 70% of patients receiving the drug (Holmes, 1987). It is difficult to assess the cognitive effects of treatment with ethosuximide in patients with absence epilepsy because 16% to 23% of these patients present comorbid mild and nonprogressive neurological abnormalities that confound interpretation. Findings of adverse effects on cognitive functioning when ethosuximide has been given in combination with other medications and in those individuals who initially are more cognitively limited have been disputed (Bourgeois, 1988).

Carbamazepine (Tegretol) has long reigned as the antiepileptic drug of choice for treatment of partial seizures, as well as generalized tonic–clonic seizures. It has a relatively low index of sedation compared with other antiepileptic drugs and no behavioral side effects, including no deleterious effects on intellectual ability. In fact, beneficial effects on alertness, visuomotor coordination, and problem solving have been reported. Some studies have found substantial improvements in the IQs of children with epilepsy who were being treated with carbamazepine. Important methodological issues diminish the potential nature of these findings, however (Trimble & Cull, 1988). Skin disorders, such as rash and pruritus (i.e., itching), are the most common side effects, leading to discontinuation of the drug in 10% of patients. Idiosyncratic hematological side effects, such as aplastic anemia, *leukopenia* (the deficiency of white blood cells), *thrombocytopenia* (the deficiency of platelets), and anemia are rare, but remain an area of focused concern with carbamazepine.

Oxcarbazepine (Trileptal) is a homologue of carbamazepine and an equally effective first-line drug for the treatment of partial seizures, as well as an effective adjunctive therapy for generalized seizures (Gaily, Granstrom, & Luikkonen, 1998). Oxcarbazepine appears to have similar benefits but fewer side effects than carbamazepine. It is less problematic when combined with valproate and may be effective in patients who were unresponsive to carbamazepine (Rutecki & Gidal, 2002). Oxcarbazepine is well tolerated by children as well as adults. Skin rash was noted in 5% of patients. *Hyponatremia* (low blood sodium concentration) is a unique side effect in children receiving the drug.

Valproic acid (Depakote) was introduced in the 1970s as the first true broad-spectrum antiepileptic drug. It is considered the drug of choice for the treatment of primary generalized tonic–clonic seizures. It also is effective in the treatment of partial seizures, absence seizures, myoclonic seizures, and Lennox–Gastaut epilepsy (Pellock, 2002). Idiosyncratic hepatotoxicity and pancreatitis are chief concerns (Bryant & Dreifuss, 1996) because they cannot be reliably anticipated by laboratory monitoring of blood levels. Early signs of hepatic failure include vomiting, nausea, loss of appetite, apathy, increased seizure activity, and fever. Leukopenia and *neutropenia* (low white blood cell count) are additional hematological concerns. In most cases, symptoms remit and hepatic failure is reversible on discontinuation of the drug. Additional side effects may include mild mental slowing with complex cognitive tasks. Valproic acid does not appear to affect attention or memory, however.

Lamotrigine (Lamictal) is currently approved for use as an adjunctive therapy for partial seizures, as well as for patients with seizures associated with Lennox–Gastaut epilepsy. The efficacy of lamotrigine in reducing seizure frequency is well studied. King, Knight, and Oommen (1996) reported that 53% of patients experienced a greater than 50% reduction. Other studies have reported similar findings (Sorensen, Mai, & Friss, 1998), including observation of seizure-free status in 15% of patients previously described as medically refractory (McKee, Sunder, & Voung, 2001). Lamotrigine is typically well tolerated with few adverse effects, although irritability and aggression have been noted (Beran & Gibson, 1998). Rash and Stevens–Johnson syndrome (a serious form of rash) have an incidence of approximately 5% and 1%, respectively, and require immediate discontinuation of the drug.

Additional side effects include dizziness, headaches, and ataxia, which typically are mild and transient.

Gabapentin (Neurontin) has efficacy rates similar to lamotrigine. Studies (e.g., Crawford, Brown, & Kerr, 2001) have indicated that between one third and one half of patients receiving gabapentin demonstrated 50% reductions in seizure activity. Gabapentin is well tolerated with few significant side effects. The most commonly reported include sleepiness, dizziness, ataxia, fatigue, and tremor. Behavior problems, in the form of aggressive behavior and hyperactivity, have been reported (Lee et al., 1996). Only 4% of patients discontinue the drug because of behavioral disturbance or intolerance of side effects. There is no rash associated with gabapentin use.

Surgical Treatment of Epilepsy

Refractory epilepsy or epilepsy with persistent seizures that cannot be effectively controlled is thought to be a progressive disease (Sutula, Hagen, & Pitkanen, 2003). The association between refractory epilepsy and cognitive dysfunction (Bjornaes, Stabell, & Henriksen, 2001), brain damage (Breillmann, Berkovic, & Syngiotis, 2002), and progressive undesirable behavior changes (Austin & Dunn, 2002), including additional seizure activity (Hauser & Lee, 2002), has gathered strength. Epilepsy is no longer considered a benign disorder where the greatest risk is injury from falling. Neuronal death, as well as sudden death (Pedley & Hauser, 2002), is a reality in patients of all ages with intractable seizures. Mortality rates are 4 to 7 times higher in children, adolescents, and adults with refractory epilepsy than in patients whose seizure disorder is well controlled (Sperling, 2004).

Approximately 20% of children, adolescents, and adults with epilepsy are resistant to antiepileptic drug therapy. Patients with mesial temporal lobe epilepsy (MTLE) comprise the vast majority of this treatment refractory group. Surgical treatment of refractory epilepsy has a well-established history (Wyler, 1989) and has emerged as a safe and effective option for patients, including children and adolescents, with persistent, uncontrolled seizure disorder (Weibe, 2004). Advances in neuroimaging (Gaillard, 2000), such as positron emission tomography, single photon emission computed tomography, and functional magnetic resonance imaging (Ng, McGregor, & Wheless, 2004), have allowed the clear assessment of mesial temporal sclerosis and congenital anatomical abnormalities (cortical dysplasia) that are viewed as predispositions to the development of intractable partial seizures. The surgical procedure, which consists of resecting the anteromesial temporal lobe, performing the removal of a focal temporal lesion (lesionectomy), or both, has enjoyed widespread success. Advances in presurgical diagnostic evaluation and microsurgical techniques have allowed 70% of children, adolescents, and adults with refractory epilepsy to be seizure-free following treatment (Engel, Weibe, & French, 2003). An additional 25% of patients demonstrate a 90% decrease in seizure activity following surgery. Significant clinical complications are few (3%), and postoperative care is routine. Only a small number of patients (1%–2%) with surgically remediable intractable epilepsy receive surgical treatment (Swarztrauber, 2004). The lack of a definition of what constitutes intractability contributes to the delay in referring patients, particularly children and adolescents, for surgical treatment (Kwan & Brodie, 2000), as does the prevailing cultural attitude that surgical intervention is a treatment of last resort (Swarztrauber, Dewar, & Engel, 2003). Current data appear to indicate that the risks of uncontrolled seizures greatly outweigh the risk of surgery and that early surgical intervention could lead to substantial improvements in the quality of life for patients with otherwise refractory epilepsy.

Vagus Nerve Stimulation

Vagus nerve stimulation (VNS) is a recently developed treatment alternative for patients of all ages with refractory seizure disorder who are not candidates for surgery and who have failed multiple antiepileptic drug trials (George, 1994). The VNS procedure involves the subcutaneous implanting of a small generator in the infraclavicular region. The generator is connected to a bipolar platinum electrode placed on the left vagus nerve and programmed by laptop computer to deliver electrical pulses on an intermittent basis (Wilfong, 2002). How VNS works, precisely, is unknown. Studies have indicated, however, that the mechanism of action related to increased seizure threshold may be secondary to extensive activation of cortical and subcortical pathways, an event that is reliably observed following stimulation of the vagus nerve (Schachter, 1998). Generally speaking, the VNS procedure is an effective treatment option for patients who have not responded to conventional antiepileptic drug therapy and continue to have seizures, as well as for those patients who experience untoward effects of antiepileptic drug treatment (Wheless, 2002). Most patients, including children and adolescents, tolerate the VNS procedure well, and it produces only mild and transient side effects (e.g., coughing, hoarseness).

The Ketogenic Diet

The ketogenic diet, first introduced in the 1920s (Freeman, Kelly, & Freeman, 1994), consists of heavy cream, butter, fats, a limited amount of protein and vegetables, and virtually no starch or sugar. The ketogenic diet is carefully calculated to simulate the metabolism of a fasting body. Fasting is a well-known means of controlling seizures. Patients receiving the ketogenic diet rely on burning their body fat for energy rather than relying on the intake of glucose. Liquids also are minimized to mimic the dehydrated state of the fasting body. Unlike true fasting, which can be tolerated only for a short period of time, the ketogenic diet allows the patient to maintain a fat-burning, partially dehydrated state for an indefinite period. Fat energy is the foundation of the ketogenic diet. By severely limiting carbohydrates and, consequently, the conversion of carbohydrates into glucose, the body is forced to burn fat as its primary energy source. In the absence of glucose, stored body fat is not burned completely and leaves a residue in the form of ketone bodies that build up in the blood. In the presence of high blood levels of ketone bodies, seizures are frequently controlled. The precise mechanism of action is not known. The ketogenic diet is known to be more effective in controlling childhood myoclonic, absence, and atonic seizures but has been used successfully to control generalized tonic–clonic seizures, as well as the seizures associated with Lennox–Gastaut epilepsy. Proponents of the diet report that it controls seizure activity in 50% of children whose seizures are otherwise persistent and refractory to treatment with antiepileptic drugs (Freeman et al., 1994). A study by Kinsman, Vining, Quaskey, Mellits, and Freeman (1992) demonstrated complete seizure control in 18 of 58 patients identified with refractory epilepsy as the result of treatment using the ketogenic diet. The diet is very labor intensive, however, and requires careful calculations, dietary manipulations, and strict adherence. Slight departures may result in seizure activity. Side effects are mild, and the diet is generally safe and without untoward effects, if conducted under the supervision of a physician.

PSYCHOSOCIAL AND PSYCHOEDUCATIONAL INTERVENTIONS

Several interventions can be helpful in addressing the psychosocial stressors associated with epilepsy and seizures. The accurate identification of seizure-related signs and symptoms leading to appropriate diagnosis and treatment is essential. In the school setting, this may include teachers noting unusual staring, eye blinking, lip smacking, head drops, changes in mood, unusual difficulties focusing, lapses in attention, or repetitive nonfunctional behaviors. Once these observations have been made, a thorough neurological evaluation is mandatory, including EEG and magnetic resonance imaging studies. Symptomatic relief through appropriate treatment will provide the individual the greatest opportunity for personal and social success, as well as an increased sense of control over the body and a more favorable self-image (Perrine, Hermann, & Meador, 1995).

For the school-age child, monitoring for the potential side effects of antiepileptic medications, such as fatigue, hyperactivity, disinhibition, confusion, ataxia, or cognitive dullness and slowing, is most often successful within the structured environment of the classroom. A multidisciplinary treatment team consisting of a pediatric neurologist, teacher, school psychologist, registered nurse, and social worker is most useful in these circumstances, both for evaluating the student's progress and educating school personnel about what should be monitored in terms of seizure activity, medication side effects, associated learning disabilities, and the sometimes underestimated academic potential of students with epilepsy. In addition, teachers and classmates of the student with epilepsy may require specific interventions, education, and support after witnessing an epileptic event. A team of professionals who are knowledgeable about the disorder and know the student personally are in the best position to be helpful.

Despite the best efforts of neurologists and pediatricians, students with epilepsy and their families often have many unanswered questions and a routine need for professional support. The school psychologist can play a critical role as liaison between students with epilepsy and their teachers, parents, doctors, and other professionals. Reviewing with students and families their concerns and expectations may evince what was not asked or left unsaid in the neurologist's office and play an important role in the student's adaptation to the disorder. Relaying these concerns to the physician or helping a student and family formulate a plan to address those issues in the future can help alleviate psychosocial stressors, improve compliance with medication regimens, and enhance the student's integration into his or her primary social setting—the school.

Individual therapy also may be indicated for a patient with epilepsy. This will usually focus on issues of chronic illness, self-esteem, loss of bodily control, and medication adherence. Irritability and depressed mood secondary to chronic illness is not uncommon and may require consultation with a child psychiatrist. Group therapy with other patients with epilepsy or chronic illnesses may be helpful in terms of social support and personal and social problem solving, such as the development of coping skills.

Family therapy may include the process of psychoeducation around the disorder, including treatment outcomes and options, prognosis, and future plans to manage foreseeable obstacles. Family therapy also may be the setting to address the underlying feelings of guilt, anger, resentment, hopelessness, and sadness that may pervade family relationships and contribute to diminished family functioning. Excessive dependency on parents, siblings, school personnel, and the medical establishment also may be a reasonable topic for family therapy. There is a fine line that distinguishes therapeutic support from that of enabling dependency. Students and their families are best served when they are taught how to help themselves in terms of identifying, managing, and overcoming the many hardships related to living with epilepsy as a lifelong illness.

CONCLUSION

Epilepsy is a disorder characterized by a chronic underlying pathology that affects central nervous system functioning. A variety of epilepsy syndromes manifest themselves in the potential for recurrent seizure events involving loss of control of motor and cognitive functioning. Epilepsy, when defined as two or more seizure events, has a prevalence rate of 5 to 10 per 1,000 individuals. Seizures resulting from epilepsy may be classified as being partial or generalized, depending on involvement of both hemispheres of the central nervous system. Epilepsy takes various forms and may be either amenable or refractory to treatment. Depending on the magnitude of the epileptic disorder and the accompanying seizures, it may be severely disabling to the afflicted person. A variety of pharmacological (antiepileptic drugs), nutritional (ketogenic diet), surgical (anteromesial temporal lobe resection), and neurophysiological (vagus nerve stimulation) treatments exist. Approximately 80% of individuals with seizure disorder respond to treatment with antiepileptic drugs. Advances in neuroimaging and microsurgery have allowed drug resistant refractory epilepsy to be addressed, typically with excellent results. Psychosocial treatments also may be required secondary to comorbid psychiatric disorder as well as adverse social and psychological sequelae related to educational achievement, employment, and quality of life. Individual or group therapy (or both), in combination with family therapy, also may be useful in helping to promote compliance with treatment protocols and decrease the stress associated with chronic illness.

REFERENCES

Aldenkamp, A., DeKrom, M., & Reijs, R. (2003). Newer antiepileptic drugs and cognitive issues. *Epilepsia, 44*(Suppl. 4), 21–29.

Annegers, J. F. (1997). Incidence rates of epilepsy by age. In E. Wyllie (Ed.), *The treatment of epilepsy: Principles and practice* (2nd ed., pp. 165–172). Baltimore: Williams & Wilkins.

Austin, J., & Dunn, D. (2002). Progressive behavioral changes in children with epilepsy. *Progress in Brain Research, 135*, 419–427.

Beghi, E., & Cornaggia, C. (2002). Morbidity and accidents in patients with epilepsy: Results of a European cohort study. *Epilepsia, 43*, 1076–1083.

Begley, C. E., Famulari, M., & Annegers, J. F. (2000). The cost of epilepsy in the United States: An estimate from population based clinical and survey data. *Epilepsia, 41*, 342–351.

Beran, R. G. (1999). The burden of epilepsy for the patient: Intangible costs. *Epilepsia, 40*(Suppl. 8), 40–43.

Beran, R. G., & Gibson, R. J. (1998). Aggressive behaviour in intellectually challenged patients with epilepsy treated with lamotrigine. *Epilepsia, 39*, 280–282.

Bishop, M., & Allen, C. (2003). The impact of epilepsy on quality of life: A qualitative analysis. *Epilepsy and Behavior, 4*, 226–233.

Bjornaes, H., Stabell, H., & Henriksen, O. (2001). The effects of refractory epilepsy on intellectual functioning in children and adults: A longitudinal study. *Seizure, 10*, 250–259.

Bourgeois, B. F. D. (1988). Problems of combination drug therapy in children. *Epilepsia, 29*(Suppl.), S20–S24.

Breillmann, R., Berkovic, S., & Syngiotis, A. (2002). Seizure-associated hippocampal volume loss: A longitudinal magnetic resonance study of temporal lobe epilepsy. *Annals of Neurology, 51*, 641–644.

Bryant, A., III, & Dreifuss, F. E. (1996). Valproic acid hepatic fatalities. III. U.S. experience since 1986. *Neurology, 46*, 465–469.

Buck, D., Baker, G. A., Jacoby, A., Smith, D. F., & Chadwick, D. W. (1997). Patients' experiences of injury as a result of epilepsy. *Epilepsia, 38*, 439–444.

Cowan, L. D., Bodensteiner, J. B., Leviton, A., & Doherty, L. (1989). Prevalence of epilepsies in children and adolescents. *Epilepsia, 30*, 94–106.

Crawford, P., Brown, S., & Kerr, M. (2001). A randomized open-label study of gabapentin and lamotrigine in adults with learning disability and resistant epilepsy. *Seizure, 10*, 107–115.

Dodrill, C. B. (1992). Neuropsychological aspects of epilepsy. *Psychiatry Clinics of North America, 15*, 383–394.

Dreifuss, F. E. (1981). Proposal for revised clinical and electroencephalographic classification of epileptic seizures. *Epilepsia, 22*, 489–501.

Dreifuss, F. E. (1989). Childhood epilepsies. In B. P. Hermann & M. Seidenberg (Eds.), *Childhood epilepsies: Neuropsychological, psychosocial, and intervention aspects* (pp. 1–13). New York: Wiley.

Engel, J. (2004). The goal of epilepsy therapy: No seizures, no side effects, as soon as possible. *CNS Spectrums, 9*, 95–97.

Engel, J., Weibe, S., & French, J. (2003). Practice parameter: Temporal lobe and localized neocortical resections for epilepsy. *Neurology, 60*, 538–547.

Epilepsy Foundation of America. (1999). *Epilepsy: A report to the nation.* Landover, MD: Author.

Epilepsy Foundation of America. (2003). *Epilepsy: A report to the nation.* Landover, MD: Author.

Forsythe, W. I., & Sills, M. A. (1984). One drug for childhood grand mal: Medical audit for three-year remissions. *Developmental Medicine and Child Neurology, 26*, 742–748.

Freeman, J. M., Kelly, M. T., & Freeman, J. B. (1994). *The epilepsy diet treatment: An introduction to the ketogenic diet.* New York: Demos.

Gaillard, W. D. (2000). Structural and functional imaging in children with partial epilepsy. *Mental Retardation and Developmental Disabilities Research Reviews, 6*, 220–226.

Gaily, E., Granstrom, M. L., & Luikkonen, E. (1998). Oxcarbazepine in the treatment of epilepsy in children and adolescents with intellectual disability. *Journal of Intellectual Disability Research, 42*, 41–45.

George, R. (1994). Vagus nerve stimulation for treatment of partial seizures: Long term follow-up on the first 67 patients exiting a controlled study. *Epilepsia, 35,* 637–657.

Gilliam, F., Kuzniecky, R., Faught, E., Black, L., Carpenter, G., & Schrodt, R. (1997). Patient-validated content of epilepsy-specific quality of life measurement. *Epilepsia, 38,* 233– 236.

Hauser, W. A., & Lee, J. R. (2002). Do seizures beget seizures? *Progress in Brain Research, 135,* 215–219.

Herranz, J. L., Armijo, A., & Arteaga, R. (1988). Clinical side-effects of phenobarbital, primidone, phenytoin, carbamazepine, and valproate during monotherapy in children. *Epilepsia, 29,* 794–804.

Holmes, G. L. (1987). *Diagnosis and management of seizures in children.* Philadelphia: W. B. Saunders.

Jokeit, H., Daamen, M., Zang, H., Janszky, J., & Ebner, A. (2001). Seizures accelerate forgetting in patients with left-sided temporal lobe epilepsy. *Neurology, 57,* 125–126.

Kim, W. J. (1991). Psychiatric aspects of epileptic children and adolescents. *Journal of the American Academy of Child and Adolescent Psychiatry, 30,* 874–886.

King, J. A., Knight, J. E., & Oommen, K. J. (1996). Efficacy of lamotrigine in the developmentally disabled. *Epilepsia, 37,* 162.

Kinsman, S. L., Vining, E. P. G., Quaskey, S. A., Mellits, E. D., & Freeman, J. M. (1992). Efficacy of the ketogenic diet for intractable seizure disorders: Review of 58 cases. *Epilepsia, 33,* 1132–1136.

Kokkonen, J., Kokkonen, E., Saukkonen, A., & Pennanen, P. (1997). Psychosocial outcome of young adults with epilepsy in childhood. *Journal of Neurology, Neurosurgery, and Psychiatry, 62,* 265–268.

Kwan, P., & Brodie, M. J. (2000). Early identification of refractory epilepsy. *New England Journal of Medicine, 342,* 314–319.

Lee, D. O., Steingard, R. J., Cesena, M., Helmers, S. L., Riviello, J. J., & Mikati, M. A. (1996). Behavioral side effects of gabapentin in children. *Epilepsia, 37,* 87–90.

McKee, J. R., Sunder, T. R., & Voung, A. (2001). Lamotrigine adjunctive therapy in patients with mental retardation and refractory epilepsy in institutional and home settings. *Epilepsia, 42,* 183.

Meador, K. J. (2002). Cognitive outcomes and predictive factors in epilepsy. *Neurology, 58*(Suppl. 5), S21–S26.

Mirsky, A. F. (1989). Information processing in petit mal epilepsy. In B. P. Hermann & M. Seidenberg (Eds.), *Childhood epilepsies: Neuropsychological, psychosocial, and intervention aspects* (pp. 51–70). New York: Wiley.

Morgan, C. L., & Kerr, M. P. (2002). Epilepsy and mortality: A record linkage study in a U.K. population. *Epilepsia, 43,* 1251–1255.

Ney, G. C., Lantos, G., Barr, W. B., & Schaul, N. (1994). Cerebellar atrophy in patients with long term phenytoin exposure and epilepsy. *Archives of Neurology, 51,* 767–771.

Ng, Y. T., McGregor, A. L., & Wheless, S. W. (2004). Magnetic resonance imaging detection in mesial temporal sclerosis in children. *Pediatric Neurology, 30,* 81–85.

Pedley, T. A., & Hauser, W. A. (2002). Sudden death in epilepsy: A wake-up call for management. *Lancet, 359,* 1790–1791.

Pellock, J. M. (2002). Treatment considerations: Traditional antiepileptic drugs. *Epilepsy and Behavior, 3*(Suppl.), S18–S23.

Perrine, K., Hermann, B. P., & Meador, K. J. (1995). The relationship of neuropsychological functioning to quality of life in epilepsy. *Archives of Neurology, 52,* 997–1003.

Roper Organization. (2000). *Living with epilepsy: Report of a Roper poll of patients on quality of life.* New York: Author.

Rutecki, P. A., & Gidal, B. E. (2002). Antiepileptic drug treatment in the developmentally disabled: Treatment considerations with the newer antiepileptic drugs. *Epilepsy and Behavior, 3,* S24–S31.

Sackellares, J. C., & Berent, S. (Eds.). (1997). *Psychological disturbances in epilepsy.* Boston: Butterworth-Heinemann.

Schachter, S. C. (1998). Vagus nerve stimulation. *Epilepsia, 39,* 677–690.

Seidenberg, M., Beck, N., & Geisser, M. (1986). Academic achievement of children with epilepsy. *Epilepsia, 27,* 753–759.

Shackleton, D. P., Kasteleijn-Nolst Trenite, D. G., De Craen, A. J., Vandenbrouke, J. P., &Westendorp, R. G. (2003). Living with epilepsy: Long term prognosis and psychosocial outcomes. *Neurology, 61,* 64–70.

Sillanpaa, M. (1992). Children with epilepsy as adults: Outcome after 30 years of follow-up. *Acta Neurologica Scandinavica, 85,* 1–75.

Smith, D. B. (1991). Cognitive effects of antiepileptic drugs. In D. Smith, D. Treiman, & M. Trimble (Eds.), *Advances in neurology* (Vol. 55, pp. 197–212). New York: Raven.

Sorensen, T., Mai, J., & Friss, M. L. (1998). Long term follow-up on lamotrigine in treatment of epilepsy in the mentally retarded. *Epilepsia, 39,* 130.

Sperling, M. R. (2004). The consequences of uncontrolled epilepsy. *CNS Spectrums, 9,* 98–109.

Sutula, T. P., Hagen, J., & Pitkanen, A. (2003). Do epileptic seizures damage the brain? *Current Opinions in Neurology, 16,* 189–195.

Suurmeijer, T. (1991). Treatment, seizure free periods, and educational achievements: A follow-up study among children with epilepsy and healthy children. *Family Practice, 8,* 320–323.

Swarztrauber, K. (2004). Barriers to the management of patients with surgically remediable intractable epilepsy. *CNS Spectrums, 9,* 146–152.

Swarztrauber, K., Dewar, S., & Engel, J. (2003). Patient attitudes about treatments for intractable epilepsy. *Epilepsy and Behavior, 4,* 19–25.

Tomson, T. (2000). Mortality in epilepsy. *Journal of Neurology, 247,* 15–21.

Trimble, M. R., & Cull, C. A. (1988). Children of school age: The influence of antiepileptic drugs on behavior and intellect. *Epilepsia, 29*, 15–19.

Tucker, G. J. (1998). Seizure disorders presenting with psychiatric symptomatology. *Psychiatric Clinics of North America, 21*, 625–635.

Weibe, S. (2004). Effectiveness and safety of epilepsy surgery: What is the evidence? *CNS Spectrums, 9*, 120–132.

Wheless, J. (2002). Interim results of a prospective study of early adjunctive vagus nerve stimulation therapy. *Neurology, 58*, 53.

Wilfong, A. A. (2002). Treatment considerations: Role of the vagus nerve stimulator. *Epilepsy and Behavior, 3*(Suppl.), S41–S44.

Wyler, A. R. (1989). The surgical treatment of epilepsy. In B. P. Hermann & M. Seidenberg (Eds.), *Childhood epilepsies: Neuropsychological, psychosocial, and intervention aspects* (pp. 141–188). New York: Wiley.

Zelnik, N., Saado, L., Silman-Stolar, Z., & Goikhman, I. (2001). Seizure control and educational outcome in childhood-onset epilepsy. *Journal of Child Neurology, 16*, 820–824.

7

INTESTINAL DISORDERS

STEVEN G. LITTLE, K. ANGELEQUE AKIN-LITTLE,
ERIC G. WALDON, AND PIERO GARZARO

Disorders of the digestive tract are among the most common medical disorders across all ages of the population (Enck & Whitehead, 1999). Major symptoms and signs of a disorder of the digestive tract include vomiting, diarrhea, constipation, and abdominal pain (Behrman, Kliegman, & Jenson, 2000). Gastrointestinal disorders in children generally fall into one of three categories: (a) conditions that involve identifiable pathophysiology such as inflammatory bowel disease (IBD) and peptic ulcer disease; (b) conditions involving psychological etiology such as irritable bowel syndrome (IBS), recurrent abdominal pain (RAP), rumination, and psychogenic vomiting; and (c) other relevant disorders involving the gastrointestinal tract such as cystic fibrosis and celiac disease. In addition to summarizing these conditions, this chapter reviews studies investigating the influence of learning on refractory (or functional) gastrointestinal pain, summarizes research on the treatment of recurrent abdominal pain, and provides practical considerations for working with children who have gastrointestinal disorders.

This chapter provides a review of various intestinal disorders including inflammatory bowel disease, ulcerative colitis, Crohn's disease, peptic ulcers, irritable bowel syndrome, recurrent abdominal pain, rumination, psychogenic vomiting, cystic fibrosis, and celiac disease (gluten-sensitive enteropathy).

After an overview of the disorder, each section concludes with a paragraph describing psychoeducational outcomes and psychological treatments, particularly for disorders with psychological etiology. A final section is dedicated to psychoeducational implications of these various disorders. The section's first portion provides evidence that learning plays a major role in some disorders. The second portion gives an overview of treatments for these learned behaviors, including relaxation training, cognitive–behavioral therapy, and reinforcement of pain-free behaviors.

OVERVIEW AND OUTCOMES OF CONDITIONS INVOLVING PATHOPHYSIOLOGY

The conditions discussed in this section involve identifiable pathophysiology. That is, they are the result of specific disease processes, and psychological factors do not play a major role in their manifestation or course.

Inflammatory Bowel Disease

Inflammatory bowel disease (IBD) is the name of a group of disorders that cause the intestines to become inflamed (Schölmerich, 2003). The inflammation can last for an extended period of time and is usually recurrent. Every year, more than 600,000 Americans have some kind of inflammatory bowel disease (American Academy of Family Physicians, 2000), and IBD is the major cause of intestinal inflammation and a major cause of chronic illness in children and adolescents in Western Europe and North America (Ulshen, 2000a). Symptoms of IBD include abdominal cramps and pain, diarrhea, weight loss, and bleeding from the intestines. IBD encompasses two distinct illnesses: ulcerative colitis and Crohn's disease. Onset typically occurs in late childhood and adolescence and is characterized by an unpredictable course of remission and exacerbation. Because of the increased incidence of these conditions and difficulty of differential diagnosis, the term IBD is used more frequently for patients with the symptoms just described, whereas the terms ulcerative colitis and Crohn's disease are reserved for those classically presenting cases as described subsequently (Rigas & Spiro, 1995).

Ulcerative Colitis

Ulcerative colitis involves an inflammation of the mucosa of the large intestine and is distinguished by the presence of bloody diarrhea, lower abdominal cramping, and fecal urgency (Gionchetti et al., 2003). Prevalence rates vary from 40 to 225 per 100,000, and approximately 20% of all cases begin in childhood or adolescence (Ulshen, 2000a). Etiology is unknown, but it is generally accepted that there is an immunological reaction triggered in genetically susceptible individuals. No evidence exists for dietary, environmental, allergic, or psychological etiologies (Ulshen, 2000a). Pharmaco-logic treatment consists of antiinflammatory medication (i.e., steroids), antimotilic agents, and the use of immunosuppressive therapies. There is no curative medical therapy available. Surgical removal of the colon is indi-cated in the most severe cases with colostomy placement (Rigas & Spiro, 1995).

Psychoeducational implications are minimal for children with ulcer-ative colitis because the disease has no direct effect on intelligence or aca-demic performance. The disease may result in frequent school absences, how-ever, and interfere with school functioning. Additionally, social adaptation may be hindered by these absences and symptom manifestation in the school environment (Lesen, 1998).

Crohn's Disease (Regional Enteritis)

Crohn's disease can affect the entire digestive tract but primarily pre-sents as an inflammatory disease of the bowel (Behrman et al., 2000; Husain, 2004; Rigas & Spiro, 1995). Onset may be relatively subtle and involves abdominal cramping and diarrhea. With a prevalence rate of 40 to 100 per 100,000, 25% to 40% of cases manifest before age 20 but rarely before age 10 (Ulshen, 2000a). Unlike ulcerative colitis, however, patients with Crohn's disease may present with general malaise, fever, growth failure, and joint pain. Any teenager with chronic malaise and growth problems, especially if accompanied by fever, should be suspected of having this condition (Ulshen, 2000a). Similar to ulcerative colitis, curative medical therapy is not avail-able, but treatment can include antiinflammatory medication, immunosup-pressive therapy, and surgical removal or widening of the intestinal lumen. Unfortunately, medical treatment has a minimal effect and psychological interventions are often recommended. The child and family should be edu-cated regarding the nature of the disease and its disabling symptoms. Therapy may focus on enabling the individual to live as full a life as possible and not consider oneself an invalid. Exercise is encouraged but not to the extent that fatigue is induced, and the diet should be complete and nutritious (Miehsler & Gasche, 2003). Similar to ulcerative colitis, psychoeducational implica-tions involve frequent school absences and social stigmatization as a result of the disease (Proctor & Kranzler, 1998).

Peptic Ulcer Disease

Although peptic ulcer is less common in children than in adults, an incidence of approximately 5 per 100,000 children is reported (Carroll & Li, 2004). Peptic ulcer disease is characterized by the presence of lesions occur-ring in the duodenum and, less commonly, the stomach. A number of etio-logical factors have been linked to the development of ulcers including ge-netic predisposition, stress, excess gastric acid, and *Helicobacter pylori* bacteria

(Okuda & Nakazawa, 2004; Wallis-Crespo & Crespo, 2004). Clinical manifestation may consist of vomiting, abdominal pain, and strong familial incidence (Wallis-Crespo & Crespo, 2004). Successful treatment is achieved through dietary modification, antacid medication, and surgical correction (Rigas & Spiro, 1995).

Approximately 70% of adolescents diagnosed with peptic ulcer disease will have recurrences as they enter adult life. It is therefore important to counsel these individuals to avoid behaviors that may exacerbate the condition. Specifically, aspirin and alcohol may increase the risk of additional ulcers forming, and tobacco use may delay healing of existing ulcers. The only dietary restriction that is typically recommended is to avoid food that causes discomfort. Bland diets and the avoidance of caffeine or spicy foods have not been demonstrated to have any effect on ulcer formation or healing.

OVERVIEW AND OUTCOMES OF CONDITIONS INVOLVING PSYCHOLOGICAL ETIOLOGY

Generally, the conditions discussed in this section are considered diagnoses of exclusion after other pathophysiology has been ruled out, thus lending themselves to psychological etiologies. Ulshen (2000b) noted that among children and adolescents, these disorders are common, perplexing problems characterized by frequent abdominal pain; the majority of the disorders have no apparent pathophysiology.

Irritable Bowel Syndrome

Irritable bowel syndrome (IBS) is typified by lower abdominal pain, cramping, constipation, and diarrhea (L. S. Walker, 2004). One in five Americans has IBS, making it one of the most common disorders diagnosed by physicians. It occurs more often in women than in men, and it usually begins around age 20 (National Digestive Diseases Information Clearinghouse, 2003), but recurrent attacks of abdominal pain are observed in 10% to 15% of school-age children (Ulshen, 2000b).

Rigas and Spiro (1995) conceptualized IBS as a complex syndrome resulting from the interaction of psychological factors, bowel contents, and bowel motility. Of primary importance to mental health professionals are the psychological factors related to personality that may be connected to this condition. In light of the fact that half of all IBS patients exhibit no underlying psychological mechanism to explain their symptoms, Rigas and Spiro concluded there is no single IBS "personality profile." IBS patients do, however, "show strikingly different responses in their small bowel motor activity from normal when subjected to prolonged stress over a lifetime" (p. 266).

In addition to pharmacological treatment and dietary changes, recommended "supportive therapy" should consist of a discussion of psychosocial factors and the interaction of life events and symptoms. Furthermore, C. E. Walker (1995) recommended the use of relaxation training, stress inoculation, and assertiveness training.

Recurrent Abdominal Pain

As with all diagnoses of exclusion, a diagnosis of recurrent abdominal pain (RAP) is not made until after other organicity is ruled out (e.g., IBD). The incidence in the general pediatric population is approximately 10%, and the female to male ratio is 4 to 3. RAP is rare before age 4 to 5 and most common between ages 8 and 10, with a second peak in girls during early adolescence (Merck, 2004). RAP is psychogenic in 80% to 90% of patients. Symptoms in RAP are generally characterized by a lack of specificity and may include abdominal tenderness, erratic bowel action, headaches, and "limb tingling" (Ulshen, 2000b). Considering this vague symptomology, Blanchard and Scharff (2002) reported that psychological and psychiatric disturbance are common among patients with RAP and early abuse may play a role in its development. Psychogenic RAP is thought to arise from stress, anxiety, or depression. Individuals susceptible to RAP appear to be easily stressed, possibly because of events at home or at school. In addition, RAP itself may cause stress by creating significant school absenteeism and lack of peer contact or by compounding preexisting problems such as sibling conflict. Disproportionate comorbidity of nocturnal enuresis, extreme shyness, excessive perfectionism, family dysfunction, and sleep disorders has been reported (Blanchard & Scharff, 2002). Ulshen (2000b), however, noted that it is useful to determine whether pain wakens the child from sleep or interrupts pleasurable activity because each of these may imply organicity rather than functionality. Behaviorally based treatment recommendations consist of differential reinforcement of well behavior, cognitive coping skills training, various generalization enhancement procedures, treatment of school refusal (if present), and extinction of the reinforcing function of RAP in the home.

Rumination

Rumination is defined in the *Diagnostic and Statistical Manual of Mental Disorders* (4th ed., text rev.; *DSM–IV–TR*; American Psychiatric Association [APA], 2000) as the "repeated regurgitation and rechewing of food for a period of at least 1 month following a period of normal functioning" (p. 106). This is a relatively uncommon condition typically occurring in the latter half of the first year of life and occurs more often in boys than in girls (APA, 2000). Although the etiology is predominantly unknown, the regurgitated material may serve as a source of self-stimulation in the absence of other adequate environmental stimuli. With regard to assessment and diagnosis, careful observation is recommended to determine the mechanisms by which vomiting occurs (i.e., by use of hands in the mouth or by mouth movements) and the conditions that tend to trigger these behaviors. A number of behavioral interventions have been proposed to treat rumination: noncontingent holding (effective in approximately 80% of cases); punishment of regurgitation including contingent time out from social interaction, and use of electrical shock (Friedrich & Jaworski, 1995). A dearth of research and methodological weaknesses plague this efficacy literature, however. In some cases rumination disorder will have a spontaneous remission, and the child returns to eating normally without treatment (PsychNet—UK, 2003).

Psychogenic Vomiting

Psychogenic vomiting is a syndrome observed in children and is characterized by repeated episodes of vomiting without an underlying organic cause. It is a diagnosis of exclusion. Most frequently, vomiting occurs after meals and without a sense of nausea. Unlike bulimia nervosa, psychogenic vomiting is not associated with a disordered perception of body image. With psychogenic vomiting, individuals usually show no weight loss or dehydration (Merck, 2005). As in rumination, stomach contents are forcibly regurgitated; however, in psychogenic vomiting, the regurgitated contents are seldom, if ever, reingested. In describing psychogenic vomiting, Friedrich and Jaworski (1995) proposed a number of etiological hypotheses in which the regurgitation of gastric contents is a learned response used to mitigate stress or signal psychological upset. Psychogenic vomiting may be self-induced or may occur involuntarily in situations that are anxiety inducing, threatening, or in some way "distasteful." With regard to treatment, Friedrich and Jaworski reported that operant and family psychotherapeutic techniques are more effective than medical intervention.

OVERVIEW AND OUTCOMES OF OTHER RELEVANT PEDIATRIC GASTROINTESTINAL DISORDERS

Cystic Fibrosis

Cystic fibrosis (CF) is a congenital disorder in which a proliferation of mucosal secretions disrupt organ system functioning. It affects approximately 30,000 children and adults in the United States (Cystic Fibrosis Foundation, 2004). A defective gene causes the body to produce an abnormally thick, sticky mucus that clogs the lungs and leads to life-threatening lung infections. Although its primary effects are on the lungs and respiratory system, the disease does affect the gastrointestinal tract. The profusion of mucus in the intestinal tract can block the secretion of digestive enzymes into the digestive lumen and disrupt the absorption of nutrients. As a result, children with CF typically need to take dietary supplements with meals and consume a high-calorie meal to help the body absorb needed nutrients (Boat, 2000). Nutritional deficiencies can result in retardation of physical growth and muscle mass (Sanchez & Guiraldes, 1995).

Psychoeducational implications focus more on factors related to the respiratory system than the digestive system. Berge and Patterson (2004) reviewed 54 studies conducted over 2 decades and concluded that a complex balance is needed between meeting the needs of a child with CF and other family responsibilities. They suggested that parental involvement in medical treatment adherence is essential when the child is young, but more responsibility needs to be given to the child when adolescence is reached. Furthermore, it is important to monitor the mental health needs of parents, particularly mothers, when they feel overwhelmed with the treatment needs of their child. In schools, the psychologist needs to be aware of the needs of children with CF to facilitate teacher awareness of the disease and the academic, social, and behavioral concerns that may arise because of the chronic nature of the disease. These concerns include maintaining grades, keeping up with the academic work, making friends and maintaining friendships, and both externalizing and internalizing behavior problems.

Celiac Disease (Gluten-Sensitive Enteropathy)

Celiac disease (CD), involving an intestinal intolerance to gluten (a protein found in wheat, rye, barley, and oats), results in serious lesions within the small intestine interfering with the absorption of nutrients (Ulshen, 2000c). The prevalence rate in the United States is approximately 1 in every 133 to 250 persons. This prevalence is relatively consistent with the 1% estimate of worldwide prevalence (Celiac Disease Foundation, 2002). Clinical manifestations in children may include pain, diarrhea, nausea, bloating, foul-smelling stools, and weight loss; however, some may present near or normal health. The only treatment for CD is the lifelong adherence to a gluten-free diet. When gluten is removed from the diet, the small intestine begins to heal, and overall health improves. Medication is normally not required; however, treatment sometimes includes use of antiinflammatory medication along with a gluten-free diet (Rigas & Spiro, 1995). Because many of the foods most common in the diet of American children contain gluten, children with CD may experience anger and depression at not being able to eat a diet similar to their peers. They may be tempted to "go along with the crowd" and eat forbidden foods and may need help coping with these environmental and social challenges (Jackson & Murray, 1998).

PSYCHOEDUCATIONAL IMPLICATIONS

A number of studies have investigated the role of learning in childhood on the course of various gastrointestinal disorders and symptom presentation in adulthood. In general, data support the notion that early learning experiences, particularly reinforcement of sick role behavior, influence coping strategies and illness conceptualization in later life, particularly with regard to symptoms with a possible psychogenic origin. For example, Bonner and Finney (1996) concluded that at the age at which children typically develop an intestinal disorder (9 to 11 years), children lack the cognitive faculties to cope with abdominal discomfort. Subsequently the child (and parents) may use (or overutilize) medical services that may inadvertently reinforce the conceptualization of external locus of control of health status. In this regard, physicians may inadvertently worsen maladaptive and dysfunctional coping and foster dependency, thereby hindering the child's ability to develop adequate coping skills.

Crane and Martin (2004) investigated the role of learning in childhood to the development of IBS versus IBD (a functional disorder vs. a disease with identifiable pathophysiology). They conducted a survey of 55 adult outpatients diagnosed with IBS ($n = 25$) or IBD ($n = 33$). Participants completed questionnaires including a retrospective survey of their parents' history of reinforcing their illnesses when they were children. Results indicated that there was a significant relationship between passive behavioral coping in adulthood and parental reinforcement of illness behavior in childhood. These results support the findings that early learning experiences (in this case, a history of reinforcement for sick role behavior) may have a significant impact on the coping strategies and illness conceptualization in later life.

Schurman and colleagues (2004) studied parental behaviors related to their child's intestinal disorder symptoms. Participants in this study were 136 children (mean age 11 years, 10 months) diagnosed with functional gastrointestinal disorders (FD) or disorders involving psychological etiology (IBS) and their mothers. Findings suggested that children with IBS reported more parental encouragement of their illness behaviors than children diagnosed with FD. This may have been due to the more unpredictable course of IBS compared with FD, however. Furthermore, children reporting more significant disability with regard to their diagnosis were more likely to report more parental encouragement of their illness behaviors (i.e., the children are "released" from their typical responsibilities such as chores or school attendance).

Sanders and colleagues (1989) evaluated the efficacy of a cognitive–behavioral treatment package for nonspecific RAP using a controlled-group, pretest–posttest design. Their treatment approach was to focus on stimulus control and teaching incompatible–alternative behaviors. A sample of 16 children was randomly assigned to either a treatment or wait-list control group. The treatment package interventions included implementation of a token economy, use of relaxation and imagery, and differential reinforcement of pain-free behaviors. Results suggested that compared with the control group, the treatment group showed improvement more rapidly, exhibited generalization to the classroom, and evidenced a significantly higher proportion of pain-free participants at a 3-month follow-up (87.5% vs. 37.5%). These data support the use of an "intervention package" when addressing intractable conditions such as abdominal pain to which there appears no organic etiology.

Campos and Fritz (2001) presented a management model for pediatric somatization, including pain resulting from intestinal disorders. They recommended that the physician be frank and direct when presenting results of the diagnosis and suggested the use of behavioral and cognitive–behavioral interventions, self-management, and aggressive treatment of comorbid psychiatric problems. Behavioral interventions include positive reinforcement for healthy behavior and extinction for somatic symptoms where the sick role is being rewarded. Cognitive–behavioral interventions have been particularly useful in the treatment of recurrent abdominal pain through the use of reinforcement of engagement in routine activities, self-monitoring of symptoms, relaxation training, and diet management.

Friedrich and Jaworski (1995) recommended a number of general, clinical practice guidelines for psychologists working with children who have gastrointestinal disorders. These included (a) consideration of the existence of somatic symptomology in other family members, (b) assessment of the quality and impact of parent marital status and the possibility of the triangulation of the affected child, (c) helping parents reframe their perceptions about their children's gastrointestinal symptoms while encouraging them to set limits with their children, (d) assisting the child and family in discovering more effective means of expression (i.e., not through physiological means), (e) educating parents on the developmental role of the functions of gastrointestinal distress in positive and negative reinforcement, and (f) assisting parents in understanding the developmental needs of their children so that they can become more responsive to those needs (especially in situations where the gastrointestinal distress can limit activity or functioning).

Overall, studies support the efficacy of behavioral and cognitive–behavioral interventions in the treatment of symptom management for children with various intestinal disorders (Campos & Fritz, 2001). These interventions need to involve the parent, the child, and possibly the teacher and may include positive reinforcement for nonsick behaviors, recognition and control of discriminative stimuli, self-monitoring, behavioral contracting, and token economies (Heiby & Frank, 2003). Using negative reinforcement (e.g., lifting behavioral restrictions imposed by the illness contingent on functional improvement) is also recommended (Campos & Fritz, 2001). Finally, cognitive–behavioral interventions involving the family are frequently needed to help all family members balance the needs of the sick child with overall family needs.

CONCLUSION

Gastrointestinal disorders have notable consequences for children that may influence their functioning in academic and social contexts. Physiological, pathological, or psychological etiologies are all possible, but, regardless of the etiology, behavioral and cognitive behavioral treatments have been demonstrated to be efficacious. These treatments may include cognitive–behavioral family therapy, positive reinforcement for nonsick behaviors, self-monitoring, behavioral contracting, and token economies but all require close collaboration among medical, psychological, and school professionals to ensure proper treatment integrity of both medical and psychological treatment regimens. This collaboration also ensures continuity of treatment across settings. Given the proper medical treatment, combined with psychological interventions when necessary, children with intestinal disorders often function well and evidence few long-term educational or psychological consequences.

REFERENCES

American Academy of Family Physicians. (2000). *Inflammatory bowel disease*. Retrieved August 30, 2004, from http://familydoctor.org/x1895.xml

American Psychiatric Association. (2000). *Diagnostic and statistical manual of mental disorders* (4th ed., text rev.). Washington, DC: Author.

Behrman, R. E., Kliegman, R. M., & Jenson, H. B. (Eds.). (2000). *Nelson textbook of pediatrics* (16th ed.). Philadelphia: W. B. Saunders.

Berge, J. M., & Patterson, J. M. (2004). Cystic fibrosis and the family: A review and critique of the literature. *Families, Systems, & Health, 22,* 74–100.

Blanchard, E. B., & Scharff, L. (2002). Psychosocial aspects of assessment and treatment of irritable bowel syndrome in adults and recurrent abdominal pain in children. *Journal of Consulting and Clinical Psychology, 70,* 725–738.

Boat, T. F. (2000). Cystic fibrosis. In R. E. Behrman, R. M. Kliegman, & H. B. Jenson (Eds.), *Nelson textbook of pediatrics* (16th ed., pp. 1315–1327). Philadelphia: W. B. Saunders.

Bonner, M. J., & Finney, J. W. (1996). A psychosocial model of children's health status. In T. H. Ollendick & R. J. Prinz (Eds.), *Advances in clinical child psychology* (Vol. 18, pp. 231–282). New York: Plenum Press.

Campos, J. V., & Fritz, G. (2001). A management model for pediatric somatization. *Psychosomatics, 42,* 467–476.

Carroll, M., & Li, B. U. (2004). *Peptic ulcer disease*. Retrieved January 10, 2005, from http://www.emedicine.com/ped/topic2341.htm

Celiac Disease Foundation. (2002). *What is CF?* Retrieved August 27, 2004, from http://www.celiac.org/cd-who.html

Crane, C., & Martin, M. (2004). Social learning, affective state and passive coping in irritable bowel syndrome and inflammatory bowel disease. *General Hospital Psychiatry, 26*, 50–58.

Cystic Fibrosis Foundation. (2004, May). *What is CF?* Retrieved August 27, 2004, from http://www.cff.org/about_cf/what_is_cf/

Enck, P., & Whitehead, W. E. (1999). *Gastrointestinal disorders*. In E. A. Blechman & K. D. Brownell (Eds.), *Handbook of behavioral medicine for women* (pp. 178–194). Elmsford, NY: Pergamon Press.

Friedrich, W. N., & Jaworski, T. M. (1995). Pediatric abdominal disorders: Inflammatory bowel disease, rumination/vomiting, and recurrent abdominal pain. In M. C. Roberts (Ed.), *Handbook of pediatric psychology* (2nd ed., pp. 479–497). New York: Guilford Press.

Gionchetti, P., Rizzello, F., Habal, F., Morselli, C., Amadini, C., Romagnoli, R., & Campieri, M. (2003). Standard treatment of ulcerative colitis. In J. Schölmerich (Ed.), *Inflammatory bowel disease* (pp. 157–167). Basel, Switzerland: Karger.

Heiby, E. M., & Frank, M. R. (2003). Compliance with medical regimens. In W. O'Donohue, J. E. Fisher, & S. C. Hayes (Eds.), *Cognitive behavior therapy: Applying empirically supported techniques in your practice*. Hoboken, NJ: Wiley.

Husain, A. (2004). Communicating with patients with inflammatory bowel disease. *Inflammatory Bowel Diseases, 10*, 444–450.

Jackson, N. E., & Murray, J. A. (1998). Celiac disease. In L. Phelps (Ed.), *Health-related disorders in children and adolescents* (pp. 131–138). Washington, DC: American Psychological Association.

Lesen, B. M. (1998). Ulcerative colitis. In L. Phelps (Ed.), *Health-related disorders in children and adolescents* (pp. 696–700). Washington, DC: American Psychological Association.

Merck. (2004, August 27). Recurrent abdominal pain. In *The Merck manual of diagnosis and therapy* (chap. 268). Retrieved November 14, 2005, from http://www.merck.com/mrkshared/mmanual/section19/chapter268/268a.jsp

Merck. (2005, January 14). Functional vomiting. In *The Merck manual of diagnosis and therapy* (chap. 21). Retrieved November 14, 2005, from http://www.merck.com/mrkshared/mmanual/section3/chapter21/21d.jsp

Miehsler, W., & Gasche, C. (2003). Standard treatment of Crohn's disease. In J. Schölmerich (Ed.), *Inflammatory bowel disease* (pp. 146–156). Basel, Switzerland: Karger.

National Digestive Diseases Information Clearinghouse. (2003, April). *Irritable bowel syndrome* (NIH Publication No. 03-693). Retrieved August 26, 2004, from National Digestive Diseases Information Clearinghouse Web site, http://digestive.niddk.nih.gov/ddiseases/pubs/ibs/

Okuda, M., & Nakazawa, T. (2004). *Helicobacter pylori* infection in childhood. *Journal of Gastroenterology, 39,* 809–810.

Proctor, B. E., & Kranzler, J. H. (1998). Crohn's disease. In L. Phelps (Ed.), *Health-related disorders in children and adolescents* (pp. 197–203). Washington, DC: American Psychological Association.

PsychNet—UK. (2003, July 22). *Rumination disorder.* In Mental health and psychology directory. Retrieved November 30, 2005, from http://www.psychnet-uk.com/dsm_iv/rumination_disorder.htm

Rigas, B., & Spiro, H. M. (1995). *Clinical gastroenterology* (4th ed). New York: McGraw-Hill.

Sanchez, I., & Guiraldes, E. (1995). Drug management of noninfective complications of cystic fibrosis. *Drugs, 50,* 626–635.

Sanders, M. R., Rebgetz, M., Morrison, M., Bor, W., Gordon, A., Dadds, M., & Shepherd, R. (1989). Cognitive–behavioral treatment of recurrent nonspecific abdominal pain in children: An analysis of generalization, maintenance, and side effects. *Journal of Consulting and Clinical Psychology, 57,* 294–300.

Schölmerich, J. (2003). Inflammatory bowel diseases 2003: From genetics to biological theory. In J. Schölmerich (Ed.), *Inflammatory bowel disease* (pp. 83–84). Basel, Switzerland: Karger.

Schurman, J. V., Danda, C. E., Friesen, C. A., Weichert, E., Andre, L., Comninellis, T., et al. (2004, July). *Parental illness encouragement in children with functional gastrointestinal disorders.* Poster session presented at the annual meeting of the American Psychological Association, Honolulu, HI.

Ulshen, M. (2000a). Inflammatory bowel disease. In R. E. Behrman, R. M. Kliegman, & H. B. Jenson (Eds.), *Nelson textbook of pediatrics* (16th ed., pp. 1150–1151). Philadelphia: W. B. Saunders.

Ulshen, M. (2000b). Recurrent abdominal pain of childhood. In R. E. Behrman, R. M. Kliegman, & H. B. Jenson (Eds.), *Nelson textbook of pediatrics* (16th ed., pp. 1176–1178). Philadelphia: W. B. Saunders.

Ulshen, M. (2000c). Gluten-sensitive enteropathy (celiac disease). In R. E. Behrman, R. M. Kliegman, & H. B. Jenson (Eds.), *Nelson textbook of pediatrics* (16th ed., pp. 1165–1167). Philadelphia: W. B. Saunders.

Walker, C. E. (1995). Elimination disorders: Enuresis and encopresis. In M. C. Roberts (Ed.), *Handbook of pediatric psychology* (2nd ed., pp. 537–557). New York: Guilford Press.

Walker, L. S. (2004). Recurrent abdominal pain: Symptom subtypes based on the Rome II criteria for pediatric functional gastrointestinal disorders. *Journal of Pediatric Gastroenterology and Nutrition, 38,* 187–191.

Wallis-Crespo, M. C., & Crespo, A. (2004). *Helicobacter pylori* infection in pediatric population: Epidemiology, pathophysiology, and therapy. *Fetal and Pediatric Pathology, 23,* 11–28.

8

KIDNEY DISEASES

SANDRA M. CHAFOULEAS, JESSICA BLOM-HOFFMAN,
AND ELEAS J. CHAFOULEAS

This chapter provides an overview of both acute and chronic kidney diseases, in addition to a discussion of related medical, psychosocial, and educational outcomes and implications for psychologists and educators working with affected children. The kidneys are essential organs that serve multiple purposes, including filtering waste products and excess water from the blood, balancing electrolytes, producing stimulatory factors in blood production, and metabolizing vitamin D. Given these important jobs, kidney failure for any person, and particularly a child, can have serious consequences. According to the National Kidney and Urologic Diseases Information Clearinghouse (NKUDIC, 2003a), the incidence of kidney failure in children is approximately 1 to 2 new cases per 100,000, with African Americans in their late teens and boys among the populations at greater risk. The risk increases substantially in adulthood (over age 19), with estimates around 30 out of 100,000.

OVERVIEW

Causes of kidney failure may be hereditary or acquired (NKUDIC, 2003a). For pediatric populations under age 14, the leading causes of kidney

The authors thank Dr. Nataliya Zelikovsky for providing feedback on a draft of this chapter.

failure are hereditary diseases and birth defects. As children enter the teenage years and then into adulthood, diseases that damage the glomeruli (a microscopic ball of blood vessels in the kidney that is involved in urine formation) become the leading cause.

Acute Kidney Disease

Acute renal failure is defined by a rapid accumulation of toxins normally cleared by the kidneys. It may or may not be reversible, based on the etiology. Acute kidney disease in children often occurs as a result of either injury with blood loss or blood poisoning. One of the most common causes of acute kidney failure, hemolytic uremic syndrome (HUS), frequently results when the child ingests food contaminated by a certain toxin producing strains of *Escherichia coli* bacterium (Davis & Avner, 2004). Symptoms include vomiting, stomach cramps, and bloody diarrhea, followed later by a listless and pale affect along with possible decrease in urine output, swelling of the body, and small bruises or bleeding from the nose or mouth. These symptoms occur because of damage to the red blood cells, which clog tiny blood vessels, including those in the kidneys. Although most cases of HUS recover within a few days, children who progress into acute kidney failure need immediate treatment to regulate salt and water levels. In severe cases, blood transfusions or short-term dialysis may be needed. Most children recover from HUS without long-term consequences. The best protection from HUS is prevention through proper handling of food and avoiding unclean swimming areas.

Acute kidney failure in children is also seen with nephrotic syndrome, although much more rarely (NKUDIC, 2003b). Nephrotic syndrome itself is not a disease but rather a constellation of symptoms that result from glomerular diseases. The most common are represented by minimal change disease and focal segmental glomerulosclerosis. Minimal change disease is the most common type of nephrotic syndrome and results when there is damage to a cell involved in urine filtration (the podocyte). Focal segmental glomerulosclerosis results when segments of some of the glomeruli become scarred. These diseases are not distinguishable without a renal biopsy, but often this is not performed in young children because many physicians will treat both diseases with prednisone, and other nephrotic diseases are rare in children. The other disorders include the following:

- *membranoproliferative glomerulonephritis*, which occurs when immunologic material is deposited in or around the membrane surrounding the blood vessels of the glomerulus (basement membrane), resulting in damage;
- *membranous glomerulonephritis*, which also has a damaged basement membrane because of deposited immunologic material; and

- *mesangial proliferative glomerulonephritis,* which has increased cellularity within the space between the blood vessels of the glomerulus. (Rose & Appel, 2004)

Children with nephrotic syndrome have swelling around the eyes, legs, and belly because of excess water and salt in the body, along with low levels of protein in the blood. Treatments for nephrotic syndrome in young children may include prednisone to stop protein leakage or a diuretic to promote urination and decrease swelling. In minimal change disease, prednisone doses are eventually tapered and the child generally recovers without permanent damage, although relapse can occur. Children with frequent relapses may be prescribed a cytotoxic agent (e.g., cyclophosphamide, chlorambucil). Membranous and focal segmental glomerulosclerosis are often more steroid resistant, which could require additional immunosuppressants. Membranoproliferative and membranous glomerulonephritis may be treated with the angiotensin-converting enzyme (ACE) inhibitor antihypertensive medications.

In rare cases, pediatric nephrotic syndrome may be caused by congenital nephropathy (i.e., present at birth), which usually requires a kidney transplant. The evaluation of suspected nephrotic syndrome begins with checking a urine sample for large amounts of protein and a blood sample for low levels of the protein albumin and high cholesterol levels.

Chronic Kidney Disease

Chronic kidney disease (CKD) is long-standing (e.g., longer than 3 months) and generally worsens over time, sometimes progressing to end-stage renal disease (ESRD). The time course of ESRD can range from months to years; it is individualized to the patient and the underlying disease process. Patients with ESRD are unable to sustain life without indefinite dialysis or transplantation. In the United States, ESRD occurs in pediatric population at approximately 13 per million each year (Furth, Gerson, Neu, & Fivush, 2001). Treatment for ESRD is costly, ranging from $14,000 (transplant) to $34,000 (dialysis) per year (Furth et al., 2001). Ongoing treatment and frequent monitoring from the child's pediatrician in consultation with a nephrologist are necessary. Fortunately, no one may be excluded for treatment of ESRD given its unique coverage by the federal government under Medicare (Furth et al., 2001). Although relatively uncommon in children, CKDs are serious.

Most cases of chronic kidney failure in children under age 14 years are due to hereditary diseases or birth defects. Birth defects can include abnormally formed kidneys or no kidneys. In addition, blocked urine flow may occur, which can damage the kidney. Finally, the child may inherit defective genes that cause kidney disease. For example, in polycystic kidney disease, genes cause the kidneys to develop cysts that replace healthy kidney tissue and prevent the kidneys from working. In another hereditary disease, Alport syndrome, the defective gene can cause hearing or vision loss along with kidney disease.

As a child gets older, the risk of kidney failure resulting from the nephritic form of glomerular diseases increases. The only symptom of nephritis that may be recognized by the patient is blood-tinged urine. Physical examination findings include hypertension and lower grade protein losses in the urine. Lupus nephritis, pauci-immune glomerulonephritis (GN), post-streptococcal GN (an acute disease), anti-glomerular basement membrane (GBM) disease, and immunoglobulin-A (IgA) nephropathy are some examples of diseases that present this way. In lupus nephritis, complexes of antibodies are deposited in various positions of the glomerulus. More severe forms of the disease are treated with steroids and cytotoxic drugs. Pauci-immune GN is another autoimmune disorder in which the body destroys small blood vessels, resulting in glomerular cell death. Treatments often include steroids and cytotoxic drugs. Post-streptococcal GN is seen following streptococcal throat infections and may be the result of the deposit of immune complexes in the glomerulus or an immune reaction to infection-related deposits in the glomerulus. The disease is rarely chronic and usually does not require therapy. Anti-GBM disease is characterized by an autoantibody (an antibody produced in the patient's body) that attacks the basement membrane. Treatment often includes plasmapheresis (the mechanical removal of the patient's blood plasma), steroids, and cytotoxic drugs. IgA nephropathy results in immune deposits largely in the messangium (material that fills the space in the glomerulus). The treatment of this disease often includes an ACE inhibitor and sometimes omega-3 rich fish oils. The definitive diagnosis of the etiology of a nephritic syndrome requires a biopsy. A presumptive diagnosis of post-streptococcal GN is often made from blood work and a history of pharyngitis, but this approach requires long-term follow-up with a physician. Blood tests are also helpful in the diagnosis of lupus nephritis, pauci-immune GN, and anti-GBM disease.

Finally, systemic diseases such as diabetes can affect the kidneys. The high levels of glucose found in diabetes can damage the glomeruli and result in kidney failure, for example. Because it usually takes many years of high blood glucose to create such damage, it is not often found in children. The increasing number of children with Type 2 diabetes suggests that the future will result in more children with chronic kidney failure, however (NKUDIC, 2003c).

OUTCOMES

Acute Medical Outcomes

Outcomes for acute, reversible kidney failure are dependent on early management. For example, acute kidney disease resulting from HUS requires immediate attention to regulation of salt and water levels, perhaps with blood transfusion or short-term dialysis. Successful treatment at this stage should preclude significant long-term medical outcomes. As previously mentioned, childhood nephrotic syndrome may be treated with medication such as prednisone, which is tapered over time. Short-term effects of prednisone include swelling, weight gain, poor healing, depression, mania, hypertension, stunted growth, and elevated blood sugars. These symptoms cease, however, when medication is discontinued. Relapses of the nephrotic syndrome are often treated with further prednisone. When the disease fails to respond adequately to prednisone, additional immunosuppressants are often considered, along with a kidney biopsy.

Chronic Medical Outcomes

If the kidneys fail completely, treatment options include dialysis and transplantation (NKUDIC, 2003c). Dialysis is used to remove waste products and excess fluid from the body and is conducted through peritoneal dialysis or hemodialysis. In peritoneal dialysis, the lining of the abdominal cavity (peritoneum) is used to filter the wastes and excess fluid from the blood. A catheter is placed in the belly, and a solution is instilled to remove the waste and fluid. Then the solution containing the wastes is drained and the cleaning process repeated. Peritoneal dialysis is the preferred method of dialysis because it can be performed at home without a health care professional and thus can be the least disruptive to a school schedule. In contrast, hemodialysis uses a machine to pump blood into a filter that cleans the blood and returns it to the body. Hemodialysis is performed in a clinic about 3 times per week under the supervision of a nurse, with each session lasting 3 to 4 hours.

Transplantation offers an improved overall prognosis and a return to the most normal life possible for those with chronic kidney failure. It is the most desired treatment option in children because of its association with better quality of life, improved growth, lower cost, and survival benefits (Furth et al., 2001). The wait for a transplant can be long, however, depending on finding an appropriate match between a child and donor. The match requires ABO blood group compatibility identical to the requirements for receiving blood (e.g., $A \neq B$, $O \rightarrow A$). In addition, a negative cross-match must be present, meaning that the recipient does not have significant preformed antibodies against the donor. Although not a requirement for transplantation, there are some advantages to a human leukocyte antigen (HLA) zero mismatch in regard to decreased rates of rejection and increased long-term transplant survival. When a kidney from a deceased donor (cadaveric) becomes available, a national databank managed by the United Network for Organ Sharing (UNOS) is searched for a list of compatible recipients. Candidate age and length of waiting time are factors used to determine the list, with children under 18 receiving extra points over adults because they are likely to receive the greatest benefit. Another option for obtaining a kidney comes from a living donor (blood relation or unrelated) who has been tested to ensure donation will not risk the donor's health and that the kidney is an appropriate blood-type match for the patient. Advantages to a kidney from a living donor include greater ability to prepare for and schedule the operation and possible better condition of the kidney because less time has been spent in transportation from the donor to the recipient. In addition, although not a requirement for transplantation, kidneys donated by a parent may be less likely to be rejected because the kidney is guaranteed to match on at least three of six proteins. Approximately half of the kidneys procured for children come from family members, who are often motivated by these factors (NKUDIC, 2003c).

Patients with CKD often require complex medication regimens ranging from antihypertensives to immunosuppressants. Side effects of some of the immunosuppressants include weight gain, unusual hair growth, and acne. Unfortunately, these effects may promote social or behavioral problems such as treatment nonadherence in the child (particularly among teenagers). A special immunization schedule is required secondary to their weakened immune system (NKUDIC, 2003c). Along with standard vaccinations, these children need additional vaccinations for pneumonia and influenza. Children with transplants should not receive vaccines containing live viruses (e.g., varicella) because this may actually cause the disease that is meant to be prevented.

Additional medical complications of CKD that have a specific impact on children include growth problems. Growth problems are most prevalent when children develop renal disease at birth or in infancy (National Institutes of Health [NIH], 2002). Bone problems and growth failure can occur when kidneys are not able to balance phosphorus and calcium levels in the blood and phosphorus levels become too high. One way to reduce growth failure is through dietary management to restrict foods with large amounts of phosphorous. Often, a synthetic form of vitamin D is used to increase absorption of calcium in combination with a dietary phosphate binder (e.g., taking a calcium-containing antacid such as Tums) to excrete excess phosphorous. In extreme cases, growth hormones may also be prescribed, although questions remain about the usefulness and safety of this treatment (NKUDIC, 2003d). Despite these interventions, short stature is likely as a long-term consequence. For example, research has suggested that almost half of long-term survivors of renal disease will not achieve a final height above the third percentile for age (Furth et al., 2001).

Children are also at risk for anemia, a low concentration of red blood cells in the blood resulting from decreased production of blood stimulatory factors by the kidney. When not corrected by supplementation of the stimulatory factors, anemia can cause fatigue and, if severe enough, shortness of breath with exertion. Blood transfusions are generally avoided because of risk of allergic reactions, infections, and buildup of antibodies that could adversely affect a transplant or chance of being transplanted.

Children on dialysis or with advanced kidney failure have strict dietary restrictions that can be understandably difficult. A low-sodium diet is often required to assist with the management of hypertension. An oral daily fluid restriction is used to prevent excessive fluid buildup and resulting swelling or when extreme fluid accumulation to the lungs occurs. A potassium restriction is often required to prevent excessive blood levels and cardiac rhythm problems. (Refer to Table 8.1, p. 132, for a description of common dietary restrictions for individuals with CKD.)

Psychosocial Outcomes

The psychosocial impact of CKD has yet to be fully understood. Symptoms such as low self-esteem, feelings of powerlessness and depression, and difficulty making and maintaining friends have been reported in children with chronic diseases (NKUDIC, 2003e). These symptoms have been suggested to occur as a result of the high intrusiveness on a child's life, including frequent medical appointments and physical changes (e.g., short stature, hair growth, acne) that make the child look different from peers. According to the NKUDIC (2003e), children with functioning transplants appear to be less at risk for psychosocial problems than those on dialysis, potentially because of a decrease in dependence on health care professionals. In fact, one retrospective cohort study using a structured telephone interview found almost three quarters of transplant recipients reported functional outcome as good or excellent, in contrast to slightly less than half of patients on dialysis (Furth et al., 2001). Overall, research has not consistently suggested the presence of increased adjustment problems in children with CKD compared with healthy children (see Soliday, Kool, & Lande, 2000).

Although some researchers have found an increased risk for internalizing and externalizing symptoms, it has been suggested that the symptoms may be a result of moderating factors such as family environment rather than the disease itself. In an effort to extend research into the interrelationships of family environment, parenting stress, and child behavior problems in children with kidney disease, Soliday and colleagues (2000) investigated the psychosocial adjustment of children with chronically relapsing nephrotic syndrome, chronic renal insufficiency, or kidney transplant. In general, they found that children with multiple types of CKD did not differ from healthy children on parent-reported measures of behavioral functioning. These findings were consistent with those of Qvist and colleagues (2004), who found parent and teacher reports of behavioral functioning within normal limits in children who had received a kidney transplant under age 5 years. Qvist and colleagues noted, however, that reports of somatic complaints and social problems were more pronounced in boys and that reports of attention problems were more frequent among both boys and girls. In contrast, Soliday and colleagues found a larger than expected number of parents whose children who had received a kidney transplant (i.e., 29%) to report clinically significant concerns related to internalizing disorders among their children. Children who are transplant recipients may have fears related to possible organ rejection, separating from their parents while in the hospital or when returning to school, and concerns about school achievement and peer acceptance (Zelikovsky & Vereb, in press). Not surprisingly, Soliday also found that family variables, including high cohesion and expressiveness and low conflict, predicted positive child adjustment. In summary, these findings yield implications for the importance of family counseling and academic interventions when appropriate.

Educational Outcomes

In addition to academic difficulties derived from frequent absenteeism because of the need for frequent medical evaluation, malfunctioning kidneys are associated with impaired cognitive functioning. Excess toxins that build up in the body as a result of malfunctioning kidneys may reduce alertness, concentration, memory, and perceptomotor coordination (Stewart & Kennard, 1999). Children who develop acute renal failure may also display such symptoms, but these will typically recede following successful treatment of the renal failure.

Significant problems with neurocognitive development have been noted when children are born with or develop CKD in infancy, with some studies suggesting severe delays in 60% to 85% of this subpopulation (NIH, 2002). Small head circumference, delayed gross motor skills, and global developmental delays are commonly described. A paucity of research exists regarding the cognitive functioning of children and adolescents who develop CKD later in childhood, although there is evidence that age of renal failure onset is positively correlated with IQ (Lawry, Brouhard, & Cunningham, 1994). In addition, when compared with healthy control children matched for age, gender, and ethnicity, children with CKD performed lower in some cognitive areas, including subtle differences in verbal abstract and visuoperceptual reasoning, showed more marked differences in visuomotor integration, and had lower scores in some aspects of memory and learning (Fennell et al., 1990). Continued research in this area is required to understand more fully the cognitive outcomes of children with CKD (NIH, 2002).

MEDICAL AND PSYCHOEDUCATIONAL IMPLICATIONS

As described earlier, the intrusiveness of medication regimens and medical interventions for children with CKD is high. For example, when children require hemodialysis, they must go to a dialysis center multiple times per week. They are often fatigued during and after their treatment, which can make it difficult for them to complete homework or be involved in extracurricular and social activities. Given this high level of intrusiveness, psychologists and educators working with children who have CKD should be familiar with several issues: (a) the importance of adherence to medical treatment, (b) the need for special guidelines related to diet and physical activity, (c) attention to school functioning, and (d) attention to psychosocial adjustment.

Adherence to Medical Treatment

Management of CKD requires careful attention to a medical regimen that can include dialysis several times per week and numerous medications taken at multiple times throughout the day. Adherence to medical regimens is affected by a number of factors, including (a) regimen characteristics (e.g., duration, complexity, and presence of negative side effects), (b) disease characteristics (e.g., family's perceptions of illness severity), and (c) patient and family variables (e.g., premorbid behavioral and emotional problems; Lemanek, Kamps, & Chung, 2001). Given the intensive medical regimen that children with CKD need to follow, there is ample opportunity for difficulties associated with treatment adherence to arise. When working with a child with CKD, it is important to assess the child and caregivers' understanding of the medical regimen. In addition, barriers to treatment adherence are critical to understand. Working with families, pediatric psychologists can assess the factors that may be impeding adherence and use these data to develop and implement strategies that improve adherence (Zelikovsky & Walsh, 2004a). Zelikovsky and Walsh recommended that interventions be individualized to suit the needs of each child and family because there is no "best fit" suited to all children. Adherence-promoting interventions may include the following: (a) educational (e.g., teaching children and their caregivers about how to follow specific aspects of the medical regimen), (b) organizational (e.g., creating a system to store and keep track of medications), and (c) behavioral (e.g., behavioral contracting, token economies; Zelikovsky & Walsh, 2004b). For example, an intervention package might first consist of explaining the disease and necessary treatment to the child and caregivers. Then, consultation to develop a way to manage the treatment protocol for the specific child could occur, such as using a chart or pillbox to keep track of appropriate medication regimens. Finally, a system for positive reinforcement for adherence to the system could be put in place, such as special activities or items the child will enjoy if she or he meets weekly preestablished goals for adherence.

TABLE 8.1
Foods Often Restricted in Patients With Advanced Renal Failure
or End-Stage Renal Disease

Foods	Examples
Sodium	Table salt, prepared and fast foods, canned foods, smoked foods
Phosphorous	Dairy products, dried beans, nuts, peanut butter, dark colas
Potassium	Potatoes, orange juice, broccoli, cantaloupe, bananas, nuts, bran cereals, dried fruit (especially figs)
All fluids (for patients on hemodialysis)	3% of weight allowed to be gained between dialysis sessions

Note. Data from the National Kidney Foundation (2001) and Gennari (1998).

Nutrition and Physical Activity

As mentioned previously, children and adolescents with CKD need to adhere to strict dietary guidelines. Examples of foods often restricted in patients with advanced renal failure or ESRD can be found in Table 8.1. These dietary restrictions can be difficult for children and adolescents to follow, particularly when they are in school, at parties, or out with friends. Children and families can receive guidance from a renal dietician to help them become knowledgeable about specific nutritional guidelines. It is also helpful for educators to know which foods children with CKD can eat and to take this information into consideration when planning school parties involving food so children with renal disease do not feel excluded.

In addition to dietary restrictions, the child's physician may restrict the types of physical activity in which the child may partake. For example, contact sports and activities that involve a high risk of injury (e.g., football, karate) are discouraged. At the same time, it is important that children with chronic kidney disease are physically active to the extent possible. Clear communication between the child's physician and school personnel is critical to clarify how and to what extent the child should be involved in physical education and recess activities.

School Functioning

Given the potential concerns regarding cognitive and academic functioning outlined earlier, educators and school psychologists should pay close attention to the academic skill development of children with chronic kidney disease. Psychoeducational assessment, including curriculum-based assessment (Shapiro, 2004), can be used to identify the child's instructional level across academic subject areas and to match the child's instructional materials to her or his level. Progress monitoring, using curriculum-based measurement (Shinn, 1989, 1997) may be helpful to ensure that the child is gaining appropriate academic skills. Problem solving and planning with the school's child study team may be necessary to develop and coordinate educational interventions to address specific educational needs. In addition to planning for academic needs, the physical and medical needs of children with chronic kidney disease while in school may be addressed through an accommodation plan under Section 504 of the Rehabilitation Act or an Individualized Education Plan under the Individuals With Disabilities Education Act.

In addition to potential cognitive difficulties caused by biological factors, children with chronic kidney disease may fall behind their classmates academically because of excessive absenteeism. Many of these children are required to go to the dialysis center three times per week or to the transplant clinic two times per week initially. Absenteeism tends to have academic as well as social implications. Academically, educational plans for tutoring are important when children are hospitalized or cannot attend school for prolonged periods of time. School personnel should communicate with educators at the hospital regarding the child's academic level and appropriate educational goals to maximize instructional opportunities when out of school.

Adults working with children with CKD must recognize the social implications that children deal with when out of school for long periods of time. These children sometimes feel they "don't fit in" with the other children because they miss the continuity of social relationships when they are not at school consistently. Some consideration should be devoted to helping students with CKD to feel connected to their peers and to the school. The widespread availability of e-mail can help children communicate with their friends and teachers when out of school. In addition, young peers may worry that they will "catch kidney disease" from their classmate with CKD (Davis, 1999), which may further serve to make the student feel excluded. With permission from the family of the student with CKD, educators may want to help the student's classmates to understand what is happening with their classmate. Furthermore, sometimes children may use their medical needs as an opportunity to miss school, and parents may be anxious about allowing their child to return to their regular routine. Therefore, periodic communication between the medical team and school staff regarding the child's ability to be in school and the importance of the child returning to school are needed (Davis, 1999).

Psychosocial Adjustment

As described earlier, physical problems of children with CKD including short stature as well as side effects from immunosuppressive medications (e.g., weight gain, acne) have potential impact on areas of psychosocial adjustment. Visible symptoms such as these may incite teasing or exclusion from

TABLE 8.2
Generic Measures of Health-Related Quality of Life for Children

Measure	Brief description	Respondent	Age appropriateness (years)
Child Health and Illness Profile—Adolescent Version (Starfield et al., 1993)	153-item measure of 6 domains of health (discomfort, satisfaction, disorders, achievements, resilience, risks). Support for reliability and validity in populations from 11–17 years has been established.	Child	11–17
Child Health Questionnaire (Eiser & Morse, 2001)	Parent and child versions available that measure 12 domains of health status. Internal consistency and concurrent validity have been reported.	Child, parent	4–19
Functional Status (II)—R (Eiser & Morse, 2001)	43-item report assessing 8 domains of health. Reliability and validity (construct, concurrent) have been reported.	Parent	0–16
Pediatric Quality of Life Questionnaire (Seid, Varni, & Kurtin, 2000)	30-item instrument measuring 5 domains of health. Internal reliability and validity (construct, clinical) have been established.	Child, parent	2–18

Note. Data from Furth, Gerson, Neu, and Fivush (2001).

other children, which in turn may cause adjustment difficulties for children with CKD. Educators and clinicians working with children with CKD may find assessment of perceived health-related quality of life (HRQL; i.e., the psychological and social aspects of a patient's health as viewed by the patient) to be useful in determining severity of adjustment difficulties (Furth et al., 2001). Measurement of HRQL may include areas such as physical, social, and role functioning as well as mental health and general health perceptions (Furth et al., 2001). Although guidelines from the National Kidney Foundation's Dialysis Outcomes Quality Initiative recommend patient-based assessment of quality of life at intervals beginning with initiation of dialysis, there is a lack of quality instruments specific to kidney disease (as opposed to generic measures of HRQL). This is especially true for children in that few psychometric evaluations of generic measures of HRQL have been conducted. Some potentially useful generic measures of HRQL in children are listed in Table 8.2. Note, however, that most studies of their psychometric properties have not been conducted specifically in children with CKD.

TABLE 8.3
Internet Resources on Kidney Failure in Children

Internet location	Brief descriptor
http://kidney.niddk.nih.gov	This Web site contains information from the National Kidney and Urologic Diseases Information Clearinghouse (NKUDIC), a service run by the National Institute of Diabetes and Digestive and Kidney Diseases (NIDDK). The Web site contains a series of articles related specifically to kidney disease in children.
http://www.ikidney.com	This Web site is sponsored through an educational grant to Watson Pharma. Along with articles written by various professionals, a section for family members contains lifestyle and adherence tips as well as renal-friendly recipes. In addition, a personal support network is promoted through patient ability to sign up to receive newsletters and post a personal profile on the Web site.
http://www.kidney.org	This Web site is maintained by the National Kidney Foundation. Tips for parents of children with chronic kidney diseases can be found on this site.
https://kidshealth.org	The Nemours Foundation supports the KidsHealth Web site, which contains articles on many topics (including kidney diseases) written specifically for parents, teenagers, and young children.

Depending on the results of a psychosocial assessment, children and adolescents may benefit from counseling to address pertinent issues. Such topics are likely to include body image dissatisfaction, treatment nonadherence, development of social skills to promote making friends and to respond to possible teasing, and other issues related to successful integration in school. In addition, opportunities to get together with other children experiencing similar problems may help promote positive self-esteem. For example, a special summer camp may be beneficial. In addition to maintaining a list of camp options, the American Kidney Fund (AKF) sponsors a Pediatric Campership Program that provides financial assistance to low-income patients to attend such camps.

Coordination of efforts, particularly as related to psychosocial adjustment, with all mental and health care providers is desirable. For example, if the child attends a dialysis or transplant center, a social worker affiliated with that center will work with the child and family. Communication with this professional may facilitate coordination of appropriate services across settings. As with other pediatric chronic illnesses, children with renal diseases should experience an environment that is as normal as possible. It is important for them to have developmentally appropriate levels of independence and control, while simultaneously respecting their treatment regimen.

CONCLUSION

Given that kidneys serve multiple important functions, kidney failure can have serious consequences, particularly for children. For children under 14, kidney failure is usually caused by hereditary diseases or birth defects and can be either acute or chronic. All forms of kidney failure require intensive treatment. Effects of kidney failure and its treatment can have a great impact on a child's daily life. Psychologists and educators working with children with CKD should be aware of a number of factors that affect these students' physical, psychosocial, and academic functioning. Knowledge of treatment adherence issues, potential academic difficulties, psychosocial adjustment issues, and special dietary and physical activity restrictions are important. Clear communication among the child's family, school, and medical team is critical to promote the child's well-being and success. Communication should focus on ways to promote the child's experience of normalcy, independence, and control, while helping the child to follow the medical regimen as closely as possible. Further Internet sources containing useful information regarding renal failure in children can be found in Table 8.3.

REFERENCES

Davis, I. D. (1999). Pediatric renal transplantation: Back to school issues. *Transplantation Proceedings, 31*(Supple.), 61S–62S.

Davis, I. D., & Avner, E. D. (2004). Hemolytic–uremic syndrome. In R. Behrman, R. Kliegman, & H. Jenson (Eds.), *Nelson Textbook of Pediatrics* (17th ed., pp. 1746–1747). St. Louis, MO: W. B. Saunders.

Eiser, C., & Morse, R. (2001). A review of measures of quality of life for children with chronic illness. *Archives of Diseases in Childhood, 84*, 205–211.

Fennell, R. S., Fennell, E. B., Carter, R. L., Mings, E. L., Klausner, A. B., & Hurst, J. R. (1990). A longitudinal study of the cognitive function of children with renal failure. *Pediatric Nephrology, 4*, 11–15.

Furth, S. L., Gerson, A. C., Neu, A. M., & Fivush, B. A. (2001). The impact of dialysis and transplantation on children. *Advances in Renal Replacement Therapy, 8*, 206–213.

Gennari, F. J. (1998). Hypokalemia. *New England Journal of Medicine, 339*, 451–458.

Lawry, K. W., Brouhard, B. H., & Cunningham, R. J. (1994). Cognitive functioning and school performance in children with renal failure. *Pediatric Nephrology, 8*, 326–329.

Lemanek, K. L., Kamps, J., & Chung, N. B. (2001). Empirically supported treatments in pediatric psychology: Regimen adherence. *Journal of Pediatric Psychology, 26*, 253–275.

National Institutes of Health. (2002). *Prospective study of chronic kidney disease in children.* Retrieved April 18, 2004, from http://grants.nih.gov/grants/guide/rfa-files/FRA-DK-03-012.html

National Kidney and Urologic Diseases Information Clearinghouse. (2003a, December). *Hemolytic uremic syndrome* (NIH Publication No. 04-4570). Retrieved June 21, 2004, from http://kidney.niddk.nih.gov/kudiseases/pubs/childkidneydiseases/index.htm

National Kidney and Urologic Diseases Information Clearinghouse. (2003b, December). *Childhood nephrotic syndrome* (NIH Publication No. 04-4695). Retrieved June 21, 2004, from http://kidney.niddk.nih.gov/kudiseases/pubs/childkidneydiseases/index.htm

National Kidney and Urologic Diseases Information Clearinghouse. (2003c, December). *Overview of kidney diseases in children* (NIH Publication No. 04-5167). Retrieved June 21, 2004, from http://kidney.niddk.nih.gov/kudiseases/pubs/childkidneydiseases/index.htm

National Kidney and Urologic Diseases Information Clearinghouse. (2003d, December). *Treatment methods for kidney failure in children* (NIH Publication No. 04-5082). Retrieved June 21, 2004, from http://kidney.niddk.nih.gov/kudiseases/pubs/childkidneydiseases/index.htm

National Kidney and Urologic Diseases Information Clearinghouse. (2003e, December). *School and family problems of children with kidney failure* (NIH Publication No. 04-5165). Retrieved June 21, 2004, from http://kidney.niddk.nih.gov/kudiseases/pubs/childkidneydiseases/index.htm

National Kidney Foundation. (2001). *Nutrition and chronic kidney disease*. New York: Author.

Qvist, E., Narhi, V., Apajasalo, M., Ronnholm, K., Jalanko, H., Almqvist, F., & Holmberg, C. (2004). Psychosocial adjustment and quality of life after renal transplantation in early childhood. *Pediatric Transplantation, 8*, 120–125.

Rose, B. D., & Appel, G. A. (2004). *Minimal change variants: Mesangial proliferations; IgM nephropathy; Clq nephropathy*. Retrieved December 26, 2004, from http://www.uptodate.com

Seid, M., Varni, J. W., & Kurtin, P. S. (2000). Measuring quality of care for vulnerable children: Challenges and conceptualization of a pediatric outcome measure quality. *American Journal of Medical Quality, 15*, 182–188.

Shapiro, E. S. (2004). *Academic skills problems: Direct assessment and intervention* (3rd ed.). New York: Guilford Press.

Shinn, M. R. (1989). *Curriculum-based measurement: Assessing special children*. New York: Guilford Press.

Shinn, M. R. (1997). *Advanced applications of curriculum-based measurement*. New York: Guilford Press.

Soliday, E., Kool, E., & Lande, M. B. (2000). Psychosocial adjustment in children with kidney disease. *Journal of Pediatric Psychology, 25*, 93–103.

Starfield, B., Bergner, M., Ensminger, M., Riley, A., Ryan, S., Green, B., et al. (1993). Adolescent health status measurement: The development of CHIP. *Pediatrics, 91*, 430–435.

Stewart, S. M., & Kennard, B. D. (1999). Organ transplantation. In R. T. Brown (Ed.), *Cognitive aspects of chronic illness in children* (pp. 220–237). New York: Guilford Press.

Zelikovsky, N., & Walsh, A. (2004). Medical adherence. In B. Kaplan & K. Meyers (Eds.), *The requisites in pediatrics: Nephrology/urology* (pp. 69–75). Philadelphia: Elsevier Mosby.

Zelikovsky, N., & Vereb, R. (2004). Psychological considerations in renal disease. In B. Kaplan & K. Meyers (Eds.), *The requisites in pediatrics: Nephrology/urology* (pp. 57–62). Philadelphia: Elsevier Mosby.

9

LANGUAGE-RELATED DISORDERS IN CHILDHOOD

LEA A. THEODORE, MELISSA A. BRAY, THOMAS J. KEHLE, AND RICHARD J. DIOGUARDI

Language, which is fundamental to the transmission of ideas, exchange of information, and expression of feelings, allows children to express their emotions, beliefs, and desires, and interact socially with others. In young children, language is a critical component for continued growth in academic, socioemotional, and behavioral development. Conversely, deficits in language may result in multiple areas of dysfunction relating to performance at home, school, and the community. This chapter reviews specific language impairment (SLI), stuttering, otitis media, and selective mutism, providing evidence-based recommendations for the treatment of each disorder in children.

SPECIFIC LANGUAGE IMPAIRMENT

Overview

Specific language impairment (SLI), also known as developmental dysphasia, refers to deficits in expressive and receptive language typically diagnosed during the preschool or early school years (Kovac, Garabedian, Souich, & Palmour, 2001). The most recent U.S. population prevalence for SLI is

7.4% in preschool children (Tomblin et al., 1997). A diagnosis of SLI requires that an impairment in speech or language (or both) be evident, scores on standardized measures of expressive or receptive language be substantially below those of nonverbal cognitive ability, and exclusion criteria be met (*Diagnostic and Statistical Manual of Mental Disorders*, 4th ed., text rev. [DSM–IV–TR]; American Psychiatric Association, 2000). Common exclusionary criteria include mental retardation, peripheral hearing impairment, and neurological disorder (Kovac et al., 2001).

Although the exact cause of SLI has yet to be established, several factors may be etiological in its development, including genetic, neuropsychological, neurobiological, and linguistic influences (Tallal & Benasich, 2002). The disorder has been shown to aggregate in families, with twin data suggesting a genetic component (Bishop, North, & Donlan, 1995; Spitz, Tallal, Flax, & Benasich, 1997). Neuropsychological research has investigated substrates (e.g., motor, attention, sensory, perceptual, and memory) hypothesized to be precursors of higher order cerebral cortex functioning, such as language (Tallal & Benasich, 2002). One such function, speed of information processing, that has been postulated to have a negative impact on various aspects of language learning has been the focus of behavioral and neuroimaging investigations. In children with SLI, processing rate deficiencies have been demonstrated in several sensory systems as well as the motor modality (Laasonen, Tomma-Halme, Lahti-Nuuttila, Service, & Virsu, 2000; Tallal, 1998). Other neuropsychological abnormalities, such as fine motor impairments, hyperreflexia, and obligatory synkinesis, have also been found in 70% of children with SLI (Trauner, Wulfeck, Tallal, & Hesselink, 2000). Additionally, approximately one third of these children exhibited atypical magnetic resonance imaging results, including enlarged ventricles, central volume loss, and anomalies in white matter. Individuals with SLI also evidence neuroanatomical abnormalities including enlarged ventricles, central volume loss, anomalies in white matter, and abnormal asymmetry in the parietal and frontal lobe brain regions, as well as size and shape abnormalities in the planum temporale of Wernicke's area and pars triangularis (Cowell, Jernigan, Denenberg, & Tallal, 1995; Gauger, Lombardino, & Leonard, 1997; Trauner et al., 2000). Linguistically, children with SLI evidence deficits in various components of language, including grammatical morphology, phonology, and syntax (Joanisse, Manis, Keating, & Seidenberg, 2000; van der Lely & Stollwerck, 1997). Such deficits result in significantly delayed progression through the normal language acquisition trajectory, which may continue into adulthood (Curtiss, Katz, & Tallal, 1992; Rissman, Curtis, & Tallal, 1990).

Outcomes

It has been well established that language disorders adversely affect academic achievement and social functioning and are commonly associated with emotional and behavioral problems. Educational implications stemming from language disorders include diminished achievement within the domains of reading and spelling (Snowling, Bishop, & Stothard, 2000; Young et al., 2002). Specifically, difficulties with phonological awareness, a particular component of language development, are commonly believed to contribute to reading deficits (Catts, Fey, Zhang, & Tomblin, 2001). Furthermore, reading difficulties have been linked to poor academic performance, greater risk of social and emotional problems, lower socioeconomic status and occupational success, and a greater likelihood of dropping out of school (Snow, Burns, & Griffin, 1998). Children with SLI also evidence difficulty with mathematics because of the high linguistic components involved, including an understanding of vocabulary, comprehension of written language, and the ability to count (Young et al., 2002). Finally, higher order functions, such as regulation and management of information processing (executive functioning) and working memory, become more critical as school-related demands increase (Young et al., 2002).

Specific language impairment also places children at higher risk for social, emotional, and behavioral difficulties. Although the most common psychiatric diagnosis for children with SLI is attention-deficit/hyperactivity disorder (Cohen et al., 2000), links have also been found between SLI and anxiety, depression, and antisocial personality disorder (Beitchman et al., 2001; Irwin, Carter, & Briggs-Gowan, 2002). It has been hypothesized that the emotional and behavioral problems stem from the child's inability to express his or her thoughts and comprehend others effectively (Willinger et al., 2003). These linguistic difficulties place children at particular risk for social impairment because of their significant contribution to social interaction (Damico & Damico, 1993). In support of this reasoning, Vallance, Cummings, and Humphries (1998) found that in children with language learning disabilities, impaired social interactional functioning (e.g., poor social discourse skills) was central to the development of their behavioral symptomatology. These students are in danger of peer rejection, which in turn may reduce their contact with language and diminish opportunities to practice and sharpen conversational skills (Willinger et al., 2003).

Medical and Psychoeducational Implications

Remediation strategies for SLI, typically provided by speech–language pathologists, special education teachers, or psychologists, have centered on teaching the child to use age-appropriate language structures in multiple situations (Tallal & Benasich, 2002). Both receptive and expressive language difficulties have been remediated with phonological awareness training programs (Gillon, 2002; Hesketh, Adams, Nightingale, & Hall, 2000; Segers & Verhoeven, 2004), which aim to enhance a child's ability to detect, segment, and manipulate phonemes within words and develop knowledge of the connection between speech and print. The growing interest in phonological awareness intervention derives from research that has demonstrated a significant link between early phonetic awareness and literacy achievement. Specifically, preschool children who exhibit early phonemic awareness have a better chance of learning to read, and their ability to rhyme may predict future spelling competency (Muter & Snowling, 1998).

The need to maximize the treatment benefits of speech and language therapy has spawned management strategies that incorporate parental participation in language development and remediation (Manolson, 1992; McDade & McCartan, 1998). These indirect styles of intervention contrast with direct, therapist-delivered didactic methods and focus on the early reciprocal dialogue between children and their parents. Such programs encourage the parent to improve the quality of interaction in spontaneous, naturalistic situations by exercising several techniques, including increased responsiveness, decreased directiveness, improved turn taking, slowed rate and repetition, exaggerated intonation, and short, simple utterances. Although there is evidence to support the model that specific parent interaction styles can enhance language acquisition in normally developing children (Baxendale & Hesketh, 2003), more research is needed to provide evidence for the successful application of this philosophy in language-impaired children.

Recently, remediation strategies have been developed that integrate knowledge of the neural basis of learning (i.e., neuroplasticity) with research on language development and disorders (Tallal & Benasich, 2002). Based on research indicating that phonological and language delays of individuals with SLI result from constraints in processing rate (e.g., processing brief, rapidly sequenced acoustic cues in verbal stimuli) and producing quick successive stimuli (Tallal, 1998), audiovisual computer training interventions have been developed to sharpen a child's ability to segment successive sensory events and adequately process critical acoustic cues within the context of fluent, ongoing speech. These computer-supported phonological awareness interventions use temporal and acoustic modifications of speech elements so as to differentially emphasize and extend them over time (Tallal & Benasich, 2002). One such program, Fast ForWard, has been used successfully in treating children with SLI and dyslexia (Habib et al., 1999; Segers & Verhoeven, 2004) and has resulted in significant gains on tasks including following auditory commands, morphology and syntax, speech–sound discrimination, and speech articulation (Tallal, Miller, & Bedi, 1996).

STUTTERING

Overview

Stuttering may be defined as the involuntary repetition of sounds, syllables, and words; sound prolongations; or blocking (i.e., inability to begin a word) that results in dysfluent speech (Perino, Famularo, & Tarraoni, 2000). Because of interruptions in the flow and rhythm of speech, stuttering is also considered a fluency disorder. Stress resulting from this disrupted flow of speech often manifests in secondary characteristics such as muscular tension in the face and upper body, blinking, grimacing, or rigid body movements. The child's struggle with dysrhythmia frequently leads to minimal eye contact, restricted use of certain words, and limited verbal interactions with others (Baker & Blackwell, 2004).

The prevalence rate of stuttering is relatively low, affecting approximately 1% of the general population (Craig, Hancock, Tran, Craig, & Peters, 2002), and with a male to female ratio of 2–3:1 in young children and 4:1 in adolescence (Craig et al., 2002). Onset typically occurs between ages 2 and 7 (*DSM–IV–TR*; American Psychiatric Association, 2000). A diagnosis of stuttering is usually made when an individual evidences 3% or more stuttered syllables or 5% stuttered words. Significantly, stuttering has been shown to remit spontaneously prior to adolescence in approximately 75% of children (Yairi & Ambrose, 1999).

Multiple factors have been implicated in the etiology of stuttering, including genetics (Baker & Blackwell, 2004; Felsenfeld, 2002), environmental variables (Baker & Blackwell, 2004), an interaction between biological and environmental influences (Conture, 2001), neurological abnormalities (Ingham, 2001), and learned behavior (Baker & Blackwell, 2004). Genetically, a high incidence of stuttering occurs among first-degree family members as well as monozygotic twins (Felsenfeld, 2002; Stagg & Burns, 1999). Environmental factors playing an etiological role include competition for turn taking in conversations and demands to speak when language is developmentally premature (Baker & Blackwell, 2004). An interaction between biological and environmental factors, such as when the coordination of muscles controlling speech deteriorates in socially stressful situations, has also been proposed. This poor muscle control, in conjunction with excessive pressure to communicate, culminates in dysfluent speech (Baker & Blackwell, 2004).

Neurologically, research has suggested that the brain structure of individuals who stutter differs from that of fluent speakers in terms of brain hemispheric function (i.e., lack of strong left cerebral dominance) and levels of neurotransmitters in specific brain regions. Specifically, atypical levels of dopamine and serotonin have been found in areas of the brain responsible for coordinating language processing and vocal chord movement (Friedlander, Noffsinger, Mendez, & Yagiela, 2004). Neuroimaging studies examining the dynamic relationships among different brain areas during normal speech and in individuals who stutter suggest that abnormalities in the timing of neural activity across several brain areas characterize stuttering (Ludlow & Loucks, 2003). For instance, abnormal temporal lobe activation during speech production is associated with a malfunction in the processing sequence among premotor regions (e.g., auditory association cortex, cerebellum, anterior insula) important in phonology (Ingham, 2001). Finally, conditioning and other learning variables seem to maintain stuttering. These factors include parents' anxious and negative reactions to their children's stuttering, which serve to exacerbate the child's dysfluent speech (Baker & Blackwell, 2004).

Outcomes

Children who stutter exhibit an array of academic and social difficulties. In the academic domain, approximately 15% of children who stutter are diagnosed with learning disabilities and 8% with literacy disorders (Arndt & Healy, 2001; Blood, Ridenour, Qualls, & Hammer, 2003). In addition, 62% of children who stutter also evidence coexisting speech and language disorders, with 33.5% and 12.7% exhibiting articulation disorders and phonological disorders respectively (Blood et al., 2003). This is particularly noteworthy in that language disorders have been linked to the etiology of stuttering. With regard to social and emotional functioning, stuttering has been associated with depression (Liu et al., 2001), anxiety (Ezrati & Levin, 2004), attentional difficulties (Blood et al., 2003), and diminished self-efficacy (Perkins, 1993). In addition, the self-imposed angst surrounding stuttering often results in disengagement from participation in social events (Arndt & Healy, 2001). As a result, these students are often perceived as reticent and withdrawn, and these peer-perceived characteristics increase the likelihood that they will experience poor peer relationships, lower sociometric standing among classmates, and victimization (Davis, Howell, & Cooke, 2002).

Medical and Psychoeducational Implications

Interventions designed to treat childhood stuttering may be categorized as direct and indirect treatment methods (Finn, 2003). Indirect treatment strategies involve having parents redirect their child's focus on the stuttering, offer sufficient positive opportunities to converse by allowing ample time to speak, and minimizing pressure from others to talk perfectly (Finn, 2003). Direct interventions incorporate positive reinforcement for fluent speech and modification of dysfluencies in a gentle, reassuring manner. This approach teaches children awareness and control of their stuttering by applying skills that foster naturally sounding, stutter-free speech. By directly addressing dysfluencies, children who stutter learn to manage avoidance behavior effectively (Finn, 2003). One intervention that incorporates these direct and indirect strategies is the Lidcombe Program, which is an operant treatment administered by parents (Jones, Onslow, Harrison, & Packman, 2000). Parents are taught to use positive reinforcement of fluent speech according to a predetermined contingency schedule and ask the child to repeat or correct stuttering (Ratner, 2004; Wilson, Onslow, & Lincoln, 2004).

Another strategy that has been used to reduce stuttering is self-modeling, which involves the presentation of edited videotapes depicting the student engaging in fluent speech, enabling the student to learn by observing and modeling him- or herself (Bray & Kehle, 2001). Finally, pharmacological treatments with antidepressant, antipsychotic, and anxiolytic medications have been used to reduce stuttering. There are, however, potentially negative side effects and adverse interactions with other medications the child may be taking (Friedlander et al., 2004).

In light of recent research indicating that children who stutter are more likely to experience peer victimization and rejection, social skills training that directly addresses coping with harassment and bullying is suggested. Social skills training would not only teach strategies to cope with victimization but also ways to establish and maintain healthy friendships. The ultimate goal would be enhanced inclusion in social events (Davis et al., 2002).

OTITIS MEDIA

Overview

Otitis media is an inflammation of the middle ear and may be categorized as either acute otitis media (AOM) or otitis media with effusion (OME). It is one of the more common chronic conditions of childhood (Roberts et al., 2004) and the most frequent presenting medical complaint to pediatricians in young children (Auinger, Lanphear, Kalkwarf, & Mansour, 2003). Otitis media generally manifests as mild hearing loss with an onset that may be sudden or gradual. AOM is typified by an onset that is sudden. Hallmark symptoms of AOM include a red and bulging eardrum, fever, pain, ear pulling, irritability, and vomiting (Darrow, Dash, & Derkay, 2003). Conversely, OME has a gradual onset and is more difficult to detect in that there are no salient symptoms other than mild hearing loss and fluid buildup (American Academy of Pediatrics, 2004).

Otitis media with effusion is caused by a collection of fluid in the middle ear behind the intact tympanic membrane without any acute signs and symptoms of infection (American Academy of Pediatrics and American Academy of Family Physicians, 2004). A myriad of factors may lead to a blocked tube, including bacterial and viral infection, impaired eustachian tube function, large adenoids, immature immune system status, and allergy (Darrow et al., 2003). In most circumstances, otitis media begins with an upper respiratory tract viral infection, leading to eustachian tube congestion and normal tube malfunction, the result of which is a disturbance of ventilation and drainage in the middle ear (Darrow et al., 2003).

Otitis media is considered a frequent health problem in children. Research has found that the prevalence of otitis media for children under age 6 is approximately 68%, with 44% and 38% of these children having had early-onset and repeated otitis media, respectively (Auinger et al., 2003). The highest incidence occurs between 6 to 12 months of age, with more than 50% of children experiencing OME. This figure increases to greater than 60% by the time the child reaches 2 years (Casselbrant & Mandel, 2003). Because of anatomical characteristics distinct to infants (e.g., short length and horizontal alignment of the eustachian tube), this age group is more likely to develop AOM compared with older children (Hoberman, Marchant, Kaplan, & Feldman, 2002). Otitis media with effusion affects 80% of preschool children at least once, with the highest risk of developing the disorder occurring before age 3 (de Ru & Grote, 2004). Risk factors for otitis media, both single-episode and recurrent, include gender (occurring more in boys), ethnic background (Native American or Alaskan and Canadian Inuit), lower socioeconomic level, attendance in center-based day care, early breast-feeding termination, bottle feeding, allergies, exposure to tobacco smoke, and number of children in the home under 12 years old (Darrow et al., 2003; Monobe, Ishibashi, Fujishiro, Shinogami, & Yano, 2003).

A diagnosis of AOM is provided when there is evidence of a history of acute onset of symptoms (e.g., ear pulling, irritability, otorrhea, or fever), signs and symptoms of middle-ear inflammation (e.g., distinct redness of the tympanic membrane and earache), and the presence of middle-ear effusion (e.g., bulging and limited mobility of the tympanic membrane, air-fluid bubble behind the tympanic membrane, and mucus discharge from the ear (American Academy of Pediatrics, 2004; American Academy of Pediatrics and American Academy of Family Physicians, 2004). Unlike the diagnosis of AOM, OME does not require a history of acute signs or symptoms, nor does it necessitate the presence of middle-ear effusion and inflammation (American Academy of Pediatrics, 2004).

Outcomes

Hearing loss is typically associated with otitis media, particularly with recurrent episodes. Research has found that a history of recurrent OME negatively affects speech and language development in the first 3 years of life, a time critical for the development of language as well as acquisition of grammar and mathematical knowledge (Keles et al., 2004; Paradise et al., 2000; Shriberg et al., 2000). It has been hypothesized that the fluctuating hearing loss occurring in children with episodes of OME may hamper the perception of auditory stimulations, as well as the discrimination and identification of sounds (Keles et al., 2004). Mody, Schwartz, Gravel, and Rubin (1999) found long-term effects of early episodes of otitis media on speech sound perception, which ultimately diminishes the infrastructure on which language is acquired. The hearing loss accompanying OME may also adversely affect academic performance by impairing the ability to develop language (Roberts, Burchinal, & Zeisel, 2002). In particular, reading and language-based tasks have been identified as academic domains most affected by otitis media because of the fundamental linguistic component required to engage successfully in these tasks (Roberts et al., 2004). Reading and language-based skills may be impacted by OME via disrupting attention to verbal learning (Roberts et al., 2002, 2004).

Despite the presumption that otitis media is linked to these psychoeducational and communication delays, the data have yielded inconsistent results. For example, research has also found that no relationship exists between OME and speech, language, and academic difficulties (Campbell et al., 2003; Rovers et al., 2000). These data echo the body of literature representing the continued controversy and debate about whether otitis media does in fact affect language and academic performance. To date, this controversy has yet to be reconciled.

Medical and Psychoeducational Implications

From a medical perspective, antibiotics are often prescribed to treat the bacterial infection for children with AOM, with amoxicillin continuing to be an appropriate primary treatment choice (Hoberman et al., 2002). Tympanocentesis, which is recommended for patients who fail pharmacological therapy, can be beneficial by relieving pressure in the middle ear cavity and encouraging drainage of the middle-ear effusion (Block, 1999). For children diagnosed with OME, the course of treatment may also include antibiotics, allowing the fluid to resolve on its own, or surgical treatment (American Academy of Pediatrics, 2004; Koopman et al., 2004). A myringotomy, which is a surgical incision in the eardrum, may be performed if the child is not responsive to antibiotics or has high fever and severe pain. Although the myringotomy allows fluid to drain from the ear, it often reappears. Therefore, ventilation tubes are often inserted under general anesthesia, which allows the fluid to drain and prevents fluid accumulation, thus restoration of hearing (Medley & Roberts, 1995). Complications that may arise from ventilation tube insertion include intermittent ear discharge, deterioration or hardening of the tympanic membrane, lasting perforation, or cholesteatoma (Koopman et al., 2004). Surgical removal of the adenoids (adenoidectomy) may also be performed given that enlarged or infected adenoids may result in recurrent otitis media (Koopman et al., 2004).

Behavioral strategies for otitis media include having affected children placed in close proximity to the individual speaking, obtaining their full attention prior to speaking to them, repeating words, and speaking in a clear and articulate manner. Teachers should consider using visual aids to reinforce orally presented information, reduce distractions by keeping doors and windows closed, and provide opportunities for games that elicit careful auditory attention such as Simon Says and Red Rover (Medley & Roberts, 1995).

SELECTIVE MUTISM

Overview

Children with selective mutism typically do not speak in the school setting, although they freely speak in other environments. Its prevalence is approximately less than 1% (Bergman, Piacentini, & McCracken, 2002) and appears to affect more girls than boys (Bergman, Holloway, & Piacentini, 1999). Selective mutism is usually noticed when the child begins school. Although it is not clear what causes selective mutism, poor knowledge of the spoken language and embarrassment about another communication disorder are unlikely etiological factors (*DSM–IV–TR*; American Psychiatric Association, 2000). It also is unrelated to abuse, neglect, or trauma (Shipon-Blum, 2002). In contrast, a genetic predisposition for the disorder or a form of social anxiety may be a contributing variable (Black & Uhde, 1995). Finally, arguments based on behavioral theory suggest that selective mutism may arise because of a pattern of learned behaviors that are shaped and maintained.

Outcomes

Selective mutism can affect both academic and social functioning. It is often associated with excessive shyness, social isolation, withdrawal, negativism, compulsions, tantrums, fear, anxiety, and oppositional behavior (*DSM–IV–TR*; American Psychiatric Association, 2000). Although some children with selective mutism may evidence a complete recovery, it is more probable that the condition will endure throughout the child's academic career, and in some cases even into adulthood (Ford, Sladeczek, Carson, & Kratochwill, 1998; Remschmidt, Poller, Herpeztz-Dahlman, Hennighausen, & Gutenbrunner, 2001). Specifically, Remschmidt et al. noted that an astounding 61% of the individuals with selective mutism continued to have symptoms 12 years after diagnosis. Individuals with selective mutism were also described as more dependent, insecure, immature, and less physically healthy. In addition to exhibiting these frequently associated dysfunctional behaviors, these children were predisposed to social isolation and diminished academic functioning.

Medical and Psychoeducational Implications

Whereas psychotherapy has proved to be relatively ineffective in treating children with selective mutism, behaviorally based interventions, including stimulus fading, contingency management, shaping, self-modeling, and combinations of treatment strategies, have been effective (Kehle, Madaus, Baratta, & Bray, 1998). In addition, pharmacological treatments such as fluoxetine have been successfully used (Black & Uhde, 1995). Stimulus fading is defined by transferring stimulus control by fading the discriminative stimulus and involves providing stimuli that result in the child speaking in school-related situations. For instance, this can be accomplished by having the child with selective mutism engage in a board game with a few people with whom he or she will speak in the school (e.g., mother). Subsequently, a few classmates are gradually introduced to play. Once the first person has played the game for a while and the child with selective mutism continues to speak, additional classmates are introduced, further fading stimuli. Another behavioral intervention, contingency management, involves reinforcing verbal behavior, and ignoring nonverbal attempts to communicate. In addition, shaping, defined as the systematic reinforcement of successive approximations toward normal verbal speech, has been used successfully. Finally, self-modeling has shown treatment effectiveness and involves the positive change in behavior (i.e., speech) that is due to repeated and spaced viewings of oneself on edited videotapes that only show exemplary behaviors (Dowrick & Dove, 1980).

Kehle, Bray, Margiano, Theodore, and Zhou (2002) suggested that self-modeling is so effective because it alters the child's self-efficacy for speaking. In addition, a complementary effect of self-modeling may exist that functions to fade the child's memory of being selectively mute. On the basis of research conducted by Loftus (1997) and Braum and Loftus (1998), it has been substantiated that memories are dynamic and rather easily altered. Repeatedly exposing a child with selective mutism to edited videotapes that depict exemplary speaking behavior in formerly problematic settings, such as in the classroom, may function to create false memories of not being selectively mute. Presenting visual information to the child is perhaps the most powerful strategy to alter memory. Further, the newly acquired memory is quite enduring and resistant to subsequent attempts at alteration (Braum & Loftus, 1998).

CONCLUSION

In sum, this chapter serves as a functional blueprint outlining the developmental outcomes of language-related disorders, as well as their medical and psychoeducational implications. Language, which is fundamental to communication, involves listening, speaking, reading, and writing. The core symptoms of language-related disorders can have an impact on multiple areas of a child's performance and are often associated with academic, social, and emotional problems, and childhood psychiatric disorders. In light of the serious implications stemming from language-related disorders, it is imperative to intervene, using evidence-based treatments. Intervention requires collaboration among human service professionals, including physicians, school psychologists, speech–language pathologists, parents, and teachers to expand on and enhance children's overall level of performance. Additionally, continued communication with parents, teachers, and other professionals involved in the child's treatment is necessary to monitor progress.

REFERENCES

American Academy of Pediatrics. (2004). Otitis media with effusion. *Pediatrics, 113*, 1412–1429.

American Academy of Pediatrics and American Academy of Family Physicians. (2004). Diagnosis and management of acute otitis media. *Pediatrics, 113*, 1451–1465.

American Psychiatric Association. (2000). *Diagnostic and Statistical Manual of Mental Disorders* (4th ed., text rev.). Washington, DC: Author.

Arndt, J., & Healy, E. C. (2001). Concomitant disorders in school-age children who stutter. *Language, Speech, and Hearing Services in Schools, 32*, 68–79.

Auinger, P., Lanphear, B. P., Kalkwarf, H. J., & Mansour, M. E. (2003). Trends in otitis media among children in the United States. *Pediatrics, 112*, 514–520.

Baker, B. M., & Blackwell, P. B. (2004). Identification and remediation of pediatric fluency and voice disorders. *Journal of Pediatric Health Care, 18*, 87–94.

Baxendale, J., & Hesketh, A. (2003). Comparison of the effectiveness of the Hanen Parent Programme and traditional clinic therapy. *International Journal of Language and Communication Disorders, 38*, 397–415.

Beitchman, J. H., Wilson, B., Johnson, C. J., Atkinson, L., Young, A., Adlaf, E., et al. (2001). Fourteen-year follow-up of speech/language-impaired and control children: Psychiatric outcome. *Journal of the American Academy of Child and Adolescent Psychiatry, 40*, 75–82.

Bergman, R. L., Holloway, J., & Piacentini, J. (1999, March). *Selective mutism questionnaire: Preliminary findings*. Paper presented at the 19th National Conference of the Anxiety Disorders Association of America, San Diego, CA.

Bergman, R. L., Piacentini, J., & McCracken, J. T. (2002). Prevalence and description of selective mutism in a school-based sample. *Journal of the American Academy of Child and Adolescent Psychiatry, 41*, 938–946.

Bishop, D. V. M., North, T., & Donlan, C. (1995). Genetic basis of Specific Language Impairment: Evidence from a twin study. *Developmental Medicine and Child Neurology, 37*, 56–71.

Black, B., & Uhde, T. W. (1995). Treatment of elective mutism with fluoxetine: A double-blind, placebo-controlled study. *Journal of the American Academy of Child and Adolescent Psychiatry, 33*, 1000–1006.

Block, S. (1999). Tympanocentesis: Why, when, and how. *Contemporary Pediatrics, 16*, 103.

Blood, G. W., Ridenour, V. J., Qualls, C. D., & Hammer, C. S. (2003). Co-occurring disorders in children who stutter. *Journal of Communication, 36*, 427–448.

Braum, K. A., & Loftus, E. F. (1998). Advertising's misinformation effect. *Applied Cognitive Psychology, 12,* 569–591.

Bray, M. A., & Kehle, T. J. (2001). Long-term follow-up of self-modeling as an intervention for stuttering. *School Psychology Review, 30,* 135–141.

Campbell, T. F., Dollaghan, C. A., Rockette, H. E., Paradise, J. L., Feldman, H. M., Shriberg, L. D., et al. (2003). Risk factors for speech delay of unknown origin in 3-year-old children. *Child Development, 74,* 346–357.

Casselbrant, M. I., & Mandel, E. M. (2003). Epidemiology. In R. M. Rosenfeld & C. D. Bluestone (Eds.), *Evidence-based otitis media* (2nd ed., pp. 147–162). Hamilton, Ontario, Canada: BC Decker.

Catts, H. W., Fey, M. E., Zhang, X., & Tomblin, J. B. (2001). Estimating the risk of future reading difficulties in kindergarten children: A research-based model and its clinical implications. *Language, Speech, and Hearing Services in Schools, 32,* 38–50.

Cohen, N. J., Vallance, D. D., Barwick, M., Im, N., Menna, R., Horodezky, N. B., et al. (2000). The interface between ADHD and language impairment: An examination of language, achievement, and cognitive processing. *Journal of Child Psychology and Psychiatry, 41,* 353–362.

Conture, E. (2001). *Stuttering: Its nature, diagnosis, and treatment.* Boston: Allyn & Bacon.

Cowell, P. E., Jernigan, T. L., Denenberg, V. H., & Tallal, P. (1995). Language and learning impairment and prenatal risk: An MRI study of the corpus callosum and cerebral volume. *Journal of Medical Speech–Language Pathology, 3,* 1–13.

Craig, A., Hancock, K., Tran, Y., Craig, M., & Peters, K. (2002). Epidemiology of stuttering in the community across the entire life span. *Journal of Speech, Language, and Hearing Research, 45,* 1097–1105.

Curtiss, S., Katz, B., & Tallal, P. (1992). Delayed vs. deviance in the language acquisition of language impaired children. *Journal of Speech and Hearing, 35,* 373–383.

Damico, J. S., & Damico, S. K. (1993). Language and social skills from a diversity perspective: Considerations for the speech–language pathologist. *Language, Speech, and Hearing Services in Schools, 24,* 236–243.

Darrow, D. H., Dash, N., & Derkay, C. S. (2003). Otitis media: Concepts and controversies. *Current Opinion in Otolaryngology and Head and Neck Surgery, 11,* 416–423.

Davis, S., Howell, P., & Cooke, F. (2002). Sociodynamic relationships between children who stutter and their non-stuttering classmates. *Journal of Child Psychology and Psychiatry, 43,* 939–947.

de Ru, J. A., & Grote, J. J. (2004). Otitis media with effusion: Disease or defense? A review of the literature. *International Journal of Pediatric Otorhinolaryngology, 68,* 331–339.

Dowrick, P. W., & Dove, C. (1980). The use of self-modeling to improve the swimming performance of spina bifida children. *Journal of Applied Behavior Analysis, 13,* 51–56.

Ezrati, V. R., & Levin, I. (2004). The relationship between anxiety and stuttering: A multidimensional approach. *Journal of Fluency Disorders, 29*, 135–148.

Felsenfeld, S. (2002). Finding susceptibility genes for developmental disorders of speech: The long and winding road. *Journal of Communication Disorders, 35*, 329–345.

Finn, P. (2003). Addressing generalization and maintenance of stuttering treatment in the schools: A critical look. *Journal of Communication Disorders, 36*, 153–164.

Ford, M. A., Sladeczek, I. E., Carson, J., & Kratochwill, T. R. (1998). Selective mutism: Phenomenological characteristics. *School Psychology Quarterly, 13*, 192–227.

Friedlander, A. H., Noffsinger, D., Mendez, M. F., & Yagiela, J. A. (2004). Developmental stuttering: Manifestations, treatment, and dental implications. *Special Care in Dentistry, 24*, 7–12.

Gauger, L. M., Lombardino, L. J., & Leonard, C. M. (1997). Brain morphology in children with specific language impairment. *Journal of Speech, Language, and Hearing Research, 40*, 1272–1284.

Gillon, G. T. (2002). Follow-up study investigating the benefits of phonological awareness intervention for children with spoken language impairment. *International Journal of Language and Communication Disorders, 37*, 381–400.

Habib, M., Espesser, R., Rey, V., Giraud, K., Bruas, P., & Gres, C. (1999). Training dyslexics with acoustically modified speech: Evidence of improved phonological performance. *Brain and Cognition, 40*, 143–146.

Hesketh, A., Adams, C., Nightingale, C., & Hall, R. (2000). Phonological awareness therapy and articulatory training approaches for children with phonological disorders: A comparative outcome study. *International Journal of Language and Communication Disorders, 35*, 337–354.

Hoberman, A., Marchant, C. D., Kaplan, S. L., & Feldman, S. (2002). Treatment of acute otitis media: Consensus recommendations. *Clinical Pediatrics, 41*, 373–390.

Ingham, R. J. (2001). Brain imaging studies of developmental stuttering. *Journal of Communication Disorders, 34*, 493–516.

Irwin, J. R., Carter, A. S., & Briggs-Gowan, M. J. (2002). The social-emotional development of "late-talking" toddlers. *Journal of the American Academy of Child and Adolescent Psychiatry, 41*, 1324–1332.

Joanisse, M. F., Manis, F., Keating, P., & Seidenberg, M. (2000). Language deficits in dyslexic children: Speech perception, phonology, and morphology. *Journal of Experimental Child Psychology, 77*, 30–60.

Jones, M., Onslow, M., Harrison, E., & Packman, A. (2000). Treating stuttering in young children: Predicting treatment time in the Lidcombe Program. *Journal of Speech, Language, and Hearing Research, 43*, 1440–1451.

Kehle, T. J., Bray, M. A., Margiano, S., Theodore, L. A., & Zhou, Z. (2002). Self-modeling as an effective intervention for students with serious emotional disturbance: Are we modifying children's memories? *Psychology in the Schools, 39,* 203–207.

Kehle, T. J., Madaus, M. M. R., Baratta, V. S., & Bray, M. A. (1998). Augmented self-modeling as a treatment for children with selective mutism. *Journal of School Psychology, 36,* 377–399.

Keles, E., Kaygusuz, I., Karlidag, T., Yalcan, S., Acik, Y., Alpay, H. C., et al. (2004). Prevalence of otitis media with effusion in first and second grade primary school students and its correlation with BCG vaccination. *International Journal of Pediatric Otorhinolaryngology, 68,* 1069–1074.

Koopman, J. P., Reuchlin, A. G., Kummer, E. E., Boumand, L. J., Rihntjes, E., Hoeve, L. J., et al. (2004). Laser myringotomy versus ventilation tubes in children with otitis media with effusion: A randomized trial. *Laryngoscope, 114,* 844–849.

Kovac, I., Garabedian, B., Souich, C., & Palmour, R. M. (2001). Attention deficit/hyperactivity in SLI children increases risk of speech/language disorders in first degree relatives: A preliminary report. *Journal of Communication Disorders, 34,* 339–354.

Laasonen, M., Tomma-Halme, J., Lahti-Nuuttila, P., Service, E., & Virsu, V. (2000). Rate of information segregation in developmentally dyslexic children. *Brain and Language, 75,* 66–81.

Liu, Y., Shi, W., Ding, B., Li, X., Xiao, K., Wang, X., et al. (2001). Analysis of correlates in the SAS, SDS, and the MMPI of stutterers. *Chinese Journal of Clinical Psychology, 9,* 133–134.

Loftus, E. F. (1997). Memories for a past that never was. *Current Directions in Psychological Science, 6,* 60–65.

Ludlow, C. L., & Loucks, T. (2003). Stuttering: A dynamic motor control disorder. *Journal of Fluency Disorders, 28,* 273–295.

Manolson, A. (1992). *It takes two to talk: A parent's guide to helping children communicate.* Toronto, Ontario, Canada: The Hanen Centre.

McDade, A., & McCartan, P. (1998). "Partnership with parents"—A pilot project. *International Journal of Disorders of Communication, 22*(Suppl.), 556–561.

Medley, L. P., & Roberts, J. E. (1995). At-risk children and otitis media with effusion: Management issues for the early childhood. *Topics in Early Childhood Education, 15,* 44–65.

Mody, M., Schwartz, R. G., Gravel, J. S., & Rubin, R. J. (1999). Speech perception and verbal memory in children with and without histories of otitis media. *Journal of Speech, Language, and Hearing Research, 42,* 1069–1079.

Monobe, H., Ishibashi, T., Fujishiro, Y., Shinogami, M., & Yano, J. (2003). Factors associated with poor outcome in children with acute otitis media. *Acta Otolaryngology, 123,* 564–568.

Muter, V., & Snowling, M. (1998). Concurrent and longitudinal predictors of reading: The role of metalinguistic and short-term memory skills. *Reading Research Quarterly, 33,* 320–337.

Paradise, J. L., Dollaghan, C. A., Campbell, T. F., Feldman, H. M., Bernard, B. S., Colborn, D. K., et al. (2000). Language, speech sound production, and cognition in three-year-old children in relation to otitis media in their first three years of life. *Pediatrics, 105,* 1119–1130.

Perino, M., Famularo, G., & Tarraoni, P. (2000). Acquired transient stuttering during a migraine attack. *Headache, 40,* 170–172.

Perkins, W. H. (1993). The early history of behavior modification of stuttering: A view from the trenches. *Journal of Fluency Disorders, 18,* 1–11.

Ratner, N. B. (2004). Caregiver–child interactions and their impact on children's fluency: Implications for treatment. *Language, Speech, and Hearing Services in Schools, 35,* 46–56.

Remschmidt, H., Poller, M., Herpeztz-Dahlman, B., Hennighausen, K., & Gutenbrunner, C. (2001). A follow-up study of 45 patients with elective mutism. *European Archives of Psychology and Clinical Neuroscience, 251,* 284–296.

Rissman, M., Curtis, S., & Tallal, P. (1990). School placement outcomes of young language impaired children. *Journal of Speech–Language Pathology and Audiology, 14,* 49–58.

Roberts, J. E., Burchinal, M. R., & Zeisel, S. A. (2002). Otitis media in early childhood in relation to children's school-age language and academic skills. *Pediatrics, 110,* 696–706.

Roberts, J., Hunter, L., Gravel, J., Rosenfeld, R., Berman, S., Haggard, M., et al. (2004). Otitis media, hearing loss, and language learning: Controversies and current research. *Journal of Developmental and Behavioral Pediatrics, 25,* 110–123.

Rovers, M. M., Straatman, H., Ingels, K., Jan van der Wilt, G., van den Broek, P., et al. (2000). The effect of ventilation tubes in language development in infants with otitis media with effusion: A randomized trial. *Pediatrics, 106,* e42.

Segers, E., & Verhoeven, L. (2004). Computer-supported phonological awareness intervention for kindergarten children with specific language impairment. *Language, Speech, and Hearing Services in Schools, 35,* 229–239.

Shipon-Blum, E. (2002, February). "When the words just won't come out"—Understanding selective mutism [Insert]. *NASP Communiqué, 30.*

Shriberg, L. D., Flipson, P., Thielke, H., Kwiatkowski, J., Kertoy, M. K., Katcher, M. L., et al. (2000). Risk for speech disorder associated with early recurrent otitis media with effusion: Two retrospective studies. *Journal of Speech, Language, and Hearing Research, 43,* 79–99.

Snow, C. E., Burns, S. M., & Griffin, P. (1998). *Preventing reading difficulties in young children.* Washington, DC: National Academy Press.

Snowling, M., Bishop, D. V., & Stothard, S. E. (2000). Is preschool language impairment a risk factor for dyslexia in adolescence? *Journal of Child Psychology and Psychiatry and Allied Disciplines, 41,* 587–600.

Spitz, R. V., Tallal, P., Flax, J., & Benasich, A. A. (1997). Look who's talking: A prospective study of familial transmission of language impairments. *Journal of Speech, Language, and Hearing Research, 40,* 990–1001.

Stagg, V., & Burns, M. S. (1999). Specific developmental disorders. In R. T. Ammerman & M. Hersen (Eds.), *Handbook of prescriptive treatments for children and adolescents* (2nd ed., pp. 48–62). Boston: Allyn & Bacon.

Tallal, P. (1998). Language learning impairment: Integrating research and remediation. *Scandinavian Journal of Psychology, 39*, 195–197.

Tallal, P., & Benasich, A. A. (2002). Developmental language learning impairments. *Development and Psychopathology, 14*, 559–579.

Tallal, P., Miller, S. L., & Bedi, G. (1996, January 5). Language comprehension in language-learning impaired children improved with acoustically modified speech. *Science, 271*, 81–84.

Tomblin, B. J., Records, N. L., Buckwalter, P., Zhang, X., Smith, E., & O'Brien, M. (1997). Prevalence of specific language impairment in kindergarten children. *Journal of Speech, Language, and Hearing Research, 40*, 1245–1260.

Trauner, D., Wulfeck, B., Tallal, P., & Hesselink, J. (2000). Neurological and MRI profiles of children with developmental language impairment. *Developmental Medicine and Child Neurology, 42*, 470–475.

Vallance, D. D., Cummings, R. L., & Humphries, T. (1998). Mediators of the risk for problem behavior in children with language learning disabilities. *Journal of Learning Disabilities, 31*, 160–171.

van der Lely, H. K. J., & Stollwerck, L. (1997). Binding theory and grammatical specific language impairment in children. *Cognition, 62*, 245–290.

Willinger, U., Brunner, E., Diendorfer-Radner, G., Mag, J. M., Sirsch, U., & Eisenwort, B. (2003). Behaviour in children with language development disorders. *Canadian Journal of Psychiatry, 48*, 607–614.

Wilson, L., Onslow, M., & Lincoln, M. (2004). Telehealth adaptation of the Lidcombe Program of early stuttering intervention: Five case studies. *American Journal of Speech–Language Pathology, 13*, 81–93.

Yairi, E., & Ambrose, N. (1999). Early childhood stuttering I: Persistency and recovery rates. *Journal of Speech, Language, and Hearing Research, 42*, 1097–1112.

Young, A. R., Beitchman, J. H., Johnson, C., Douglas, L., Atkinson, L., Escobar, M., & Wilson, B. (2002). Young adult academic outcomes in a longitudinal sample of early identified language impaired and control children. *Journal of Child Psychology and Psychiatry, 43*, 635–645.

10

NEUROCUTANEOUS SYNDROMES

DAVID E. McINTOSH AND MEGAN M. MORSE

The neurocutaneous syndromes consist of about 40 disorders that exhibit various forms of cutaneous stigmata (i.e., abnormalities on the skin, including bumps, spots of various sizes and colors, and abnormal freckling) visible at birth or shortly thereafter. The majority of these disorders are considered to be inherited through autosomal dominant transmission, although expressivity is variable. This means that the symptoms of a particular syndrome may be more severe in a child than in the parent from whom it was transmitted. The involvement of the central and peripheral nervous systems in these syndromes suggests that they begin to evolve between the 8th and 24th month of gestation (Hynd & Willis, 1988). Common among these disorders is the presence of seizures and behavioral and cognitive problems. Three of these disorders, neurofibromatosis, Sturge–Weber syndrome, and tuberous sclerosis, make up a significant proportion of the referrals of neurocutaneous syndromes to pediatric neurological clinics (Hynd & Willis, 1988) and are therefore the focus of this chapter. The chapter includes general information on each of the disorders as well as outcomes, medical implications, psychoeducational implications, and psychological implications related to the disorders.

NEUROFIBROMATOSIS

Overview

Friedrich von Recklinghausen first noted neurofibromatosis in 1882 when he discovered tumors that originated from nerve cells. Neurofibromatosis is considered an autosomal dominant genetic disorder that results in both benign and malignant tumors; these increase in frequency within both the central and peripheral nervous systems. When mothers are affected by neurofibromatosis, the disorder takes a more severe course and develops earlier than when fathers are the transmitters (Miller & Hall, 1978). Although many people inherit this disorder, 30% to 50% of cases arise from spontaneous mutations in an individual's genes. Neurofibromatosis occurs in both sexes and across all racial and ethnic groups.

Clinical manifestations of this syndrome include café au lait macules (coffee-brown pigmented spots), primarily on the trunk; cutaneous and subcutaneous tumors; focal brain lesions (a wound or injury resulting in changes in brain tissue) frequently observed in the basal ganglia; cerebellum, brain stem, and subcortical white matter; freckling in areas not exposed to sunlight; and Lisch nodules (slightly raised tumors on the iris). Two types of the disorder are commonly noted, although others may exist. Neurofibromatosis Type 1 (NF1) occurs more frequently (1 in 4,000 live births) and has been studied in greater detail than neurofibromatosis Type 2 (NF2) 1 in 40,000; Nilsson & Bradford, 1999).

NF1 consists of abnormal nerve cell growth in the peripheral nervous system, although brain tumors and other lesions within the brain are also present as well. Symptoms are typically present during childhood, but the disorder may become more pronounced during puberty, pregnancy, or hormonal changes (Nilsson & Bradford, 1999). Although the disorder has been heavily researched, diagnosis of NF1 is still based on clinical criteria. The National Institutes of Health (NIH) directs physicians diagnosing this disorder to look for changes in skin appearance, tumors, or bone abnormalities, or a parent, sibling, or child with NF1 (National Institute of Neurological Disorders, 2005).

NF2 is characterized by bilateral (occurring on both sides of the body) tumors on the eighth cranial nerve, which cause pressure damage to neighboring nerves. Diagnostic criteria for NF2 include bilateral eighth nerve tumors and similar signs and symptoms in a parent, sibling, or child. Other symptoms may include hearing loss, tinnitus (ringing noise in the ear) and poor balance as early as the teen years, headaches, facial pain, or facial numbness, caused by pressure from the tumors (Nilsson & Bradford, 1999).

Outcomes

The clinical expression, severity of symptoms, and progression of NF1 vary greatly among individuals (Nilsson & Bradford, 1999). Because of the varied manifestations of NF1, it is difficult to discern the medical, socioemotional, and behavioral outcomes and generalize these to all individuals with NF1. Physically, individuals with more severe manifestations of the disease may experience pain. Nilsson and Bradford (1999) noted that the severity depends greatly on the location, type of neurofibromas (benign tumors), and sometimes their size. Neurofibromas can develop at any time; however, their size and number often increase after puberty. Plexiform neurofibromas (diffuse soft tissue or nerve enlargements) are considered common; however, the prognosis is considered poorer if they develop prior to age 10 and on the head, face, or neck (Needle et al., 1997). Gutmann (1999) also reported a 3% to 5% risk of malignant degeneration with plexiform neurofibromas.

The prognosis of individuals with NF depends greatly on the severity of the symptoms. In most cases, symptoms of NF1 are mild. Therefore, individuals with mild NF typically live healthy, productive lives with minimal disability (Grostern, 2004). According to Grostern (2004), individuals with more severe aspects of NF1 may experience a shorter life expectancy. He also noted that CNS tumors, malignant tumors, mental retardation, or severe seizures could lead to a shorter life expectancy if associated with NF1. With NF2, the risk of damage to critical structures within the brain (e.g., cranial nerves, brain stem) can be life threatening.

The general cognitive functioning of individuals with NF1 is typically in the low average range (Hofman, Harris, Bryan, & Denckla, 1994; Mazzocco, 2001; Moore, Ater, Needle, Slopis, & Copeland, 1994; North et al., 1997). There does appear to be an increased risk of mental retardation among individuals with NF1 (4%–8%) compared with the general population. Although prior cross-sectional research has suggested individuals with NF1 may demonstrate increases in general cognitive functioning from childhood to adulthood (Riccardi & Eichner, 1986), more recent research does not support such a general conclusion (Hyman et al., 2003). In their longitudinal study, Hyman et al. did, however, find increases in cognitive ability among older individuals (15 years old on average at the start of the study) with NF1, but the increases were similar to the normal control group. They indicated that their results supported Riccardi and Eichner's (1986) finding that cognitive abilities of adults with NF1 are similar to normal adults. Hyman et al. also found a strong relationship between the presence of hyperintensities (bright areas found in the brain) prior to age 18 and lower cognitive functioning. Specifically, they found that the presence of hyperintensities were good predictors of lowering IQ up until the age of 18 (Hyman et al., 2003).

A large number of studies have been published substantiating the presence of learning disabilities (LDs) among children with NF1 (Brewer, Moore, & Hiscock, 1997; Cutting, Koth, & Denckla, 2000; Gutmann, 1999; Mazzocco, 2001). The comorbid incidence of LDs with NF1 has been reported to range from 25% to 61% (North et al., 1997; Riccardi, 1981; Stine & Adams, 1989).

It is clear that the incidence of LDs among children with NF1 is considerably higher compared with the 2% to 15% prevalence among healthy children. A neuropathological basis of LDs among children with NF1 has been proposed (Brewer et al., 1997), given the strong association found between the presence, location, and number of hyperintensities and the occurrence of an LD (Hofman et al., 1994; Moore, Slopis, Schomer, Jackson, & Levy, 1996; North et al., 1997). Preliminary research also suggests significant diversity in the types of LDs identified among children with NF1 (Brewer et al., 1997). Although studies have been published demonstrating that a large percentage of children with NF1 have visuospatial and motor deficits (Cutting et al., 2000; Eliason, 1986; Varnhagen et al., 1998), recent studies also have shown that both verbal and nonverbal LD is common among children with NF1 (Cutting et al., 2000; Hofman et al., 1994; Mazzocco, 2001).

Medical Implications

The primary focus of medical treatment for NF1 and NF2 is to control symptoms. Surgery to remove cutaneous neurofibromas may be considered if they are painful, result in loss of function, become infected, or are disfiguring. There is a risk that tumors may reoccur and in greater numbers after surgery, however. Surgery also may be needed at times to address bone deformities depending on their size and location. Malignant tumors may require radiation treatment, chemotherapy, or surgery.

Treatment options for individuals with NF2 include complete or partial removal of tumors on the auditory nerves; however, completely removing tumors may result in hearing loss. Use of radiation also may be an option. In many cases, monitoring the growth rate of tumors and taking a conservative approach toward treatment is preferred (Grostern, 2004). With both NF1 and NF2, parents may be referred to ophthalmologists, neurosurgeons, orthopedists, or dermatologists depending on the systemic manifestations of the syndrome.

STURGE–WEBER SYNDROME

Overview

Sturge–Weber syndrome was first described by Sturge in 1879 in a patient with partial epilepsy. Sturge believed that the epilepsy was due to a lesion (a wound or injury that changes brain tissue) of the vasomotor center (an area of the brain responsible for some motor processes) and that the neurological problems were related to hemiplegia (paralysis affecting one side of the body) and a facial naevus flammeus (port-wine stain, often present at birth) the patient also exhibited. Weber (1922, 1929) described another early case of the syndrome, calling it "encephalotrigeminal angiomatosis."

Sturge–Weber syndrome is characterized by a port-wine stain on the face, which is usually unilateral (on one side of the face) but may be bilateral (on both sides of the face), caused by an overabundance of capillaries just beneath the surface of the affected skin. The primary neurological symptom is angioma (excessive blood vessel growth on the surface of the brain). In about 30% to 50% of cases, hemiparesis (a weakening or loss of use of the side of the body opposite the port-wine stain) or homonymous hemianopsia (loss of vision in the same part of the visual field of each eye) exists. Other indications include glaucoma (increased pressure within the eye), oculocutaneous melanosis (increased pigmentation [melanin] resulting in darker coloration in and around the eyes), intracranial calcification (the hardening of tissue in the skull caused by the deposit of calcium salts), atrophied cerebral hemisphere (shrinkage of brain tissue caused by loss of brain cell processing), intracerebral calcifications (the deposit of calcium in brain tissue), vascular lesions (overgrown enlarged blood vessels or multiple small vessels), and abnormalities in blood-flow patterns (Hynd & Willis, 1988).

Unlike neurofibromatosis and tuberous sclerosis, Sturge–Weber syndrome has no known genetic cause. It occurs less frequently than the other two disorders, although because of the variations in clinical presentation that exist, the true prevalence and incidence remain unknown. It is estimated that Sturge–Weber syndrome occurs in 1 in 6,000 births. Physicians diagnosing the syndrome should refer to Roach's (1988) diagnosing scheme, which divides the syndrome into three classifications. Type I (classic) is characterized by a facial birthmark and leptomeningeal angioma (tumors of the blood vessels in the membranes covering the brain and spinal cord). Type II exhibits only the facial angioma (birthmark), and Type III exhibits only the leptomeningeal angioma (Cody & Hynd, 1998).

Outcomes

As with NF, the symptoms of Sturge–Weber syndrome vary greatly among individuals. Although the syndrome itself is not considered fatal, associated seizures can place individuals at risk. Roach (2002) indicated that the risk for developing seizures is highest during the first 2 years of life, although seizures can begin at anytime from birth to adulthood. In fact, Sujansky and Conradi (1995) found that 75% of individuals with Sturge–Weber syndrome have seizures within the first year of life. Overall, 80% of individuals with Sturge–Weber syndrome who have unilateral lesions and 93% who have bihemispheric lesions develop seizures (Bebin & Gomez, 1988; Roach, 2002; Rochkind, Hoffman, & Hendrick, 1990). There also is the tendency for seizures to start acutely with corresponding hemiparesis.

An estimated 50% of individuals with Sturge–Weber syndrome are also classified with mental retardation (Aicardi, 1992; Bodensteiner & Roach, 1999). There appears to be a strong correlation between age of onset of seizures and level of cognitive functioning (Arzimanoglou & Aicardi, 1992; Rochkind et al., 1990). The probability of mental retardation increases significantly if seizures occur prior to age 1 (Arzimanoglou & Aicardi, 1992) or 2 (Roach, 2002). Therefore, children with Sturge–Weber syndrome who do not experience seizures prior to age 3 are more likely to display normal cognitive functioning (Roach, 2002). In contrast, Kramer, Kahana, Shorer, and Ben-Zeev (2000) found cognitive impairment among individuals with unilateral Sturge–Weber syndrome was more highly correlated with seizure intensity than age of onset of seizures. This preliminary research suggests that seizure intensity among young children may serve as a prognostic marker for cognitive deterioration.

According to Sujansky and Conradi (1995), early development is typically normal; however, mild to profound mental retardation eventually emerges in approximately 50% of children with Sturge–Weber syndrome. The prognosis of children with bilateral brain involvement is poorer, with approximately 8% falling within the normal range of cognitive functioning (Bebin & Gomez, 1988).

Sturge–Weber syndrome is usually limited to the skin, eyes, and brain and rarely involves other body organs. Neurological deficits are often related to the location of excessive blood vessel growth on the surface of the brain (i.e., angiomas). Although angiomas can occur anywhere on the brain, they typically develop on the posterior or occipital lobes of the brain. Angiomas usually cause seizures and contribute to motor delays and cognitive impairment. Strokes also may occur. According to Roach (2002), not all individuals with Sturge–Weber syndrome have enduring specific neurological signs.

Glaucoma may be present at birth but usually develops within the first 10 years (Roach, 2002). Roach (2002) did indicate that glaucoma sometimes develops later among young adults. In addition, glaucoma is often restricted to the eye with the port-wine stain. If untreated, glaucoma can lead to blindness. Enlargement of the coatings of the eye (buphthalmos) involved with port-wine stain also may occur. *Amblyopia* (i.e., lazy eye) may be present at birth.

Medical Implications

Medical treatment of Sturge–Weber syndrome often focuses on the presenting symptoms. Laser treatments are available to remove or decrease coloration of port-wine stains, even among children as young as 1 month old. For glaucoma, surgery or eyedrops are common forms of treatment. Corrective lenses may be used to correct vision.

Anticonvulsant medication is commonly used to treat and control seizures. Individuals with refractory seizures may be considered for epilepsy surgery. Considerable controversy exists, however, as to when or if to conduct epileptic surgery (Kramer et al., 2000). Therefore, surgery is only pursued when clinically significant seizures are nonresponsive to medical treatment (Roach et al., 1994).

TUBEROUS SCLEROSIS

Overview

Bournville first recognized tuberous sclerosis in the late 1800s in a young patient who was experiencing the effects of epilepsy, mental retardation, and hemiplegia (paralysis of one side of the body). The name *tuberous sclerosis* was given to reflect the potatolike lesions (wounds or injuries causing changes in the tissue), known as tubers, found in the cerebral cortex of patients with this disorder (Harrison & Bolton, 1997).

Like neurofibromatosis, tuberous sclerosis is an autosomal-dominant genetic disorder that occurs across all sex, ethnic, and racial groups. Sixty-six percent of cases may result as a spontaneous mutation (not based on genetic factors). It is estimated that 1 in 10,000 individuals are born with tuberous sclerosis.

Tuberous sclerosis is characterized by adenoma sebaceum (red bumps on the skin) that may resemble acne. These lesions may become large and wartlike in appearance and will increase in number over time so that by age 35, close to 100% of individuals with tuberous sclerosis will be affected. Tuberous sclerosis affects the central nervous system and the organs in the viscera, which means that the kidneys, heart, lungs, and bones may be affected. Other symptoms include amelanotic naevus (white spots) on trunk and limbs and occasionally on the face, shagreen patch (an uneven, rough patch of skin), subungual fibromas (fleshy overgrowth of fibrous tissue on finger or toenail), and, in rare cases, some café au lait spots (Hynd & Willis, 1988).

Seizure disorders frequently co-occur with tuberous sclerosis (85%–95% of individuals), causing seizures to become a core characteristic of tuberous sclerosis (Curatolo et al., 1991). These seizures may start out as infantile spasms and evolve into true seizure disorders in older children and adults (Smalley, Burger, & Smith, 1994).

Like Sturge–Weber syndrome, the diagnosis of tuberous sclerosis is complicated by the variability of disease expression. Diagnosis may be confirmed through a physical examination, including brain and kidney scan investigations. It is believed that 1 in 12,000 children are affected by tuberous sclerosis (Sampson, Scahill, Stephenson, Mann, & Conner, 1989), and 1 in 14,500 people among all age groups are affected (Shepherd, Beard, Gomez, Kurland, & Whisnant, 1991).

Outcomes

The National Institute of Neurological Disorders and Stroke ([NINDS], 2004) indicates that the prognosis for individuals with tuberous sclerosis is highly dependent on the severity of symptoms. Symptoms can "range from mild skin abnormalities to varying degrees of learning disabilities and epilepsy to severe mental retardation, uncontrollable seizures, and kidney failure" (NINDS, 2004). The NINDS Web site notes, however, that people with tuberous sclerosis who have mild symptoms often live long and productive lives, whereas those with severe symptoms may have significant disabilities. The Web site further reports that "in rare cases, seizures, infections, or tumors in vital organs may cause complications in some organs such as the kidneys and brain that can lead to severe difficulties and even death." With suitable health care, the majority of individuals with tuberous sclerosis will live to normal life expectancies (NINDS, 2004).

The prevalence of LDs among individuals with tuberous sclerosis has been estimated to range from 50% to 65% (Hunt & Lindenbaum, 1984; Shepherd & Stephenson, 1992; Webb, Fryer, & Osborne, 1996; Wiederholt, Gomez, & Rurland, 1985). There are uncertainties regarding the etiology of LDs among individuals with tuberous sclerosis, however. Harrison and Bolton (1997) noted that it is unclear whether cognitive impairments are a result of a general decline in intellectual abilities or whether specific deficits in verbal and nonverbal skills are related to the location of tubers. A wide variety of LDs seem to be identified among individuals with tuberous sclerosis. Dyspraxia, speech delay, dyscalculia, visuomotor deficits, expressive language difficulties, and auditory processing problems are a few identified in the literature (Ferguson, McKinlay, & Hunt, 2002; Jambaque et al., 1991). Given the lack of systematic research using control groups, it has been difficult to determine whether individuals with tuberous sclerosis who display normal intelligence have LDs similar to those of lower functioning individuals with TSC (Harrison & Bolton, 1997). There do appear to be links between the presence of early-onset epilepsy, a history of infantile spasms, and refractory seizures and an increased likelihood of learning disabilities (Shepherd & Stephenson, 1992; Webb et al., 1996).

Although past research has consistently estimated the incidence of mental retardation among individuals with tuberous sclerosis to range between 50% and 60% (Gillberg, Gillberg, & Ahlsen, 1994; Shepherd & Stephenson, 1992; Webb et al., 1996), some researchers are now questioning the accuracy of these estimates because of the lack of studies that used standardized measures of IQ (Harrison & Bolton, 1997; Joinson et al., 2003). There is also research that suggests a bimodal distribution of IQ scores among the tuberous sclerosis population, with individuals falling either within the mental retardation or normal ranges (Hunt & Lindenbaum, 1984; Shepherd & Stephenson, 1992; Webb et al., 1996). Although the results of these studies have been questioned because they failed to use standardized measures of intelligence, Joinson et al. (2003) found a bimodal distribution of IQ scores in a large sample (n = 108) of individuals with tuberous sclerosis. Specifically, Joinson et al. found the majority (55.5%) of individuals with tuberous sclerosis fell within the normal range, with 14% falling within the mild to moderate range of intelligence and 30.5% falling within the profound range. The mean IQ (M = 93.6) for the tuberous sclerosis sample was significantly lower compared with the normal comparison group (M = 105.6). These results (44.5%) are close to prior estimates in which individuals with tuberous sclerosis fell within the mental retardation range of intelligence.

A high comorbidity rate seems to exist between tuberous sclerosis and autism (Asano et al., 2001; Smalley, 1998; Weber, Egelhoff, McKellop, & Franz, 2000). The range of autism among individuals with TSC has been estimated to be between 17% and 68% (Gillberg et al., 1994; Gonzalez, Welsh, & Sepulveda, 1993; Hunt & Shepherd, 1993; Smalley, Tanguay, Smith, & Gutierrez, 1992). Smalley et al. (1992) provided a more reasonable estimate of 25%, and when combining autism and pervasive developmental disorders, the estimate raises to 40% to 45%. In contrast, tuberous sclerosis is comorbid only approximately 1% to 4% among individuals with autism (Smalley et al., 1992).

Although research has shown correlations between the total number of tubers and the degree of intellectual impairment (Goodman et al., 1997), a higher number of tubers has not been found to be a good predictor of autistic behaviors (Weber et al., 2000). Instead, the number of tubers within the cerebellum was found to be more predictive of autistic behaviors (Weber et al., 2000). This finding was consistent with prior research.

Medical Implications

The need for and extent of medical treatment vary greatly among individuals with tuberous sclerosis. Medications to control seizures as well as other problems (e.g., attention deficits, hyperactivity, anger) are available. In addition, medication may be used to assist in controlling psychiatric symptoms (e.g., depression, hallucinations, delusions, anxiety, obsessive–compulsive features) that are secondary features related to the organic nature of tuberous sclerosis (Harvey, Mahr, & Balon, 1995). Surgery to remove tumors found in the kidneys, brain, or heart may be necessary, especially if tumors grow large or are causing significant pain. Although most skin lesions are not problematic (NINDS, 2004), surgery, dermabrasion, and laser treatments are available if warranted.

Enhancing the self-help and daily living skills of many individuals with tuberous sclerosis should also be a focus of treatment. A study conducted to survey the care needs of adolescents and young adults with tuberous sclerosis found adaptive behavior was often not addressed (Ferguson et al., 2002). Parents who completed the survey raised concerns related to talking, walking, shaving, menarche, bathing, and toileting, indicating a need to assist parents in preparing them to address these self-help skills as their children matured. During puberty, individuals with tuberous sclerosis may benefit from sex education. Parents also would benefit in learning about birth control methods. Assisting parents in learning effective methods for coping with the daily stress of raising a child with tuberous sclerosis is essential (Tunali & Power, 1993), and providing respite care should be considered.

Psychoeducational Implications of Neurocutaneous Syndromes

Depending on severity of the syndrome, special education services and related services may be needed to address the educational, physical, and emotional needs of children and adolescents with a neurocutaneous syndrome. Prior to receiving services, a student must be evaluated and determined eligible for special education. Therefore, a comprehensive psychoeducational evaluation by a multidisciplinary team is recommended and should include a measure of intelligence, achievement, adaptive behavior, personality, classroom observation, review of educational records, and review of medical records. Evaluation of a student's speech, language, vision, hearing, motor skills, physical development, and learning style may also be warranted depending on a specific child's disabilities. The multidisciplinary team should include the school psychologist, regular education teacher, and special education teacher(s). The special education teacher(s) must have specific training in the student's primary area(s) of disability. To receive services, a student also must be found eligible within one of the following categories: autism spectrum disorder, communication disorder, deaf–blind, developmental disorder, emotional disability, hearing impairment, learning disability, mental disability, multiple disabilities, orthopedic impairment, other health impairment, traumatic brain injury, or visual impairment (Individuals With Disabilities Education Act [IDEA], 1997). Given the multitude of symptoms, the case conference committee may use any of the aforementioned categories to meet the needs of students with neurocutaneous syndromes.

For students with mild forms of a neurocutaneous syndrome who do not meet the classification criteria under IDEA, parents may wish to pursue services under Section 504 of the Rehabilitation Act of 1973. According to Section 504, an individual with disabilities is one who

1. has a physical or mental impairment that substantially limits one or more major life activities;

2. has a record of such an impairment; or
3. is regarded as having such an impairment.

To qualify for services under Section 504, the disabling condition must substantially limit one major life activity, which includes caring for oneself, performing manual tasks, walking, seeing, hearing, speaking, breathing, learning, and working. Note, however, that students may qualify for services under Section 504 but may not qualify for special education services. In contrast, students who are eligible for special education services are automatically eligible for services under Section 504.

Section 504 also applies to postsecondary programs and employment settings. Postsecondary institutions must make reasonable modifications or accommodations, which may include additional time to complete a degree, books on tape, interpreters, tape recorders, note takers, additional testing time, testing in a quiet location, and special equipment. Employers are required to make "reasonable accommodations" for individuals with physical or mental disabilities.

The Americans With Disabilities Act of 1990 (ADA; Pub. L. 101-336) also affords individuals with disabilities protections against discrimination. As with Section 504, ADA applies to postsecondary and employment settings. Specifically, public institutions and private institutions with more than 15 employees that receive federal money must provide accommodations for individuals with disabilities. Therefore, ADA and Section 504 should be considered when developing an educational program to meet the needs of children with neurocutaneous syndromes who do not meet the criteria for services under IDEA.

Although there is a lack of research specifically focused on discussing educational interventions for students with neurocutaneous syndromes, Nilsson and Bradford (1999) recommended that many of the intervention needs of students with less severe forms of NF are adaptive and compensatory rather than remedial. Therefore, accommodations within the regular classroom should be considered. Untimed tests, oral versus written exams, additional time to complete work, use of a calculator, access to a computer, and shorter assignments may be considered (Nilsson & Bradford, 1999).

Psychological Implications

The use of functional behavioral assessment (FBA) in developing viable interventions for problem behaviors has been well documented (Lentz & Shapiro, 1986; Lewis & Sugai, 1996; O'Neill et al., 1997). FBA can be used to help develop interventions to address aggression or poor social skills, enhance communication skills, increase daily living skills, and so on. FBA uses a problem-solving approach that focuses on identifying the variables that influence behavior (Knoster & McCurdy, 2002). The essential feature of FBA compared with other behavior management techniques is the focus on developing an intervention that has a high likelihood of being successful. FBA incorporates several characteristics of a good behavioral program, which include operationally defining problem behavior, identifying antecedents that predict behavior, identifying consequences that maintain behavior, identifying the functional aspects of behavior, collecting baseline data, writing specific goals, and progress monitoring (Knoster & McCurdy, 2002; Nilsson & Bradford, 1999). Another key feature of FBA is the emphasis placed on conducting interviews with the goal of identifying variables that affect problem behavior. Therefore, it is not uncommon for behavior specialists to interview the client, parents, and teachers when conducting FBA.

Counseling for individuals with neurocutaneous syndromes should be considered to address social and emotional symptoms secondary to the syndromes. Grostern (2004) suggests counseling for adolescents with NF1 in particular, as they often struggle with body-image issues related to physical disfigurement. Adolescents who are struggling with poor self-esteem related to body image may struggle with slipping grades, a lack of desire to leave the house, or social withdrawal. Left untreated, poor body image may even cause suicidal ideation (Wild, Flisher, & Lombard, 2004).

Body-image issues may be addressed through the use of supportive therapy to help children and adolescents come to terms with poor self-image and judgment (e.g., teasing) by peers. Cognitive–behavioral interventions to question irrational beliefs related to these issues may also be helpful. Group therapy for children and adolescents with self-esteem issues may provide individuals with positive peer feedback.

Another issue that may be commonly addressed in counseling for patients with neurocutaneous syndromes is pain management, which may involve short-term therapy that integrates clinical techniques drawn from cognitive therapy, hypnotherapy, behavior therapy, and desensitization therapies. Patients may be taught relaxation techniques, for example, to relieve tension and anxiety related to pain.

Supportive therapy for comorbid conditions such as attention-deficit/hyperactivity disorder, involving education of the family, increasing support at school, and the use of cognitive–behavioral techniques to reduce irrational beliefs and increase self-esteem and reduce aggression and anxiety may also be helpful (Warren, 2002).

Finally, depression related to dealing with a chronic illness may be treated by focusing on the behaviors, emotions, and ideas that contribute to the patient's depression, understanding and identifying the life problems or events that contribute to depression, and helping patients understand which aspects of those problems they may be able to solve or improve to regain a sense of control and pleasure in life. The use of antidepressant medications may also be warranted.

The use of psychopharmacologic medication for the treatment of mental illness in patients with neurocutaneous syndromes has not been strongly addressed in the research. Sedky, Hughes, Yusufzie, and Lippmann (2003), for example, reported on the lack of treatment recommendations for patients with tuberous sclerosis and psychosis. In general, it is recommended that mental health issues be treated as they would minus the presence of neurological disorders, but with careful monitoring of symptoms.

CONCLUSION

This chapter provided an overview of three of the most common neurocutaneous syndromes: neurofibromatosis, Sturge–Weber, and tuberous sclerosis. Neurofibromatosis and tuberous sclerosis disorders are considered predominantly inherited through autosomal dominant transmission, although spontaneous mutations also occur. There is no known genetic cause for Sturge–Weber syndrome. The clinical expression, severity of symptoms, and progression of each syndrome vary greatly among individuals. Therefore, the prognosis depends greatly on the severity of symptoms displayed. The more common symptoms presented across all three syndromes include cognitive delays, seizures, learning disabilities, and problems with social interactions. Many people with mild symptoms can lead normal and productive lives, however.

Depending on severity, medical treatments and monitoring of symptoms may be a lifelong endeavor. In general, medical treatments often focus on the presenting symptoms. Surgery, anticonvulsant medication, and laser treatments are some of the more common medical treatments cited. Enhancing self-help and daily living skills of those with moderate to severe involvement should be part of a comprehensive treatment plan. Educational interventions may need to be more adaptive and compensatory rather than remedial. Parents are also encouraged to become familiar with the federal and educational law (e.g., Section 504, IDEA) to assist them in advocating for their children within the school setting. Lastly, behavioral management and counseling should be considered to address behavior, social, and emotional problems that are secondary to neurocutaneous syndromes.

REFERENCES

Aicardi, J. (1992). *Diseases of the nervous system in childhood*. London: MacKeith Press.

Americans With Disabilities Act of 1990, Pub. L. No. 101-336, USCA § 12101 *et seq*. (West 1993).

Arzimanoglou, A., & Aicardi, J. (1992). The epilepsy of Sturge–Weber syndrome: Clinical features and treatment in 23 patients. *Acta Neurologica Scandinavica, 140*(Suppl.), 18–22.

Asano, E., Chugani, D. C., Muzik, O., Behen, M., Janisse, J., Rothermel, R., et al. (2001). Autism in tuberous sclerosis complex is related to both cortical and subcortical dysfunction. *Neurology, 57,* 1269–1277.

Bebin, E. M., & Gomez, M. R. (1988). Prognosis in Sturge–Weber disease: Comparison of unihemispheric and bihemispheric involvement. *Journal of Child Neurology, 3,* 181–184.

Bodensteiner, J. B., & Roach, E. S. (Eds.). (1999). *Sturge–Weber syndrome.* Mt. Freedom, NJ: Sturge–Weber Foundation.

Brewer, V. R., Moore, B. D., & Hiscock, M. (1997). Learning disability subtypes in children with neurofibromatosis. *Journal of Learning Disabilities, 30,* 521–533.

Cody, H., & Hynd, G. W. (1998). Sturge–Weber syndrome. In L. Phelps (Ed.), *Health-related disorders in children and adolescents* (pp. 624–628). Washington, DC: American Psychological Association.

Curatolo, P., Cusmai, R., Cortesi, F., Chiron, C., Jambaque, I., & Dulac, O. (1991). Neuropsychiatric aspects of tuberous sclerosis. *Annals of the New York Academy of Sciences, 615,* 8–16.

Cutting, L. E., Koth, C. W., & Denckla, M. B. (2000). How children with neurofibromatosis Type 1 differ from "Typical" learning disabled clinic attenders: Nonverbal learning disabilities revisited. *Developmental Neuropsychology, 17,* 29–48.

Eliason, M. J. (1986). Neurofibromatosis: Implications for learning and behavior. *Journal of Developmental Pediatrics, 7,* 175–179.

Ferguson, A. P., McKinlay, I. A., & Hunt, A. (2002). Care of adolescents with severe learning disability from tuberous sclerosis. *Developmental Medicine and Child Neurology, 44,* 256–262.

Gillberg, I. C., Gillberg, C., & Ahlsen, G. (1994). Autistic behavior and attention deficits in tuberous sclerosis: A population-based study. *Developmental Medicine and Child Neurology, 36,* 50–56.

Gonzalez, R. C., Welsh, J. T., & Sepulveda, A. C. (1993, November 3). Autismo en la esclerosis tuberosa. *Leido,* 374–379.

Goodman, M., Lamm, S. H., Engel, A., Shepherd, C. W., Houser, O. W., & Gomez, M. R. (1997). Cortical tuber count: A biomarker indicating neurologic severity of tuberous sclerosis complex. *Journal of Child Neurology, 12,* 85–90.

Grostern, R. J. (2004, September 22). Neurofibromatosis-1. *Edmedicine.* Retrieved December 12, 2004, from http://www.edmedicine.com/oph/topic338.htm

Gutmann, D. H. (1999). Learning disabilities in neurofibromatosis 1: Sizing up the brain. *Archives of Neurology, 56,* 1322–1323.

Harrison, J. E., & Bolton, P. F. (1997). Annotation: Tuberous sclerosis. *Journal of Child Psychology and Psychiatry and Allied Disciplines, 38,* 603–614.

Harvey, K. V., Mahr, G., & Balon, R. (1995). Psychiatric manifestations of tuberous sclerosis. *Psychosomatics, 36,* 314–315.

Hofman, K. J., Harris, E. L., Bryan, N., & Denckla, M. B. (1994). Neurofibromatosis type 1: The cognitive phenotype. *Pediatrics, 124,* S1–S8.

Hunt, A., & Lindenbaum, R. H. (1984). Tuberous sclerosis: A new estimate of prevalence within the Oxford region. *Journal of Medical Genetics, 24*, 272–277.

Hunt, A., & Shepherd, C. (1993). A prevalence study of autism in tuberous sclerosis. *Journal of Autism and Developmental Disorders, 23*, 323–339.

Hyman, S. L., Gill, D. S., Shores, E. A., Steinberg, A., Joy, P., Gibikote, S. V., & North, K. N. (2003). Natural history of cognitive deficits and their relationship to MRI T2-hyperintensities in NF1. *Neurology, 60*, 1139–1145.

Hynd, G. W., & Willis, W. G. (1988). *Pediatric neuropsychology.* Orlando, FL: Grune & Stratton.

Individuals With Disabilities Education Act, 20 U.S.C. Ch. 33, Sec. 1400 (1997).

Jambaque, I., Cusmai, R., Curatolo, P., Cortesi, F., Perrot, C., & Dulac, O. (1991). Neuropsychological aspects of tuberous sclerosis in relation to epilepsy and MRI findings. *Developmental Medicine and Child Neurology, 33*, 698–705.

Joinson, C., O'Callaghan, F. J., Osborne, J. P., Martyn, C., Harris, T., & Bolton, P. F. (2003). Learning disability and epilepsy in an epidemiological sample of individuals with tuberous sclerosis complex. *Psychological Medicine, 33*, 335–344.

Knoster, T. P., & McCurdy, B. (2002). Best practices in functional behavioral assessment for designing individualized student programs. In A. Thomas & J. Grimes (Eds.), *Best practices in school psychology IV* (Vol. 2, pp. 1007–1028). Bethesda, MD: NASP.

Kramer, U., Kahana, E., Shorer, Z., & Ben-Zeev, B. (2000). Outcome of infants with unilateral Sturge–Weber syndrome and early onset seizures. *Developmental Medicine & Child Neurology, 42*, 756–759.

Lentz, F., & Shapiro, E. (1986). Functional assessment of the academic environment. *School Psychology Review, 15*, 346–357.

Lewis, T. J., & Sugai, G. (1996). Functional assessment of problem behavior: A pilot investigation of the comparative and interactive effects of teacher and peer social attention on students in general education settings. *School Psychology Quarterly, 11*, 1–19.

Mazzocco, M. M. (2001). Math learning disability and math LD subtypes: Evidence from studies of Turner syndrome, fragile X syndrome, and neurofibromatosis type 1. *Journal of Learning Disabilities, 34*, 520–533.

Miller, M., & Hall, J. G. (1978). Possible maternal effect on severity of neurofibromatosis. *Lancet, 2*, 1071–1073.

Moore, B. D., Ater, J. L., Needle, M. N., Slopis, J., & Copeland, D. R. (1994). Neuropsychological profile of children with neurofibromatosis, brain tumor, or both. *Journal of Child Neurology, 9*, 368–377.

Moore, B. D., Slopis, J. M., Schomer, D., Jackson, E. F., & Levy, B. M. (1996). Neuropsychological significance of areas of high signal intensity on brain MRIs of children with neurofibromatosis. *Neurology, 6*, 1660–1668.

National Institute of Neurological Disorders and Stroke. (2004, December 3). *NINDS Sturge–Weber syndrome information page.* Retrieved December 12, 2004, from http://www.ninds.nih.gov/disorders/sturge_weber/sturge_weber.htm

National Institute of Neurological Disorders and Stroke. (2005, June 10). *NINDS neurofibromatosis information page.* Retrieved June 15, 2005, from http://www.ninds.nih.gov/disorders/neurofibromatosis/neurofibromatosis.htm

Needle, M. N., Cnaan, A., Dattilo, J., Chatten, J., Phillips, P. C., Shochat, S., Sutton, L. N., et al. (1997). Prognostic signs in the surgical management of plexiform neurofibromas: The Children's Hospital of Philadelphia experience, 1974–94. *Journal of Pediatrics, 131*, 678–682.

Nilsson, D. E., & Bradford, L. W. (1999) Neurofibromatosis. In S. Goldstien & C. R. Reynolds (Eds.), *Handbook of neurodevelopmental and genetic disorders in children* (pp. 350–367). New York: Guilford Press.

North, K. N., Riccardi, V., Samango-Sprouse, C., Ferner, R., Moore, B., Legius, E., et al. (1997). Cognitive function and academic performance in neurofibromatosis Type 1: Consensus statement from the NF-1 cognitive disorders task force. *Neurology, 48*, 1121–1127.

O'Neill, R. E., Horner, R. H., Albin, R. W., Sprague, J. R., Storey, K., & Newton, J. S. (1997). *Functional assessment and program development for problem behavior: A practical handbook.* Pacific Grove, CA: Brooks/Cole.

Rehabilitation Act of 1973, 29 U.S.C. § 974(a) (1973).

Riccardi, V. M. (1981). Von Recklinghausen neurofibromatosis. *New England Journal of Medicine, 305*, 1617–1627.

Riccardi, V. M., & Eichner, J. E. (1986). *Neurofibromatosis: Phenotype, natural history, and pathogenesis.* Baltimore: Johns Hopkins University Press.

Roach, E. S. (1988). Diagnosis and management of neurocutaneous syndromes. *Seminars in Neurology, 8*, 83–96.

Roach, E. S. (2002). Neurocutaneous syndromes. In A. K. Asbury, G. M. Mckhann, W. I. McDonald, P. J. Goadsby, & J. C. McArthur (Eds.), *Diseases of the nervous system* (pp. 2061–2081). Cambridge, England: Cambridge University Press.

Roach, E. S., Riela, A. R., Chugani, H. T., Shinnar, S., Bodensteiner, J. B., & Freeman, J. (1994). Sturge–Weber syndrome: Recommendations for surgery. *Journal of Child Neurology, 9*, 190–192.

Rochkind, S., Hoffman, H. J., & Hendrick, E. B. (1990). Sturge–Weber syndrome: Natural history and prognosis. *Journal of Epilepsy, 3*(Suppl.), 293–304.

Sampson, J. R., Scahill, S. J., Stephenson, J. B. P., Mann, L., & Conner, J. M. (1989). Genetic aspects of tuberous sclerosis in the west of Scotland. *Journal of Medical Genetics, 26*, 28–31.

Sedky, K., Hughes, T., Yusufzie, K., & Lippmann, S. (2003). Tuberous sclerosis with psychosis. *Psychosomatics, 44*, 521–522.

Shepherd, C. W., Beard, M., Gomez, M. R., Kurland, L. T., & Whisnant, J. P. (1991). Tuberous sclerosis complex in Olmsted County, Minnesota, 1950–1989. *Archives of Neurology, 48*, 400–401.

Shepherd, C. W., & Stephenson, J. B. (1992). Seizures and intellectual disability associated with tuberous sclerosis complex in the West of Scotland. *Developmental Medicine and Child Neurology, 34*, 766–774.

Smalley, S. L. (1998). Autism and tuberous sclerosis. *Journal of Autism and Developmental Disorders, 28,* 407–414.

Smalley, S. L., Burger, F., & Smith, M. (1994). Phenotypic variation of tuberous sclerosis in a single extended kindred. *Journal of Medical Genetics, 31,* 761–765.

Smalley, S. L., Tanguay, P. E., Smith, M., & Gutierrez, G. (1992). Autism and tuberous sclerosis. *Journal of Autism and Developmental Disorders, 22,* 339–355.

Stine, S. B., & Adams, W. V. (1989). Learning problems in neurofibromatosis patients. *Clinical Orthopedics and Related Research, 245,* 43–48.

Sturge, W. A. (1879). A case of partial epilepsy, apparently due to a lesion of the vaso-motor centres of the brain. *Transactions of the Clinical Society of London, 12,* 162.

Sujansky, E., & Conradi, S. (1995). Sturge–Weber syndrome: Age of onset of seizures and glaucoma and the prognosis for affected children. *Journal of Child Neurology, 10,* 49–58.

Tunali, B., & Power, T. G. (1993). Creating satisfaction: A psychological perspective on stress and coping in families of handicapped children. *Journal of Child Psychology and Psychiatry, 34,* 943–957.

Varnhagen, C. K., Lewin, S., Das, J. P., Bowen, P., Ma, K., & Klimek, M. (1998). Neurofibromatosis and psychological processes. *Journal of Developmental and Behavioral Pediatrics, 9,* 257–265.

Warren, M. P. (2002). *Behavioral management guide: Essential treatment strategies for the psychotherapy of children, their parents, and families.* Northvale, NJ: Aronson.

Webb, D. W., Fryer, A. E., & Osborne, J. P. (1996). On the incidence of fits and mental retardation in tuberous sclerosis: A population study. *Developmental Medicine and Child Neurology, 38,* 146–155.

Weber, A. M., Egelhoff, J. C., McKellop, J. M., & Franz, D. N. (2000). Autism and the cerebellum: Evidence from tuberous sclerosis. *Journal of Autism and Developmental Disorders, 30,* 511–517.

Weber, P. F. (1922) Right-sided hemi-hypertrophy resulting from right-sided congenital spastic hemiplegia with a morbid condition of the left-side of the brain, revealed by radiograms. *Journal of Neurology and Psychopathology, 3,* 134.

Weber, P. F. (1929). A note of the association of extensive haemangiomatosus naevus of the skin with cerebral (meningeal) hemangioma. *Proceedings of the Royal Society of Medicine, 22,* 431.

Wiederholt, T. W., Gomez, M. R., & Rurland, L. T. (1985). Incidence and prevalence of tuberous sclerosis in Rochester, Minnesota, 1950 through 1982. *Neurology, 35,* 600–660.

Wild, L. G., Flisher, A. J., & Lombard, C. (2004). Suicidal ideation and attempts in adolescents: Associations with depression and six domains of self-esteem. *Journal of Adolescence, 27,* 611–625.

11

NEUROLOGICAL AND CENTRAL NERVOUS SYSTEM IMPAIRMENTS

FREDERIC J. MEDWAY

This chapter provides an overview of neurological and central nervous symptom impairments that affect children and adolescents. A description is provided of congenital conditions, head size and shape abnormalities, inflammatory and infectious conditions, vascular malformations, and trauma. Prevalence rates and medical, behavioral, and educational outcome are outlined. Medical and psychoeducational options are provided for these neurological impairments that include children's treatment, rehabilitation, and long-term community integration.

OVERVIEW AND OUTCOMES

Neurological impairments of a chronic nature pose a special challenge because monitoring and management involve cognitive, affective, and physical domains. These conditions and syndromes comprise disorders, diseases, and trauma affecting the central nervous system (CNS) and peripheral nervous system (PNS). The brain controls thinking, memory, emotion, motor performance, sensory processing, and basic bodily processes such as hunger, thirst, breathing, and temperature; therefore, any damage or impairment to the brain may simultaneously disrupt multiple areas (sensory, motor, intellectual, and emotional). The spinal cord consists of nerve fibers extending from the base of the brain to the lower back that carry messages from the brain to other parts of the body; therefore, any spinal cord damage or impairment directly affects sensory and motor functioning and indirectly influences cognitive and emotional processes. The PNS consists of cranial and spinal nerves exiting the CNS and terminating in peripheral structures (e.g., the eyes, ears, sensory organs, receptors); thus, PNS damage will primarily affect sensory and motor processes.

The extent and course of neurological damage vary widely from general diminishment of abilities to localized impairment (Silver, McAllister, & Yudofsky, 2004) with functional impact depending on preimpairment neurological development. Congenital defects and those in which the brain is shaken against the skull cause diffuse damage, whereas external trauma (head injuries) tends to be localized. For diffuse brain impairments, the longer symptoms go untreated, the more severe, irreversible, and possibly fatal the damage will be. Regardless of the cause of neurological dysfunction, the presenting symptoms and impairments tend to be similar. These include cognitive, memory, and thinking impairments; changes in activity level and impaired attention; problems with gross and fine motor movement, reflexes, and coordination; muscular rigidity, tics, seizures, and tremors; headaches; and sensory impairments such as loss of sight, sensitivity to light, hearing loss, speech problems, and paralysis or tingling in extremities. In addition, children and adolescents with chronic neurological illnesses often have poor social adjustment and exhibit increased levels of anxiety, irritability, lethargy, behavioral problems, and poor self-image (Nassau & Drotar, 1997; Thompson & Gustafson, 1996). As they age, these individuals are less independent than peers, have difficulty with employment, and often are reliant on government support. For many specific neurological disorders reviewed in this chapter, however, the exact symptoms and behavioral signs overlap and diagnosis is not always precise until a variety of tests are performed. Furthermore, research on cognitive, learning, and developmental outcomes of neurological impairments is fragmented and is "largely discipline specific, with studies of genetics, development, brain imaging, and cognitive outcomes conducted in parallel rather than integrated fashion" (Liptak, 2003, p. 20).

Depending on the particular condition, the various disorders described in this chapter are diagnosed through a variety of methods and at a variety of times (e.g., in utero, at birth, or at the start of schooling). The methods include (a) standard physical exams and blood analysis; (b) neurological examinations of mental status, head size and shape, motor function and balance, sensory processes, reflexes, and cranial nerve activity; (c) ratings of functioning such as the Glasgow Coma Scale; (d) genetic studies (as in Huntington's disease); and (e) various procedures that assess the brain's electrical activity (electroencephalograph [EEG]), produce images of brain structure, function, and processes (e.g., computerized tomography [CT] scan, magnetic resonance imaging [MRI], magnetic resonance angiography [MRA], arteriogram, positron emission tomography [PET] scan) and that provide information on spinal fluid pressure and spinal cord functioning and properties (myelogram). Chronic neurological impairments usually have two major origins: (a) congenital conditions (e.g., genetic diseases, birth defects and injuries) and (b) postnatal conditions caused by trauma (e.g., car accidents, falls); and disease (e.g., infections, tumors, malformations).

In this chapter, the impairments are grouped into five categories: congenital conditions, head size and shape abnormalities, inflammatory and infectious conditions, vascular malformations, and trauma. Within each category, specific neurological impairments are described; prevalence rates are presented; physiological, social, and educational outcomes are reviewed; and maintenance or treatment procedures are summarized. Finally, the chapter overviews neurological impairment treatment procedures, primarily of a psychological nature, that have the greatest empirical support to date.

CONGENITAL AND GENETIC CONDITIONS

Among the most common congenital and hereditary neurological impairments of children are neural tube defects (anencephaly and spina bifida), Chiari malformation, hydrocephalus, craniosystosis, and microcephaly. An important, although less common, genetic condition is Huntington's disorder.

Neural Tube Defects

The neural tube is a hollow cylindrical embryonic structure in early fetal development that eventually will close to form the brain and spinal cord. Neural tube defects involve failure of this structure to develop properly and close within 4 to 5 weeks after conception. Causes of neural tube defects include environmental toxins, infections, dietary and nutritional deficiencies (particularly folic acid deficiency), maternal alcohol and drug ingestion, and genetic inheritance, although the basis of the latter is not fully established. The two most common neural tube defects are anencephaly (open skull) and spina bifida (open spine). These defects occur in 1 out of every 1,000 pregnancies in the United States, although the incidence of neural tube defects has dropped markedly in the last 25 years because of public health efforts to monitor women's folic acid intake. Anencephaly results when the head end of the neural tube fails to develop, causing incomplete development of brain, skull, and scalp. Anencephalic infants are born without a forebrain or cerebrum (responsible for thinking, vision, hearing, touch, and movement); are usually blind, deaf, unconscious; and live only a few days.

Unlike anencephaly, spina bifida (literally cleft spine) is a chronic condition that involves a birth defect of the spinal column including the backbone, spinal cord, surrounding nerves, and spinal fluid in which the bottom end of the spinal cord fails to close. This results in leg and feet paralysis, bowel and bladder control limitations, and severe developmental disabilities including learning disabilities and other cognitive delays. Spina bifida prevalence rates vary with ethnicity, geography, and sex. More females than males have spina bifida; there are higher rates among Hispanics and Whites than among Asians and African Americans; and some countries (e.g., Ireland) have had unusually high rates. Spina bifida is thought to result from multiple genetic (from both parents) and environmental factors (i.e., multifactorial trait inheritance). Multifactorial traits often affect one sex more than another. The severity of spina bifida varies with the spinal lesion level and associated complications resulting in three major types of spina bifida of increasing severity: spina bifida occulta, meningocele, and myelomeningocele. Spina bifida occulta is a mild condition characterized by an opening in one or more bones of the spinal column without damage to the spinal cord and often without symptoms. In meningocele, the protective covering of the spinal cord (meninges) pushes out through a vertebral sac. The spinal cord remains intact, and this condition can be repaired through surgery with few chronic complications. Myelomeningocele, the most severe condition, is the type most often present when the term *spina bifida* is used. It is one of the most common birth defects of the CNS and affects as many as 1 in 800 infants. In myelomeningocele, the bones of the spine do not form completely, and the spinal canal is incomplete, allowing the spinal cord and its covering to protrude out of the child's back.

Myelomeningocele results in muscle weakness, partial or complete loss of sensation, or paralysis below the spinal area where the incomplete closure (or cleft) occurs. These children may have varying limitations in walking and mobility, as well as problems with incontinence. Myelomeningocele also results in the associated complications of Chiari malformation, hydrocephalus, and meningitis (reviewed later). Hydrocephalus (fluid buildup in the brain) occurs in 70% to 90% of children with myelomeningocele (those with higher level lesions) and can lead to seizures, blindness, and low intellectual functioning (Barf et al., 2003). The public health impact of spina bifida is substantial because, until recently, most spina bifida children died shortly after birth. Now many of these children grow up with the condition, attend school, and are, to varying degrees, dependent on parents and teachers for assistance with many basic life functions. In comparison with able-bodied peers, children with spina bifida are more socially immature, lonely, less physically active, more passive, and more likely to have problems with attention. Compared with peers, these children (especially girls) are more depressed and have lower self-worth, particularly in academic, athletic, and social domains (Appleton et al., 1997; Holmbeck et al., 2003). Buran, Sawin, Brei, and Fastenau (2004) found that adolescents with myelomeningocele, although hopeful and positive about the future, reported engaging in fewer peer activities and having poorer decision-making skills compared with other children. Spina bifida further affects cognitive development such that these children tend to have lower IQs, deficits in executive functioning and abstract reasoning, and problems with specific academic skills such as arithmetic. In the home, these children are often noncompliant, with less involvement in familial interactions. Likewise, their parents report high levels of stress because of the magnitude of caregiving required (Holmbeck et al., 1997). The treatment of spina bifida involves surgical closure of the spinal cord and procedures to control the hydrocephalus such as surgical installation of a shunt. Counseling and support groups help families to cope with the emotional reactions that accompany the disorder.

Chiari Malformation

This structural condition (also called Arnold Chiari malformation) occurs when the lower part of the cerebellum crowds the outlet of the brain stem–spinal cord and protrudes into the spinal canal (see Greenlee, Donovan, Hasan, & Menezes, 2002; Speer et al., 2003). This causes poor circulation of cerebrospinal fluid from the brain to the spinal cord. Chiari malformation occurs during early embryonic development of the CNS and may be of genetic origin (Speer et al., 2003); however, symptoms may not appear until the adolescent and early adult years. Arnold Chiari Type I is the most common and often associated with syringeomyelia in which a tubular cavity develops in the spinal canal. Arnold Chiari Type II is found almost exclusively with children with myelomeningocele and hydrocephalus. Chiari malformation can result in hydrocephalus or can be made worse because of it. The disorder has a prevalence rate in the United States of 1 in 1,000 births, and about a third of the cases die prior to starting school. Diagnosis is typically done using MRI. Initial symptoms of Chiari malformation are head and neck pain followed by stiffness, unusual sensations in the arms and legs, occasional difficulty with swallowing or gagging, and vision problems. Other common symptoms include headache in the back of the head, clumsiness and coordination problems, double vision, difficulty with breathing, and irritability. For those who reach school age, the major symptoms involve visual focusing difficulties, extremity weakness, and pneumonia and respiratory problems. In severe cases, and when untreated surgically, crowding of the brain stem damages the spinal cord and leads to paralysis and mental impairment. Chiari malformation is extremely disruptive to learning processes because it involves chronic sensory deficits (e.g., listening, speaking, hearing, etc.), balance and coordination ability, and can produce dizziness, pain, and bowel and bladder difficulties.

Hydrocephalus

Hydrocephalus is an abnormal accumulation of cerebrospinal fluid (CSF) within the four ventricles of the brain that causes the ventricles to dilate and pressure inside the skull to increase. Hydrocephalus occurs in 2 out of 1,000 births and may result from either environmental or genetic–congenital factors such as stenosis (obstruction of the cerebral aqueduct between the third and fourth ventricle), enlargement of the fourth ventricle (Dandy–Walker syndrome), head trauma, ventricle hemorrhage, tumors, cysts, and trauma or head injury (referred to as hydrocephalus ex vacuo). Hydrocephalus often co-occurs with spina bifida and with infectious disorders such as meningitis and encephalitis (Cinalli, Maixner, & Sainte-Rose, 2004).

The symptoms of hydrocephalus vary with the child's ability to tolerate fluid buildup, age, and disease progression. Beyond increased head circumference, other symptoms include headache, nausea, damage to the optic nerve, failure to feed, motor and coordination problems, verbal memory retrieval impairment, dyscalculia, attention difficulties, irritability, social and behavior problems, poor adaptive behavior, personality changes, and perceptions of self as less physically competent. Left untreated hydrocephalus can be fatal. Treatment consists of surgically relieving the brain pressure by establishment of a tube or shunt that drains CSF to another part of the body (often the abdominal cavity or chamber in the heart) or making a hole in a ventricle to establish normal flow (ventriculostomy).

Craniosynostosis and Microcephaly

Craniosynostosis and microcephaly are two abnormalities involving deviations in the shape and size of the head that lead to chronic life problems. Craniosynostosis (see Cohen & Maclean, 2000) is a primarily genetic condition occurring in 1 out of 1,800 live births in which the joints (or sutures) found between the bony plates in the skull close prematurely, thus increasing the pressure inside the head and changing its shape from symmetrical to asymmetrical. There are several types of craniosynostosis (and more than 150 craniosynostosis syndromes) depending on which sutures fail to develop normally. The most common, occurring in 1 in 300 live births, is plagiocephaly, involving premature closing of the coronal suture (left or right side) that runs from ear to ear. This causes a flattening of the brow and forehead on the affected side, noticeable scalp veins, increased head circumference, and bulging eyes that prevent the child from looking upward.

Craniosynostosis causes seizures and can result in sleepiness and lethargy, irritability, and feeding problems. The initial diagnosis is made by routine physical examination (e.g., clinically viewing and measuring the infant's head) and subsequently confirmed by CT scan. Corrective surgery is necessary and is performed prior to the child's first birthday (best between 3 and 9 months of age) when scalp bones are still soft. Depending on the severity of the condition, craniosynostosis is considered a chronic illness that can result in developmental, visuoperceptual, and cognitive problems requiring future management.

Microcephaly is associated with numerous conditions that cause an abnormally small head size (<5th percentile for children) circumference on the basis of age and gender. Microcephaly can result from several factors including chromosomal and genetic causes, as well as environmental causes such as exposure to viral infections, meningitis, encephalitis, and toxins (fetal alcohol syndrome and phenylketonuria). It is usually identified through routine cerebral ultrasound or MRI, typically occurs in 1 in 6,200 to 8,500 births, and has no specific treatment. Abnormal head size can result in severe developmental delays in the cognitive, motor, and speech areas, hyperactivity, poor feeding, seizures, and frequently is associated with mental retardation, particularly when there are other complications such as lung disease and extended use of ventilation (Chiriboga et al., 2003).

Huntington's Disease

Huntington's disease is a genetic-based progressive disorder involving degeneration of the nerve cells (basal ganglia and caudate nucleus) in the brain. As a result, this disease causes a marked loss of gamma aminobutyric acid (GABA; a neurotransmitter associated with anxiety disorders), decreases in neuropeptides such as substance p (associated with depression), and decreases in endorphins such as enkephalin (associated with pain and mood regulation). Huntington's disease affects approximately 1 in 100,000 and is characterized by abnormalities of movement, coordination, emotions, and dementia. A child has a 50% chance of inheriting the disease if it is present in the biological parent. Huntington's disease and its severity are linked to multiple genetic copies of a single gene on chromosome 4, and the number of genetic copies or repeats is linked to the speed of disorder progression.

Huntington's disease involves a progressive loss of mental functioning, including personality changes such as apathy, irritability, and depression with suicide risk, as well as motor and speech impairments. Specific problems include slowed thinking and poor judgment, speech impairment, memory loss, executive function damage (organization, resolution, and awareness), sudden, unpredictable, and jerky movements, visuospatial problems, and reading disorders (e.g., letter fluency and object recall; Snowden, Craufurd, Griffiths, Thompson, & Neary, 2001). Cognitive deficits begin with memory disorders and eventuate in more widespread intellectual deterioration. Eventually the capacity for self-care may be lost, and the individual may be prone to injure themselves and others. Huntington's disease cannot be cured and is often fatal within 15 to 20 years. The treatment options focus on symptom control and maximizing individual functioning. Medications used to treat symptoms include dopamine blockers (haloperidol, phenothiazine) to reduce abnormal and unpredictable movements and reserpine to reduce agitation. Tetrabenazine, another dopamine-depleting drug used for tardive dyskinesia and Tourette syndrome, also is useful in treating hyperkinetic movements of Huntington's disease. Some evidence indicates that coenzyme Q10, a vitaminlike antioxidant involved in cell energy production, slows disease progression.

INFLAMMATIONS AND INFECTIONS

Infections reach the brain via the bloodstream or are spread along the peripheral nerves. Common childhood neurological infections are encephalitis, flaccid paralysis (limb weakness often caused by Guillain–Barré syndrome), meningitis, Reye syndrome brain abscesses, and HIV/AIDS.

Encephalitis

Encephalitis is an inflammation (irritation and swelling) of the brain related to infections, toxins, autoimmune processes, and other conditions that destroy brain nerve cells, cause bleeding within the brain, and have the potential for permanent brain damage. Encephalitis can be caused by a wide variety of viruses (e.g., insect transmitted, poliovirus, herpes simplex infection, varicella [chickenpox or shingles], measles, mumps, rubella, adenovirus, rabies, and West Nile) and, in rare cases, by vaccinations. These viral agents either attack the brain directly or cause damage to the body's immune system. Encephalitis affects primarily infants and the elderly at a rate of approximately 1,500 cases a year.

Encephalitis symptoms are varied and many resemble the symptoms of meningitis (discussed later). The early and initial symptoms include headache, fever and other flulike symptoms, neck stiffness, abnormal reflexes, and skin problems (rash and mouth ulcers). Diagnosis relies on several tests including examination of cerebrospinal fluid, blood and serology tests, and occasionally EEG, CT scan, and MRI examinations. The medical complications of encephalitis vary from mild problems with full recovery to severe, permanent impairment (multiple handicaps) or death depending on the child's age (with poorer prognosis for younger children), extent of brain damage and specific brain area damage, and the degree of cognitive and motor skill development prior to infection. Complications particularly relevant to the educational setting include fatigue, vision and hearing problems, sleeplessness or sleeping at odd times, seizures, loss of attention and concentration, distractibility, memory and information processing deficits (such as remembering directions or remembering visual stimuli better than auditory stimuli), speech and language disorders (such as expressive language deficits), impaired decision making, friendship difficulties, frustration, depression, and obsessive–

compulsive behavior (Caruso et al., 2000). Research indicates that anterograde memory (learning new information and facts) is most severely affected by encephalitis (Utley, Ogden, Bigg, McGrath, & Anderson, 1997). No specific medications are available to cure viral infections, but complications can be prevented. Supportive care, including the use of sedatives for patient comfort, can be provided until the disease runs its course. The antiviral drug acyclovir (Zovirax) is useful in treating the pain and itching of herpes simplex encephalitis and varicella zoster virus encephalitis. Steroids and diuretics are used to reduce brain swelling, intravenous fluids are given to reduce dehydration, and anticonvulsant medications are prescribed to prevent seizures.

Acute Flaccid Paralysis and Guillain–Barré Syndrome

Acute flaccid paralysis (AFP; Thacker & Shendurnikar, 2004) is associated with poliomyelitis in undeveloped countries (e.g., Nigeria, India, Pakistan) and, in countries generally free of polio, with Guillain–Barré syndrome (Roos, 2005). The global AFP rate is approximately 1.9 per 100,000 children under age 15. Guillain–Barré syndrome involves the immune system (cellular and humoral mechanisms) attacking the myelin sheath of peripheral nerve cells such that signals to and from the brain and extremities are disrupted. Guillain–Barré syndrome typically occurs in approximately 1.5 per 100,000 children under age 15 after a viral or bacterial infection (gastrointestinal and respiratory), surgery, or vaccination. The initial symptoms include weakness or tingling sensations in the extremities and, in severe cases, paralysis. Other symptoms include loss of reflexes, muscle pain, and difficulty walking and breathing. Diagnosis is by physical (blood and urine tests) and neurological examination, often aided by a test of nerve conduction velocity and a spinal tap to assess the amount of protein in the cerebrospinal fluid. There is no known cure, but several medical procedures serve to reduce the symptom severity including blood plasma exchange, immunoglobulin procedures, and the use of a ventilator to aid in breathing. Most individuals with Guillain–Barré syndrome eventually show complete recovery, but approximately 15% of cases have chronic problems that include muscle aches, pain and weakness, fatigue, and psychological problems of withdrawal, depression, and embarrassment. The mortality rate of Guillain–Barré syndrome for children age 15 and below is less than 1%.

Meningitis and Other Infections

Meningitis is a viral or bacterial infection of the membranes (menges) covering the spinal cord and the brain and of the cerebrospinal fluid. Acquired viral meningitis occurs in 3.5 per 100,000 people and is a less severe condition that may resolve without treatment, whereas bacterial meningitis can be very severe and may result in brain damage and mental retardation, seizures (epilepsy), hearing and vision loss, hydrocephalus, or learning disability. Language and executive skills are particularly impaired when the disease is contracted before 12 months of age (Anderson, Anderson, Grimwood, & Nolan, 2004). Severe meningitis must be treated immediately with a combination of antibiotics.

Brain Abscesses and Reye Syndrome

Other infectious neurological conditions that are often mistaken initially for either encephalitis or meningitis are brain abscesses and Reye syndrome. Brain abscesses are infections caused by bacteria or fungi that attack brain cells, including those associated with HIV infections. These infections result in inflammation and blockage of blood vessels. Brain abscesses cause headache, muscle weaknesses, vision difficulties, seizures, impaired balance and coordination, decreased mental capacity, irritability, inattention, and drowsiness. Treatment involves the use of antibiotics to address infections and surgery (shunts) to relieve cranial fluid pressure (Kanev & Sheehan, 2003). Reye syndrome, another viral infection, also results in a swelling of brain tissue. This condition generally affects children between the ages of 6 and 15 and has been strongly linked to aspirin use (Young, Torretti, Williams, Hendriksen, & Woods, 1984). The symptoms include vomiting, listlessness, irritability, loss of consciousness, and confusion. If left untreated, Reye syndrome causes brain damage and death. Treatment includes the use of various drugs to reduce brain swelling and use of a mechanical ventilator to aid breathing.

HIV/AIDS

Most of the 700,000 children under age 15 with HIV/AIDS acquire this infectious disorder through the mother in a variety of ways both in the womb and after birth. HIV/AIDS causes neurological and cognitive deficits such as memory and attention problems, language disorders, decreased head circumference (MacMillan et al., 2001), spatial ability problems, and occasionally mental retardation, anxiety, depression, and conduct problems (Loveland et al., 2000). There are no curative treatments; however, various medications are prescribed for the physical symptoms of pain, infections, and gastrointestinal and respiratory problems, as well as to slow down viral replication (e.g., nucleoside analog reverse transcriptase inhibitors, nonnucleoside reverse transcriptase inhibitors, and protease inhibitors). Various psychotherapeutic approaches are used to improve quality of life, provide emotional support, reduce stress, reduce absenteeism, and develop language, phonological, and literacy skills.

VASCULAR MALFORMATIONS OF THE BRAIN

These conditions affect the arteries, veins, capillaries, and blood-filled spaces in the brain, and the symptoms vary with the type and severity of the disorder. The most common disorders affecting children are aneurisms, moya moya, and arteriovenous malformations (AVM). Brain aneurisms are arterial lesions usually at a point where a large artery branches off into several smaller ones, causing intracranial hemorrhage in subarachnoid crevices of the brain. The primary symptoms are similar to those of meningitis, hydrocephalus, and brain cysts—headache, weakness, stiff neck, vomiting, light sensitivity, and seizures.

Cerebral artery dissection and moya moya disease are two of the leading causes of strokes in children. Cerebral artery dissection (see deVeber, 2002; Fullerton, Johnston, & Smith, 2001) involves a tear in the lining of the major arteries (carotid and vertebral arteries) that reduces or blocks the flow of blood to the brain. This can occur for unknown reasons or can result from head trauma. Cerebral artery dissection that occurs spontaneously most commonly affects arteries within the brain, whereas dissection caused by trauma typically affects an artery in the neck. The latter may result from neck turning, various sports activities (e.g., swinging a golf club, inline skating), and roller coaster rides, to name a few causes. Boys tend to experience spontaneous arterial dissection more often than girls. Minor neck trauma may be asymptomatic, or symptoms may be delayed. Often the only initial symptom is headache and neck pain. Vertebral artery dissection accounts for 20% of the strokes in children and adolescents. These strokes may result in temporary or permanent neurological effects on motor movements, speech, behavior, and learning, and in some cases are fatal. Moya moya disease also involves a blocking of the blood vessels to the brain as they enter the skull. Moya moya can result in seizures, strokes, mental retardation, and permanent brain damage. It is treated using surgical procedures and medications that relieve headache symptoms (calcium channel blockers) and prevent blood clots.

AVMs are the primary cause of brain hemorrhage and strokes in children age 9 and older. An AVM is a type of vascular malformation in which there is abnormal growth and tangling of brain arteries and veins during embryogenesis that may occur in any part of the CNS. AVMs reduce the amount of oxygen brain tissues receive and tend to be associated with epilepsy. Although their origins are not well understood, AVMs are thought to result from genetic factors. They occur equally in males and females. AVM symptoms include seizures; headaches, nausea, and vomiting; paralysis of extremities; memory problems; and vision and speech problems. AVMs are treated through microsurgery, proton-beam irradiation, and embolization and can be controlled using antiseizure medications (e.g., phenytoin [Dilantin]).

TRAUMA AND HEAD INJURIES

It is estimated that 70,000 to 90,000 individuals have chronic physical, intellectual, and psychological impairment because of traumatic injuries, about half of them children, in which their head strikes an object resulting in an open head wound (a fast moving object penetrating the skull) or closed head wound (damage caused by the brain moving against the skull). These injuries vary in severity, visibility, and the degree to which they result in dependence on caregivers. Even mild injuries can result in neurological impairment lasting a year or more. Those head injuries that affect children's education and learning are subsumed under the "traumatic brain injury" category of IDEA, thus guaranteeing these children access to multidisciplinary school-based services, an individualized education plan, and appropriately trained teachers. Although the prevalence of traumatic neurologic injury peaks in adolescence because of the large numbers of cases caused by vehicle, boating, and sport injuries, many children suffer brain and spinal cord injuries as a result of bicycle accidents, falls, violent crime, and child abuse. Traumatic brain injuries can result in many cognitive, physical, and psychological problems depending on the degree of impairment and damage. Damage can occur at the focal point of injury and can result from the brain being damaged as it moves back and forth against the skull. In mild cases, there is skull and scalp injury; in more serious cases, there may be brain concussion, loss of memory, and loss of consciousness. The frontal and temporal brain lobes, centers of speech and language, are often damaged by brain shifting, resulting in aphasias and expressive language problems. Other problems include hearing impairments; seizures; communication and voice difficulties; problems in swallowing; walking, balance, motor skills, strength, and coordination problems; paralysis on one or more sides of the body; changes in information processing and memory; impaired concentration, attention span, planning, and judgment; changes in social and personality functioning including lethargy, lack of motivation, and poor emotional control; inappropriate emotions; sexual dysfunction; and difficulty relating to others (Bruce & Selznick, 2002). The child with a brain injury also may have difficulty dressing, bathing, and performing other age-appropriate self-help skills. These outcomes are influenced by the severity of the brain injury, preinjury functioning, and socioeconomic status (Schwartz et al., 2003). Spinal cord injuries may result from trauma or disease (e.g., spina bifida) and often cause loss of feeling and movement below the point of injury. More than 85% of individuals with spinal cord injuries have chronic conditions, and many children with these injuries also are prone to respiratory problems and heart disease.

MEDICAL AND PSYCHOEDUCATIONAL IMPLICATIONS

Neurological impairments in children usually involve so many perceptual and sensory systems that a team approach involving physicians, nurses, psychologists, and various rehabilitation professionals (physical and occupational therapists, speech therapists) are often involved in treatment, rehabilitation, and long-term adaptation (Barnes, 2003). Interventions aim first to stabilize the condition and symptoms (e.g., stop infections, reduce brain swelling and damage to brain cells, ensure an adequate amount of oxygen), then move to rehabilitation and family, school, and community reintegration (e.g., controlling seizures, infections, and muscle contractions; controlling agitation, restlessness, and impulsivity), and finally provide for long-term treatment of the chronic impairment (e.g., reducing the risk of infections). At all stages, it is essential that caregivers and family members are involved and comfortable with the treatment plan. As indicated earlier, a number of neurological impairments require surgical options (e.g., shunts) for stabilization. In addition, some individuals may receive tendon transfers to improve arm and leg functioning, nerve stimulators to improve muscle firing, and devices that allow paralyzed limbs to be activated for aerobic exercise. A primary goal of intervention is to address mobility limitations, improve coordination, address sensory deficits, and reduce reliance on others. To meet these goals, teams of relevant specialists, including physical and occupational therapists, and social workers, often work together using a case management approach. For example, hydrotherapy, physical therapy, and exercise regimens may be used to both relieve pain and improve movement in affected limbs.

Most pharmacological treatment is used for symptom reduction and management, primarily the physical symptoms of headache and pain, and seizures. Headache symptoms are responsive to a variety of medication including analgesics (acetaminophen, antiinflammatory drugs [e.g., ibuprofen], and triptans [selective serotonin antagonists); they may also respond to antidepressants and antianxiety medications. Seizures are treated by a variety of anticonvulsive agents known as either first-generation agents (e.g., phenytoin [Dilantin], carbamazepine [Tegretol, Carbatrol], and valproate [Depakote]) or second-generation agents (e.g., topiramate [Topamax], oxcarbazepine, [Trileptal], and primidone [Mysoline]). Abnormal muscle tone and spasticity are treated using various oral medications. Those most commonly prescribed are baclofen [Lioresal] and diazepam [Valium], which act on the CNS, and dantrolene [Dantrium], which acts on the muscles themselves to prevent tightening. Problems with muscle sensations can be treated using anticonvulsants and antidepressants. The management of chronic attention problems is effectively treated with stimulant medications, often used in combination with behavioral therapy (Brown & Sammons, 2002). Memory loss is treated with medications that have had limited success in patients with Alzheimer's disease. Several of the new memory drugs are still in experimental stages, however, or not yet approved for use in the United States (e.g., nootropics designed to treat memory loss; memantine [Akatinol] designed to promote nerve cell growth; and galantamine [Reminyl] designed to raise brain levels of acetylcholine). Neuromuscular deficits and paralysis often require the use of various devices to aid functioning. These may include breathing ventilators, phrenic nerve pacemakers (breathing pacemakers), functional electrical stimulation systems, and ambulatory devices (e.g., wheelchairs, braces, treadmills) to aid or retrain walking and locomotion.

Psychological treatment and intervention options for children's chronic neurological impairment can take three forms: (a) reduction of the child's suffering and other residual problems and concerns (e.g., interpersonal issues) through direct counseling and treatment, (b) improvement of the child's familial and social support system, and (c) addressing the child's educational and occupational needs. In regard to symptom alleviation and control, a broad range of physical and behavioral outcomes associated with neurological damage will respond to psychological treatments. Treatments for neurological impairment symptoms with the most empirical support are cognitive and cognitive–behavioral programs for chronic pain, cognitive and relaxation therapies for anxiety, and cognitive therapy for depression (Hays et al., 2002). Strong evidence exists for the efficacy of biofeedback, relaxation training, and cognitive therapy in treating headache (Blanchard & Diamond, 1996; Holden, Deichmann, & Levy, 1999). Side effects are few, results are relatively long lasting, and children and adolescents in the age range of 8 to 16 respond well to these treatments. Treatment with cognitive–behavioral therapy is highly effective for youth as demonstrated in numerous studies and research reviews (Velting, Setzer, & Albano, 2004). The major components of these programs, such as Kendall's (2000) Coping Cat program, include providing information about the nature of the anxiety, managing arousal symptoms, teaching realistic and coping-focused thinking, developing active problem solving, and increasing self-reliance to manage anxiety. More recently, multicomponent pain management programs have been developed that combine cognitive–behavioral strategies, parent training, and medical procedures (Schiff, Holtz, Peterson, & Rakusan, 2001). Finally, other nonbehavioral therapies focus on allowing the child to accept his or her limitations and deal with life issues in a constructive problem-solving manner. These approaches focus on self-care, socialization, optimizing self-determination and independence, addressing sexual concerns, and maximizing mental health.

Familial issues are important in chronic neurological conditions (Barakat & Kazak, 1999) and psychologists should address these through family counseling and consultation. For example, caregivers of these children have high rates of psychological distress (Bachanas et al., 2001; Weiner, Vasquez, & Battles, 2001) and personal strain (Hunfeld, Tempels, Passchier, Hazebroek, & Tibboel, 1999). This is particularly true of single-parent and low-income families (Liptak, 2003). Compared with families without chronically ill children, families in which children have neurological impairments are less cohesive, and children are viewed as vulnerable, increasing child anxiety (Anthony, Gil, & Schanberg, 2003; Holmbeck et al., 2002). Therefore, interventions are necessary that focus on parental coping and parenting behaviors, increasing parental support, and recognizing family competencies compared with deficits (Lemanek, Jones, & Lieberman, 2000). Few interventions of this type have been evaluated for empirical support, however.

A final concern for psychological intervention is how to increase the skills and confidence of community caregivers, particularly educational personnel, in working with children with chronic neurological conditions. To date, there have been no well-controlled studies of school-based interventions for children with the major conditions such as spina bifida (Liptak, 2003). In schools, these children may be served under varying federal education programs such as IDEA or Section 504 of the Rehabilitation Act. Another complicating factor is that, with the exception of seizure monitoring, educators have not been trained to work with children with chronic neurological impairments, and close contact with medical specialists is often necessary (Mukherjee, Lightfoot, & Sloper, 2000). This can involve connecting educational personnel with key resources (e.g., Nielsen, 2002), providing teacher training within school districts (Duggan, Medway, & Bunke, in press), or creating statewide multidisciplinary teams for educator training and consultation and family support (Glang, Singer, & Todis, 1997).

CONCLUSION

This chapter reviewed a variety of conditions that result in damage to the central and peripheral nervous systems of children and adolescents. Because these systems are so critical to adequate sensory, emotional, motor, and cognitive functions, their impairment results in problems in several areas of functioning. The resulting functional damage is often severe and occasionally life threatening, particularly if the damage goes undetected and treated. For many of these conditions, however, there are surgical, pharmacological, mechanical and electrical, psychological, and educational interventions that improve quality of life. The most effective interventions are those that involve multiple treatment components and include case management approaches coordinating the contributions of professionals in various medical, educational, and mental health fields; community-based agencies, including schools; and the active participation of children's caregivers.

REFERENCES

Anderson, V., Anderson, P., Grimwood, K., & Nolan, T. (2004). Cognitive and executive function 12 years after childhood bacterial meningitis: Effect of acute neurologic complications and age of onset. *Journal of Pediatric Psychology, 29,* 67–81.

Anthony, K. K., Gil, K. M., & Schanberg, L. E. (2003). Parental perceptions of child vulnerability in children with chronic illness. *Journal of Pediatric Psychology, 28,* 185–190.

Appleton, P. L., Ellis, N. C., Minchom, P. E., Lawson, V., Boll, V., & Jones, P. (1997). Depressive symptoms and self-concept in young people with spina bifida. *Journal of Pediatric Psychology, 22,* 707–722.

Bachanas, P. J., Kullgren, K. A., Schwartz, K. S., McDaniel, J. S., Smith, J., & Nesheim, S. (2001). Psychological adjustment in caregivers of school-age children infected with HIV: Stress, coping, and family factors. *Journal of Pediatric Psychology, 26,* 331–342.

Barakat, L. P., & Kazak, L. E. (1999). Family issues. In R. T. Brown (Ed.), *Cognitive aspects of chronic illness in children* (pp. 333–354). New York: Guilford Press.

Barf, H. A., Verhoef, M., Jennekens-Schinkel, A., Post, M. W. M., Gooskens, R. H. J. M., & Prevo, A. J. H. (2003). Cognitive status of young adults with spina bifida. *Developmental Medicine and Child Neurology, 45,* 813–820.

Barnes, M. P. (2003). Principles of neurological rehabilitation. *Journal of Neurology, Neurosurgery, and Psychiatry, 74,* 3–7.

Blanchard, E. B., & Diamond, S. (1996). Psychological treatment of benign headache disorders. *Professional Psychology: Research and Practice, 6,* 541–547.

Brown, R. T., & Sammons, M. T. (2002). Pediatric psychopharmacology: A review of new developments and recent research. *Professional Psychology: Research and Practice, 33,* 135–147.

Bruce, S., & Selznick, L. (2002). The role of functional behavior assessment in children's brain injury rehabilitation. *Brain Injury Source, 6,* 32–37.

Buran, C. F., Sawin, K. J., Brei, T. J., & Fastenau, P. S. (2004). Adolescents with myelomeningocele: Activities, beliefs, expectations, and perceptions. *Developmental Medicine and Child Neurology, 46,* 244–252.

Caruso, J. M., Tung, G. O., Gascon, G. G., Rogg, J., Davis, L., & Brown, W. D. (2000). Persistent preceding focal neurologic deficits in children with chronic Epstein–Barr virus encephalitis. *Journal of Child Neurology, 15,* 791–796.

Chiriboga, C. A., Kuban, K. C. K., Durkin, M., Hinton, V., Kuhn, L., Sanocka, U., & Bellinger, D. (2003). Factors associated with microcephaly at school age in a very-low-birthweight population. *Developmental Medicine and Child Neurology, 45,* 796–801.

Cinalli, G., Maixner, W. J., & Sainte-Rose, C. (Eds.). (2004). *Pediatric hydrocephalus.* London: Springer-Verlag.

Cohen, M. M., Jr., & Maclean, R. E. (Eds.). (2000). *Craniosynostosis: Diagnosis, evaluation, and management.* Oxford, England: Oxford University Press.

deVeber, G. (2002). Stroke and the child's brain: An overview of epidemiology, syndromes, and risk factors. *Current Opinion in Neurology, 15,* 133–138.

Duggan, D. D., Medway, F. J., & Bunke, V. L. (in press). Assisting educators to provide services to chronically ill students. *Canadian Journal of School Psychology.*

Fullerton, H. J., Johnston, S. C., & Smith, W. S. (2001). Arterial dissection and stroke in children. *Neurology, 57,* 1155–1160.

Glang, A., Singer, G. H. S., & Todis, B. (Eds.). (1997). *Children with acquired brain injury: The school's response.* Baltimore: Paul H. Brookes.

Greenlee, J. D. W., Donovan, K. A., Hasan, D. S., & Menezes, A. H. (2002). Chiari I malformation in the very young child: The spectrum of presentations and experiences in 31 children under age 6 years. *Pediatrics, 110,* 1212–1219.

Hays, K. A., Rardin, D. K., Jarvis, P. A., Taylor, N. M., Moorman, A. S., & Armstead, C. D. (2002). An exploratory survey on empirically supported treatments: Implications for internship training. *Professional Psychology: Research and Practice, 33,* 207–211.

Holden, E. W., Deichmann, M. M., & Levy, J. D. (1999). Empirically supported treatments in pediatric psychology: Recurrent pediatric headache. *Journal of Pediatric Psychology, 24,* 91–109.

Holmbeck, G. N., Coakley, R. M., Himmeyer, J. S., Shapera, W. E., & Westhoven, V. C. (2002). Observed and perceived dyadic and systemic functioning in families of preadolescents with spina bifida. *Journal of Pediatric Psychology, 27,* 177–189.

Holmbeck, G. N., Gorey-Ferguson, L., Seefeldt, T., Shapera, W., Turner, T., & Uhler, J. (1997). Maternal, paternal, and marital functioning in families of pre-adolescents with spina bifida. *Journal of Pediatric Psychology, 22,* 167–181.

Holmbeck, G. N., Westhoven, V., Phillips, W. S., Bowers, R., Gruse, C., Nikolopoulos, T., et al. (2003). A multimethod, multi-informant, and multidimensional perspective on psychosocial adjustment in preadolescents with spina bifida. *Journal of Consulting and Clinical Psychology, 71,* 782–796.

Hunfeld, J. A., Tempels, A., Passchier, J., Hazebroek, F. W., & Tibboel, D. (1999). Parental burden and grief one year after the birth of a child with a congenital anomaly. *Journal of Pediatric Psychology, 22,* 167–181.

Kanev, P. M., & Sheehan, J. M. (2003). Reflections on shunt infection. *Pediatric Neurosurgery, 39,* 285–290.

Kendall, P. C. (2000). *Cognitive–behavioral treatment of anxious children: Therapist manual.* Ardmore, PA: Workbook.

Lemanek, K. L., Jones, M. L., & Lieberman, B. (2000). Mothers of children with spina bifida: Adaptational and stress processing. *Children's Health Care, 29,* 19–35.

Liptak, G. S. (Ed.). (2003). *Evidence-based practice in spina bifida.* Retrieved August 24, 2004, from http://sbaa.convio.net/site/DocServer/Evidence-based_practice_in_SB1.pdf?docID=121

Loveland, K. A., Stehbens, J. A., Mahoney, E. M., Sirois, P. A., Nichols, S., Bordeaux, J. D., et al. (2000). Declining immune function in children and adolescents with hemophilia and HIV infection: Effects on neuropsychological performance. *Journal of Pediatric Psychology, 25,* 309–322.

MacMillan, C., Magder, L. S., Brouwers, P., Chase, C., Hittelman, J., Lasky, T., et al. (2001). Head growth and neurodevelopment of infants born to HIV-1-infected drug-using women. *Neurology, 57,* 1402–1411.

Mukherjee, S., Lightfoot, J., & Sloper, P. (2000). The inclusion of pupils with a chronic health condition in mainstream school: What does it mean for teachers? *Educational Research, 42*, 59–72.

Nassau, J. H., & Drotar, D. (1997). Social competence among children with central nervous system-related chronic health conditions: A review. *Journal of Pediatric Psychology, 22*, 771–793.

Nielsen, L. B. (2002). *Brief reference of student disabilities with strategies for the classroom.* Thousand Oaks, CA: Corwin Press.

Roos, K. L. (2005). *Principles of neurologic infectious diseases.* New York: McGraw-Hill.

Schiff, W. B., Holtz, K. D., Peterson, N., & Rakusan, T. (2001). Effect of an intervention to reduce procedural pain and distress for children with HIV infection. *Journal of Pediatric Psychology, 28*, 251–263.

Schwartz, L., Taylor, G., Drotar, D., Yeates, K. O., Wade, S., & Stancin, T. (2003). Long-term behavior problems following pediatric traumatic brain injury: Prevalence, predictors, and correlates. *Journal of Pediatric Psychology, 28*, 251–263.

Silver, J. M., McAllister, T. W., & Yudofsky, S. C. (Eds.). (2004). *Textbook of traumatic brain injury.* Arlington, VA: American Psychiatric Association.

Snowden, J. S., Craufurd, D., Griffiths, H., Thompson, J., & Neary, D. (2001). Longitudinal evaluation of cognitive disorder in Huntington's disease. *Journal of the International Neurological Society, 7*, 33–44.

Speer, M. C., Enterline, D. S., Mehltretter, L., Hammock, P., Joseph, J., Dickerson, M., et al. (2003). Chiari Type I malformation with and without syringomyelia: Prevalence and genetics. *Journal of Genetic Counseling, 12*, 297–311.

Thacker, N., & Shendurnikar, N. (2004). Current status of polio eradication and future prospects. *Indian Journal of Pediatrics, 71*, 241–245.

Thompson, R. J., & Gustafson, K. E. (1996). *Adaptation to chronic childhood illness.* Washington, DC: American Psychological Association.

Utley, T. F. M., Ogden, J. A., Gibb, A., McGrath, N., & Anderson, N. E. (1997). The long-term neuropsychological outcomes of herpes simplex encephalitis in a series of unselected survivors. *Neuropsychiatry, Neuropsychology, & Behavioral Neurology, 10*, 180–189.

Velting, O. N., Setzer, N. J., & Albano, A. M. (2004). Update on and advances in assessment and cognitive–behavioral treatment of anxiety disorders in children and adolescents. *Professional Psychology: Research and Practice, 35*, 42–54.

Weiner, L. S., Vasquez, M. J. P., & Battles, H. B. (2001). Fathering a child living with HIV/AIDS: Psychosocial adjustment and parenting stress. *Journal of Pediatric Psychology, 26*, 353–358.

Young, R. S., Torretti, D., Williams, R. H., Hendriksen, D., & Woods, M. (1984). Reye's syndrome associated with long-term aspirin therapy. *Journal of the American Medical Association, 251*, 754–756.

12

NEUROMUSCULAR DISEASES

JONATHAN SANDOVAL

This chapter presents an overview of diseases of the muscles (particularly focusing on several types of muscular dystrophies), diseases of the peripheral nerves, diseases of the myoneural junction, and diseases of the motor neurons. It discusses the symptoms, causes, medical treatments, and outcomes of the conditions. The implications of these outcomes for supporting children with neuromuscular diseases in schools are also highlighted.

Neuromuscular diseases (NMDs) are a group of acquired or inherited conditions that affect the neuromuscular organ system. This organ system includes (a) the muscles themselves, (b) the peripheral motor nerves, (c) the myoneural junctions between the nerves and muscles, and (d) the anterior horn cells in the spinal cord. All of the neuromuscular diseases result in muscular weakness and fatigue. Secondary effects brought on by muscular weakness and deterioration include limb contractures (the shortening of muscle or connective tissue surrounding a joint resulting in a restricted range of movement in the shoulder, elbow, wrist, ankle, hip, and knee), scoliosis (spinal deformity with lateral deviation of the spine), restrictive lung disease, and cardiac dysfunction (Karpati, Hilton-Jones, & Griggs, 2001). These dis-

This work was supported by Research and Training Center Grant H133B80016 from the National Institute on Disability and Rehabilitation Research, United States Department of Education.

eases are relatively rare, with less than 100,000 cases of all forms of NMDs prevalent in the United States (Emery, 1991). The majority of these cases are adults.

This chapter focuses on diseases that manifest during childhood or adolescence. The most common neuromuscular diseases affecting children are Duchenne muscular dystrophy, Becker muscular dystrophy, spinal muscular atrophy, and Charcot–Marie–Tooth syndrome. Other conditions seen in childhood are also discussed. Some diseases are usually fatal in infancy (e.g., infantile spinal muscular atrophy) and are not covered in this chapter.

OVERVIEW

Neuromuscular diseases can be roughly categorized by the locus of the pathology. The following sections describe childhood conditions by location.

Myopathies: Diseases of the Muscles

Muscular Dystrophies

The most common muscle diseases are the muscular dystrophies. These diseases result from irregularities in the muscle structural protein dystrophin, along with a series of glycoproteins that play a critical role in maintaining the structural integrity of muscle fibers. The dystrophin–glycoprotein complex in unaffected individuals protects the muscle membrane during muscle contraction and extension.

Duchenne Muscular Dystrophy (DMD). DMD, also called pseudohypertrophic muscular dystrophy and Meryon disease, is a sex-linked recessive genetic disease. The genetic basis for the disease is a disturbance in the dystrophin gene resulting in a deficiency in, or the absence of, dystrophin (Emery, 2001). This gene is the largest yet identified in the human genome, making up 1% of the X chromosome (den Dunnen, 2001). Because of its size and complexity, a number of areas of musculature of the body may be affected. In addition, the gene spontaneously mutates, accounting for one third of all DMD cases (Emery, 2001; Roberts, Bobrow, & Bentley, 1992). As a result of the disease, the substance dystrophin is absent from the muscles of children and fat cells and connective (scar and other nonmuscle) tissue gradually replaces muscle cells in the body.

DMD occurs in 63 in 1 million children (Emery, 1991). The symptoms are noticeable soon after a child begins to walk, and the disease may be positively identified as early as 3 years. Almost all boys with DMD are identified by age 6 (McDonald, Abresch, Carter, Fowler, Johnson, Kilmer, & Sigford, 1995). The most pervasive symptom is muscular weakness, particularly evident in the leg muscles. Symptoms observed early in children with DMD include difficulty rising (using hands pushing on the knees to stand, or using arms to rise from lying on the back, called the Grower maneuver). Walking is delayed, and one quarter of these children do not walk before age 2 years; virtually no affected boys learn to run properly (Emery, 2001). Preschoolers have trouble climbing stairs, walk on tiptoes or with a waddling gait, and display lordosis (sway back). As children develop, their muscles, particularly their calves, often appear large and overdeveloped. This condition, called calf hypertrophy (swelling), results when fat has replaced muscle in this region.

As the disease progresses and muscle structures fail, there is an increase in the backward curvature of the spine. Contractures occur, especially in the ankles but also in the hips and knees. Three quarters of children will ultimately develop severe contractures. Weakness continues until children cannot walk, even with the help of braces, and need the assistance of a wheelchair. Full-time wheelchair use may occur as early as age 7 or as late as age 14, with a mean age of 10 (Bushby & Gardner-Medwin, 1993).

In adolescence, as muscles weaken further and are unable to support the body, continued scoliosis results. Because the lungs are crowded in the chest, the most serious problem caused by curvature of the spine is difficulty breathing, which in turn makes respiratory infection a particular hazard. Cardiac muscles can also be affected, and thus approximately one third of late adolescents with the disease show symptoms such as chest pain and palpitations, and 90% show electrocardiogram abnormalities (Griggs, Mendell, & Miller, 1995; McDonald, Abresch, Carter, Fowler, Johnson, Kilmer, & Sigford, 1995). The muscle disease itself is not painful, but the child can experience muscle cramps.

Becker Muscular Dystrophy (BMD). BMD may be viewed as a mild form of DMD. It is sex-linked, caused by mutation of the same gene that causes DMD at Zp21 (de Visser & Hoogerwaard, 2001), and has a later onset, with only 20% identified before age 5 (McDonald, Abresch, Carter, Fowler, Johnson, & Kilmer, 1995). Also called benign juvenile MD and progressive tardive MD, the incidence is about 25 cases in 1 million (de Visser & Hoogerwaard, 2001). BMD is slower in progressing, and some dystrophin is present in muscles. All of the symptoms and signs of DMD are present, although not as strikingly. Half of those children with the condition have mild contractures, but only about one fifth have spinal deformity. Cardiac muscles may be affected. Children with BMD are often able to walk unaided beyond age 15 (Griggs et al., 1995).

Facioscapulohumeral Muscular Dystrophy (FSHMD). Also known as Landouzy–Dejerine dystrophy, FSHMD is not sex linked and consequently is found in both sexes. Autosomal dominant, its genetic location has not yet been identified (Upadhyaya & Cooper, 2001). It is unusual to identify this disease before age 20, although its onset may occur as early as age 7 (Kilmer et al., 1995), and early onset is associated with more severe symptoms (Upadhyaya & Cooper, 2001). This disease shows up as weakness in the muscles of the upper torso and head. Individuals with the condition lack facial mobility and have an unlined face, a pouting appearance of lips, difficulty closing the eyes, an inability to whistle, some indistinct speech, and, in the shoulder girdle muscles, difficulty raising arms overhead. As the disease progresses, it leads to a forward slope of the shoulders and the slow spread of weakness to the hip girdle muscles. Late in the disease's progression, arm and hand muscles are affected, but contractures are rare and mild (Kilmer et al., 1995). The prevalence of FSHMD is 15 in 1 million (Emery, 1991), although this may be an underestimate (Upadhyaya & Cooper, 2001).

Myotonic Muscular Dystrophy (MMD). MMD is also referred to as Steinert disease, Curschmann–Batten–Steinert syndrome, or myotonia atrophica. Two forms of MMD are usually discriminated: a congenital form, present at birth (MMD1), and a noncongenital form (MMD2). The prevalence of both forms is 50 per million. The myotonin protein kinase appears to be involved in MMD1 with a dominant mutation on chromosome 19q (Harper, 2001). It may be found in both sexes because it is autosomal dominant. This disease is usually not noted until adolescence or early adulthood, but progressive general muscle weakness can be seen at birth or shortly thereafter in about 20% of those affected (Johnson et al., 1995). MMD2 is the most common adult-onset muscular dystrophy. A striking feature of this condition is myotonia (inability to relax muscles followed in time by weakness). Grip myotonia in the hands is clearly recognizable during a handshake. Face muscles are most noticeably affected (Harper, 2001). Children with congenital MMD exhibit hypotonia (flaccid muscles) at birth, postnatal difficulties, delayed motor development, and bilateral facial weakness (Johnson et al., 1995). About half of these children may develop mild, nonprogressive scoliosis and contractures at the ankles. Conduction system (electrical impulse) problems may be found in the majority of MMD patients (Griggs et al., 1995).

Emery–Dreifuss Muscular Dystrophy (E-DMD). Clinicians distinguish two types of E-DMD (also termed humeroperoneal dystrophy) depending on the genetic abnormality. The first of these inherited conditions (E-DMD1) is caused by recessive mutations to the gene that encodes the protein emerin (Bione et al., 1994). This form occurs in males and may be termed X-EMD (Toniolo, 2001). The second, E-DMD2, is caused by a dominant or recessive mutation to the lamin gene. The onset of symptoms ranges from early childhood to adolescence. E-DMD affects the elbows and neck and results in prominent contractures. The Achilles tendon may become shortened, and there may be marked weakness in the biceps and triceps of the arms and the peroneal (calf) muscles in the legs. Associated with the disease are cardiac conduction problems, particularly atrial arrhythmias (abnormal heart rhythms), which are potentially life threatening. The symptoms of E-DMD2 tend to be more severe than those in E-DMD1. Most school-age children with the disease do not need assistance in walking (Griggs et al., 1995).

Congenital Muscular Dystrophies (CMD). This heterogeneous group of autosomal recessive conditions has recently been delineated into at least seven diseases in which the gene loci have been identified (Mercuri & Muntoni, 2001). CMD may be identified at birth or within the first few months. Some of the CMDs are characterized by significant mental retardation, and some are not (Topaloglu et al., 2003). Other variable symptoms are motor developmental delay, and muscle pathology similar to the other MDs. Some forms cause eye problems, and many forms result in the inability to walk.

Limb–Girdle Syndrome (LGMD). As a result of recent advances in genetics and molecular biology, Limb–Girdle is coming to be called a syndrome, rather than seen as a single form of muscular dystrophy. Four genes for glycoproteins seem to be responsible for various subtypes of LGMD (Worton, 1995). and at least 14 genetically defined subgroups of the disease have been identified (Bushby, 2001). The form most often seen in children is autosomal recessive muscular dystrophy of childhood (ARMDC) or severe childhood autosomal recessive muscular dystrophy (SCARMD). The various types, which together have a prevalence of 30 per million individuals, have in common a primary loss of strength in the shoulder or pelvic girdle muscles and a varying rate of progression (McDonald, Johnson, Abresch, Carter, & Fowler, 1995). There is no involvement of the facial muscles and there is a slow to moderate progression. The proximal muscles of the legs (thighs and hips) are affected before the trunk and arm muscles. Scoliosis is common. The age of onset of symptoms is between 4 and 15 with a mean of age 9 (McDonald, Johnson, et al., 1995). Mild contractures are somewhat common but not disabling.

Metabolic Myopathies

The metabolic myopathies result from abnormal muscle metabolism. Often a recessive genetic cause results in disorders of glycogen and fatty acid metabolism. The primary problem is poor exercise tolerance rather than fixed weakness, although progressive weakness is present (Moxley, Chinnery, & Turnbull, 2001). Some metabolic myopathies occur before age 10. Children appear normal but cannot participate in physical activities and are often thought to be lazy. They usually have muscle pain and cramps (Griggs et al., 1995). With heavy exertion, an observer may note dark red urine as a sign of muscle breakdown. These conditions may not become severe until teenage or adult years. Fasting and infection exacerbate the condition (Moxley et al., 2001).

Myophosphorylase Deficiency. This condition, also known as McArdle disease or carnitive palmityl transferase deficiency, is usually autosomal recessive, likely caused by a gene on chromosome 11 that codes muscle phosphorglycerate mutase (Moxley et al., 2001). In this disease, fatigue often follows intense exercise. Other symptoms include myalgia (muscle pain) and muscle stiffness. Recovery follows rest. In other respects, the child appears normal.

Myopathic Carnitine Deficiency. This is the most common of the lipid storage myopathies. The absence of substance carnitine leads to the buildup of lipids (fats) in the muscles, which results in progressive weakness, particularly in the proximal muscles (Moxley et al., 2001). It is an autosomal recessive condition and may be treated with a low-fat diet and doses of supplemental L-carnitine.

Polymyositis and Dermatomyositis Syndromes

These diseases are acquired and are among the most common of the inflammatory myopathies, with an incidence of 1 in 100,000 (Dalakas & Karpati, 2001). They are characterized by the presence of inflammatory cells, but the causes of the condition are not well known. They often occur with other diseases, such as rheumatoid arthritis and systemic lupus erythematosus.

Childhood Polymyositis. This is a rare, acquired disease, more common in girls than boys, that results in severe weakness of anterior neck and throat (pharyngeal) neck muscles and proximal limb (shoulder, hip, and thigh) flexor muscles (Dalakas & Karpati, 2001). Dysphagia (difficulty swallowing) is often seen. Muscles become swollen and sore, and the condition is painful, leading to muscle atrophy. Fifty percent of those affected have pain or muscle tenderness, and 33% have arthritic features. Facial and other skin rashes are common. A reddish-purple "butterfly" rash may be found across the nose, eyes, and forehead. Fluid may collect around the eyes. Abnormal calcium deposits (calcifications) may develop in muscle and skin tissues, and the gastrointestinal tract can be affected. The causes are not known, but the diseases seem to result from an autoimmune reaction causing inflammation of the blood vessels in the skin and muscles.

Childhood Dermatomyositis. This disease is characterized by skin rashes of the face, neck, back of hands, knees, and elbows. Particularly affected are the knuckles, which often develop papules (bumps), and the fingernails, which are discolored (Dalakas & Karpati, 2001). Children often complain of muscle pain and tenderness accompanied by progressive weakness, initially affecting the proximal muscles. One third of those affected develop dysphagia (Griggs et al., 1995). Contractures, particularly of the elbows, wrists, and shoulders are common. Occasionally children who get this disease also may develop necrotizing vasculitis (dead blood vessels). In addition, they are at increased risk for cancer. Corticosteroids are an effective treatment that often results in remission. In addition, a low-sodium, low-sugar, and low-calorie diet is recommended (Dalakas & Karpati, 2001), and physical therapy is used to reduce contractures.

Diseases of Peripheral Nerves and Motor Nerve Roots

Most of the peripheral nerve and motor nerve root diseases are hereditary but not life threatening. Many of the peripheral nerve diseases can also be acquired as a result of physical injury to the muscle or from infectious diseases, such as herpes zoster, leprosy, HIV, and Lyme disease, or from systemic diseases, such as diabetes mellitus (Schaumburg, Berger, & Thomas, 1992).

Hereditary Motor Sensory Neuropathies (HMSN)

There are at least eight types of this hereditary motor sensory neuropathy (HMSN), associated with a number of chromosomes (Kwon et al., 1995). The most frequently occurring types are simply termed Types I, II, and III.

HMSN Type 1. HMSN Type I is more commonly called Charcot–Marie–Tooth syndrome (CMT) or peroneal muscular atrophy and is the hypertrophic form of the disease. It results in abnormally slow conduction velocities in peripheral motor and sensory nerves. A variant, Roussy–Levy syndrome, also includes a tremor. The effects are a slowly progressing muscle atrophy and severe weakness. The disease attacks nerves in arms from the elbow down and legs from knee down. The calf muscles are often small, and the hand may have cocked fingers and a weak thumb. Feeling and movement in these areas may be lost. Ankle sprains are a problem for these children. Pes cavus (exaggerated height in the arch of the foot) is common, but scoliosis is rare. Approximately 10% of the children with this disease experience some pain (i.e., muscle cramping or burning nerve pain). Progression of the disease is slow. HMSN I is usually autosomal dominant genetically, but recessive forms exist with more severe symptoms. It has an estimated prevalence of 100 cases per million (Emery, 1991), but this figure may be an underestimate because in its mildest forms HMSN 1 may not be diagnosed or misdiagnosed as orthopedic foot disorder (Schaumburg et al., 1992). There are two subtypes, both linked to genes for myelin proteins on chromosome 17 and 1 (de Visser, 1994; Hayasaka, Himoro, Sato, et al., 1993).

HMSN (CMT) Type II. HMSN Type II is the neuronal form of the disease. It results in a loss of axons in motor and sensory nerves that causes impairment but is less debilitating than Type I. It is more commonly found during adolescence. Clinically it is difficult to distinguish from Type I because the same symptoms are present, although the upper extremities are less seriously affected (Schaumburg et al., 1992). The gene involvement for this type is unknown.

HMSN (CMT) Type III. Type III is also called Dejerine–Sottas disease. This rare type of HMSN is congenital, with symptoms appearing at infancy. It is also associated with disturbances in the myelin P0 gene (Hayasaka, Himoro, Sawaishi, et al. 1993). This disease is characterized by severe hypomyelination and demyelination (abnormal nerve development of the exterior of the nerve) in the peripheral nerves. The effects on children are delays in motor development. Weakness progresses from the feet and hands to the legs and arms. Areflexia (slow or missing reflexes) is noted, and sensory loss involving touch, position, vibration, and hearing can occur. Many children remain short in stature, have kyphoscoliotic (backward and lateral curvature of the spine), and develop deformed hands and feet.

Friedreich Ataxia (FA)

FA is a degeneration of the cerebral and spinal nerves and the motor nerve roots, but has effects similar to the peripheral nerve disorders. FA is hereditary, and the incidence among French Canadians is unusually high. It is autosomal recessive with a likely location on chromosome 9 (Carvajal et al., 1995). FA has an onset between ages 7 and 13 and results in a slow, progressive loss of muscle strength, leading to shaky movements and unsteadiness. With FA the brain does not properly regulate posture and muscular coordination. As the disease progresses, cognitive deficits, such as decreased motor and mental reaction times, reduced verbal span, deficits in letter fluency, and impaired acquisition and consolidation of verbal information, have been noted in adults (Wollmann, Barroso, Monton, & Nieto, 2002). People with FA exhibit clumsiness in walking and have weakness in legs. Limb movements are uncoordinated, and the tendon reflexes are reduced. Other symptoms include dysarthria (difficulty in articulation), nystagmus (rapid and involuntary eye movements, usually from side to side), scoliosis, pes cavus, hammertoe, clubfoot, and loss of sensation, particularly sense of position and vibratory sense. Three quarters of children affected with this condition have heart problems (Hewer, 1968), and between 10% and 40% contract diabetes.

Guillain–Barré Syndrome (GBS)

This acquired syndrome is characterized by progressive weakness in the limbs, pain, aparesthesias (tingling and numbness) in the feet and hands, and areflexia or hyporeflexia (no or poor reflexes) in all limbs. In some forms of the disease, there is diminished sensation and numbness. Other forms involve the muscles of the face and neck (Ropper, Wijdicks, & Truax, 1991). The disease is an inflammatory reaction related to the destruction of peripheral myelin in the nerve cells of the muscles. It may be a reaction to foreign antibodies. The yearly incidence of the disease is .6 to 1.9 cases per 100,000 across all ages. There have been "outbreaks" of GBS following widespread inoculation with the swine flu vaccine and a Finnish polio vaccine (Kinnunen, Farkkila, Hovi, Juntunen, & Weckstrom, 1989). About 70% to 80% of young patients have a good recovery with little or no residual neurological signs.

Diseases of the Myoneural Junction

The myoneural junction is where the axon of a motor neuron makes a synaptic connection with a muscle fiber. This connection may become disrupted.

Myasthenia Gravis

These diseases have a genetic source, but it is believed they may also be acquired. The disease process is autoimmunity (Newsom-Davis & Beeson, 2001). Myasthenia gravis is more common in female than male individuals. The major indicators of this disease are muscle fatigue or intermittent weakness; with rest, however, strength will recover. Most notable is weakness of the eye muscles. This weakness shows up as ptosis (drooping eyelid) or diplopia (double vision). Patients also report difficulty chewing, dysarthria, and dysphagia. Those affected with myasthenia gravis have a normal life expectancy, and the disease can be controlled with medication. The progression of the disease in individual patients varies greatly. Most do not generally require a wheelchair. Myasthenia gravis can occur in childhood, but the peak age of onset is the third decade in women and the fifth decade in men. In children, prolonged speaking and writing can provoke weakness. Myasthenia can be acquired, as can other diseases of the myoneural junction. Botulism, for example, introduces a toxin that can affect nerve cells, as can viral infections.

Lambert–Eaton Myasthenic Syndrome

Lambert–Eaton syndrome is an acquired disease (although a rare congenital form exists as well) that results in proximal muscle weakness, especially in the legs but also in the arms. Those afflicted have difficulty walking and a characteristic rolling gait (Newsom-Davis & Beeson, 2001). Lamber–Eaton myasthenic syndrome is a disorder of the distal nerve terminal where there is inadequate release of acetylcholine. Other symptoms include a dry mouth and areflexia (poor reflexes). The usual cause of this syndrome is a tumor, often of the lung, and the disease precedes cancer 80% of the time (Griggs et al., 1995).

Diseases of the Motor Neurons (Anterior Horn Cells)

Motor neuron diseases affect the anterior horn cells of motor neurons of the spinal cord. The most common inherited diseases of this kind are amyotrophic lateral sclerosis (ALS, or Lou Gehrig disease) and the spinal muscular atrophies (SMA). ALS does not usually manifest itself until adulthood and is not discussed here. SMAs are similar to a myopathy but are distinguished by a tremor, minipolymyoclonus (spasms), or fasciculations (twitches; Griggs et al., 1995). Multiple genes located on chromosome 5 seem to be involved in the condition (Thompson et al., 1995); SMAs are autosomal recessive in inheritance. Although there are three common types of spinal muscular atrophy, SMA Type I, present in infants, is fatal prior to entry into school.

Previously, the most common acquired motor neuron disease was poliomyelitis. With the development of a vaccine, this disease has been drastically curtailed. Nevertheless, as parents and others have lost their awareness of the danger of this disease, laxness in reimmunization may bring about an unwelcome return.

Intermediate Spinal Muscular Atrophy, Type II (SMAII)

Also called chronic Werding–Hoffmann disease, this condition usually manifests its first symptoms between 6 months and 2 years of age. SMAII results in delayed motor development, particularly of the legs. A progressive loss of strength occurs as muscles atrophy, usually resulting in loss of ambulation. Approximately 65% of those afflicted have significant contractures, and 78% have spinal deformity (Carter et al., 1995a). Restrictive lung disease is a linked condition.

Juvenile Spinal Muscular Atrophy, Type III (SMAIII)

SMAIII, which is know as Kugelberg–Welander disease, is identified between 1 and 15 years, but later than SMAII. Type III is a mild form of Type II with a slower progression, a lower incidence of and less severe contractions, and lower incidences of spinal deformity, lung disease, or heart involvement. As with most other neuromuscular diseases, there is weakness in leg and hip muscles with resulting difficulty in standing up and climbing stairs. Calf muscles falsely appear enlarged, and respiratory muscles weaken. Those inheriting this condition usually walk for 10 years after the first appearance of symptoms before needing assistance.

OUTCOMES

Physical

The principal outcome of almost all of the neuromuscular diseases is pervasive weakness and fatigue. In addition, changes in physiology from contractures and scoliosis or from muscles that do not develop properly usually occur. As a result, many children (e.g., those with DMD, SMA) come to use orthopedic appliances such as braces or walkers and wheelchairs while in elementary school. Children also miss school because of respiratory, cardiac, and other illness and because of hospitalization from surgery. The most common clinical complaint heard by physicians is persistent muscle pain (Abresch, Carter, Jensen, & Kilmer, 2002; Karpati et al., 2001). Many of the diseases shorten life expectancies, particularly DMD, for which the life expectancy is mid-20s.

Other MMDs, such as the diseases of the peripheral nerves and motor nerve roots and of the myoneural junctions, have less severe outcomes. Weakness and fatigue with attendant awkwardness are the major outcomes.

Cognitive

Mental retardation may also co-occur with some NMDs, particularly MMD1 (Johnson et al., 1995). The average Wechsler Adult Intelligence Scale score for adults with this condition was approximately 2 standard deviations below the mean. The prevalence of mental retardation is also higher in children with DMD than in the general population (Cotton, Voudoris, & Greenwood, 2001). Poor working memory across intellectual levels contributes to lower academic achievement in DMD (Hinton, De Vivo, Fee, Goldstein, & Stern, 2004; Hinton, De Vivo, Nereo, Goldstein, & Stern, 2000). In the DMD population, full scale IQ scores are normally distributed around a mean of 80, 1.3 standard deviations below the average for age peers. Subgroups of children have lower verbal scores than performance scores (Dorman, Hurley, & D'Avignon, 1988; McDonald, Abresch, Carter, Fowler, Johnson, Kilmer, & Sigford, 1995). Nevertheless, the full range of intellectual ability, from gifted to severely retarded, may be found among children with DMD. Children with BMD seem to fall in the normal range, as do adults with LGS, FSHD, HMSN, and SMA. The distributions for these NMD conditions are skewed, however (Carter et al., 1995a, 1995b; Johnson et al., 1995; Kilmer et al., 1995; McDonald, Johnson, et al., 1995). The percentage of individuals scoring below two standard deviations was larger than would be expected (between 10% and 20%). Performance on the Halstead–Reitan Neuropsychological Test Battery mirrors that on the Wechsler: Severe impairment for congenital muscular dystrophy (CMD), some impairment for individuals with DMD, and none for most of the other conditions. The exceptions were for SMA (Carter et al., 1995b), for which subjects demonstrated a relatively high degree of impairment despite normal functioning on the Wechsler. There is no clear mechanism connecting substances related to muscle and nerve function, such as dystrophin, to brain function. Nevertheless, fatigue can be related to attention and learning.

Social and Emotional

Researchers looking at cognitive performance have also collected personality test data on a number of hereditary conditions. Personality assessment can be misleading in that, for normal subjects, somatic complaints can suggest pathology, whereas for individuals with neuromuscular disease, somatic complaints are reality. As a result it is unreasonable to interpret typically elevated Minnesota Multiphasic Personality Inventory Hysteria, Hypochondriasis, and Depression scales as abnormal. With this allowance, little pathology was observed for those with BMD, FSHMD, and HMSN.

The adjustment of children with DMD has been assessed using the Personality Inventory for Children. Scores on this test indicate a high degree of pathology in these children (McDonald, Abresch, Carter, Fowler, Johnson,

Kilmer, & Sigford, 1995). As a group, children with chronic illnesses and physical disabilities are at risk for experiencing socioemotional difficulties. In a review of the clinical literature that principally focuses on MMD, Livneh and Antonak (1994) reported that children with MD experience several psychosocial reactions to their disease, including (a) dependency related to overprotectiveness of parents; (b) social isolation because of negative attitudes of peers and shame about their physical appearance; (c) negative body image and self-concept; (d) feelings of helplessness because of increasing dependency on others; (e) anxiety over impending death; (f) depression; and (g) anger toward parents and peers without disabilities. This research on MMD does not necessarily reflect the psychosocial experiences of all children with an NMD. Nevertheless, when adults with HMSN1 were interviewed about their school and social experiences, many reported that they became more introverted in school and that their relationships with peers were negatively affected (Goldfarb & Shapiro, 1991).

MEDICAL AND PSYCHOEDUCATIONAL IMPLICATIONS

Medical Implications

There are no proven treatments to prevent or cure the diseases of the muscles or most other NMDs. Possible new treatments involving gene therapy are in their infancy (Dunckley & Dickson, 2001; Leiden, 1995). The genetic basis for most diseases is known, but methods of gene transfer in skeletal muscle are not yet efficient. The future may bring in utero gene transfer to prevent the disease (Dunckley & Dickson, 2001). The use of immunosuppressive therapy for some conditions in which the immune system is overactive is another possible treatment (Barohn, Amato, Sahenk, Kissel, & Mendell, 1995).

Palliative approaches can moderate the effects of the diseases. The use of corticosteroids such as prednisone may prolong the ability to walk and is widely used in treating inflammations, but these medications have serious side effects. Newer pharmacological strategies for MD seem to be promising and clinical trials are under way (Khurana & Davies, 2003). Recently investigators have been examining anabolic steroids as a means of increasing muscle strength. Creatine, which some athletes use to enhance performance, shows promise for use with MD. Some new drugs, such as the aminoglycoside gentamicin, work to increase dystrophin levels and may also work to delay the onset of some of the symptoms. The protein utrophin, which is related to dystrophin and may be functionally redundant with it, has been suggested as a drug that might address early developmental effects in DMD.

Medical interventions for children include physical therapy aimed at retaining muscle tone and joint flexibility, surgery to lengthen tendons, leg braces to aid walking, and aggressive treatment of respiratory infections. Physicians must also monitor and treat pain. Because so few direct therapies for curing these diseases are available, attention must be directed toward achieving and maintaining an optimum quality of life.

Psychoeducational Implications

Children with NMD have a wide range of educational needs, depending on the type of NMD. Comorbidity with learning disabilities may occur with some conditions. Children with Duchenne muscular dystrophy and myotonic muscular dystrophy are most at risk and should be monitored closely. They should be screened for learning disabilities and their possible phonological processing problems (Dorman et al., 1988). Many, but certainly not all, children with NMD will have difficulty learning for a variety of reasons, including poor attendance.

Retardation may also be present, particularly in CMD, and children with this condition will need help in school. Many children with NMD will not have learning difficulties, however. Because of the wide range of educational needs of children with NMD, an individualized assessment will be useful in the development of an appropriate educational plan.

Research indicates that children with chronic illnesses and physical disabilities experience more depressive symptoms when there are inadequate levels of social support from family, peers, and teachers. However, when these children receive adequate levels of social support, they exhibit significantly fewer symptoms. In one study, mothers of 153 children (aged 4–16) with a chronic physical illness were asked about their children's behavior and the family environment. Low family and low peer support were related to higher disruptive behavior problems, and low peer support was related to higher depression and anxiety problems (Wallander & Varni, 1989). Teachers, parents, and peers play a critical role in the promotion of protective factors and in enhancing coping strategies for all children, especially those in greater need of emotional and social support.

Research by Strong (1998) indicates that children with NMD have fewer opportunities to interact with their peers because of several factors. Children with NMD experience more solitary play and activities than their peers, and they engage in fewer social interactions with their peers. In addition, their peers do not engage in social interactions with them as often as with other children in their classrooms. Children with NMD also use fewer strategies to enter successfully into a peer group or to join in play with another child (Strong, 1998). Other research with children with physical disabilities also indicates that, as a group, these children experience fewer successful peer interactions and often lack critical social skills (Odom, Peterson, McConnell, & Ostrosky, 1990).

Parents of children with NMD report that their child is often left out of social events, such as birthday parties and field trips because of lack of awareness by parents and schools and because of fears of dealing with the disability. Many parents try to provide alternative social activities, such as Special Olympics and other community activities that provide access and accommodations for disabilities. The lack of social support that they and their children may receive is often a great source of parental distress, however (Strong & Sandoval, 1999).

Although children with NMD are more at risk for having difficulties forming healthy peer relations, they do not appear to have more problematic behaviors, such as aggressive or disruptive behaviors. In general, children with NMD are more solitary and tend to experience social activities on the periphery, rather than within the social group (Strong, 1998). Children with NMD tend to have more internalized socioemotional difficulties rather than externalized or disruptive behaviors and often are not targeted for socioemotional interventions because they do not cause problems in their classrooms (Strong & Sandoval, 1999). Nevertheless, because of the importance of social support for improved emotional well-being, and because children with NMD are at risk for reduced social support from peers, school-based social skills interventions are an important component in the child's educational programming. Children may be helped to become more assertive and to learn how to join peer groups (Strong, 1998).

Classroom Accommodation

The goal of assistive technology and classroom accommodation is to promote access to the curriculum and school environment, as well as to increase independence. Areas to consider for assistive technology include communication, mobility, self-help and activities of daily living, fine-motor performance, as well as cognitive or learning needs. Because mobility is impaired for children with neuromuscular diseases, the first need to be addressed is physical accessibility. Most schools have now been modified with ramps for wheelchairs, accommodations in plumbing, and special furniture. Electronic aids such as wheelchairs and computers may need extra power supplies. Increasingly, children with NMD are successfully mainstreamed into regular education classes. With special education legislation and the Americans with Disabilities Act, public buildings have become accessible, and state and federal monies are available to support educating children with disabilities along with their peers.

Weakness and fatigue are perhaps more difficult to address. Children with NMD may need extra time to finish assignments because of muscular difficulties with writing or seeing. They may need more rest periods than other children. Children with NMD should be expected to perform to the best of their capabilities, but expectations should be realistic. Children with NMD will tire more easily than other children, but not expecting effort can lead them to become dependent and lazy (Strong & Sandoval, 1999). When aids are used, they must understand that they are to help the child with physical, but not mental tasks.

Physical education must be modified for children with NMD (Hutzler, Flies, Chacham, & Van den Auweele, 2002). Exercise that facilitates flexibility and does not contribute to muscle damage must be planned with the help of physicians (Block, 2000). Alternate roles in team activities, such as umpire or scorekeeper can keep children involved. Adaptations to games to get around a weakness (allowing more time or a pinch runner) may also be successful.

Recess and lunch times may also require extra accommodations. Dietary and nutritional needs may need to be addressed. The spontaneous social activities that take place during these periods may be difficult for children who lack mobility (Strong, 1998). Strategies such as peer helpers and the planning of attractive leisure activities that do not require strength and speed can help facilitate the social development of children with NMD.

Parent Involvement

It is important to be sure to use the parent as a resource in educational planning. A parent may have better knowledge of a child's abilities and be more aware of recent changes in a child's condition that could influence classroom functioning. Parents also may know much more about these unusual conditions than will the typical special educator. The demands that are imposed on children and families at any particular point in time depend on the course of the illness. Although NMDs are progressive in nature, at times children will experience more or less illness-related stress. Because of these changes, regular and systematic communication between parents and educators is essential (Strong & Sandoval, 1999). There may be conflicts between educators who have low expectations of children with NMD (e.g., they do not require children to finish assignments or do not insist on their participation in group activities) and parents who wish their children to finish the same amount of work that "normal" children do or who push their children to do even more than what would be expected. The expectations must be mediated and altered so that the child receives the best education possible.

CONCLUSION

NMDs are relatively rare conditions affecting the neuromuscular organ system. Most of them, such as muscular dystrophy, have a genetic origin. They result in varying degrees of muscle weakness, which limit mobility, cause fatigue, and may lead to serious and irreversible physical deformities. The contracting of muscles results in pain and problems with the heart and lungs. Medical treatment focuses on extending and improving the quality of life for children with these diseases. Children can be successfully accommodated in the classroom by attending to their physical, academic, and socioemotional needs.

REFERENCES

Abresch, R. T., Carter, G. T., Jensen, M. P., & Kilmer, D. D. (2002). Assessment of pain and health-related quality of life in slowly progressive neuromuscular disease. *American Journal of Hospice & Palliative Care, 19,* 39–48

Barohn, R. J., Amato, A. A., Sahenk, Z., Kissel, J. T., & Mendell, J. R. (1995). Inclusion body myositis: Explanation for poor response to immunosuppressive therapy. *Neurology, 45,* 1302–1304.

Bione, S., Maestrini, E., Rivella, S., Mancini, M., Regis, S., Romeo, G., & Toniolo, D. (1994). Identification of a novel X-linked gene responsible for Emery–Dreifuss muscular dystrophy. *Nature Genetics, 8,* 323–327.

Block, M. E. (2000). A teacher's guide to including students with disabilities in regular physical education (2nd ed.). Baltimore: Brookes Publishing.

Bushby, K. M. D. (2001). The limb–girdle muscular dystrophies. In A. E. H. Emery (Ed.), *The muscular dystrophies* (pp. 109–136). Oxford, England: Oxford University Press.

Bushby, K. M. D., & Gardner-Medwin, D. (1993). The clinical, genetic and dystrophin characteristics of Becker muscular dystrophy: I. Natural history. *Journal of Neurology, 240,* 98–104.

Carter, G. T., Abresch, R. T., Fowler, W. M., Jr., Johnson, E. R., Kilmer, D. D., & McDonald, C. M. (1995a). Hereditary motor and sensory neuropathy, Types I and II. *American Journal of Physical Medicine and Rehabilitation, 74*(Suppl.), S140–S149.

Carter, G. T., Abresch, R. T., Fowler, W. M., Jr., Johnson, E. R., Kilmer, D. D., & McDonald, C. M. (1995b). Spinal muscular atrophy. *American Journal of Physical Medicine and Rehabilitation, 74*(Suppl.), S150–S159.

Carvajal, J. J., Pook, M. A., Doudney, K., Hillerman, R., Wilkes, D., Al-Mahdawi, S., et al. (1995). Friedreich's ataxia: A defect in signal transduction? *Human Molecular Genetics, 4,* 1411–1419.

Cotton, S., Voudouris, N. J., & Greenwood, K. M. (2001). Intelligence and Duchenne muscular dystrophy: Full-Scale, Verbal and Performance intelligence quotients. *Developmental Medicine and Child Neurology, 43,* 497–501.

Dalakas, M. C., & Karpati, G. (2001). Inflammatory myopathies. In G. Karpati, D. Hilton-Jones, & R. C. Griggs (Eds.), *Disorders of voluntary muscle* (7th ed., pp. 636–659). New York: Cambridge University Press.

de Visser, M. (1994). Hereditary motor and sensory neuropathy Type Ia. In A. E. H. Emery (Ed.), *Diagnostic criteria for neuromuscular disorders* (pp. 55–61). Baarn, the Netherlands: European Neuromuscular Centre.

de Visser, M., & Hoogerwaard, E. M. (2001). Becker muscular dystrophy. In A. E. H. Emery (Ed.), *The muscular dystrophies* (pp. 72–94). Oxford, England: Oxford University Press.

den Dunnen, J. T. (2001). Point mutation detection in the dystrophin gene. In K. M. D. Bushby & L. V. B. Anderson (Eds.), *Muscular dystrophy: Methods and protocols* (pp. 85–110). Totowa, NJ: Humana Press.

Dorman, C., Hurley, A. D., & D'Avignon, J. (1988). Language and learning disorders of older boys with Duchenne muscular dystrophy. *Developmental Medicine and Child Neurology, 30,* 316–327.

Dunckley, M. G., & Dickson, G. (2001). Options for development of gene-based therapy for muscular dystrophy. In K. M. D. Bushby & L. V. B. Anderson (Eds.), *Methods in molecular medicine, Vol. 43. Muscular dystrophy: Methods and protocols* (pp. 409–434). Totowa, NJ: Humana Press.

Emery, A. E. H. (1991). Population frequencies of inherited neuromuscular diseases: A world survey. *Neuromuscular Disorders, 1,* 19–29.

Emery, A. E. H. (2001). Duchenne muscular dystrophy or Meryon's disease. In A. E. H. Emery (Ed.), *The muscular dystrophies* (pp. 55–71). Oxford, England: Oxford University Press.

Goldfarb, L. P., & Shapiro, H. K. (1991). Psychosocial aspects of Charcot–Marie–Tooth disease in childhood. *Loss, Grief & Care, 4,* 109–124.

Griggs, R. C., Mendell, J. R., & Miller, R. G. (1995). *Evaluation and treatment of myopathies.* Philadelphia: F. A. Davis.

Harper, P. S. (2001). Myotonic dystrophy. In G. Karpati, D. Hilton-Jones, & R. C. Griggs (Eds.), *Disorders of voluntary muscle* (7th ed., pp. 541–559). New York: Cambridge University Press.

Hayasaka, K., Himoro, M., Sato, W., Takada, G., Uyemura, K., Schimizu, N., et al. (1993). Charcot–Marie–Tooth neuropathy Type Ib is associated with mutations of the myelin P0 gene. *Nature Genetics, 5,* 31–34.

Hayasaka, K., Himoro, M., Sawaishi, Y., Nanao, K., Takahashi, T., Takada, G., et al. (1993). De novo mutation of the myelin P0 gene in Dejerine–Sottas disease (hereditary motor and sensory neuropathy type III). *Nature Genetics, 5,* 266–268.

Hewer, R. L. (1968). Study of fatal cases of Friedreich's ataxia. *British Medical Journal, 3,* 649–652.

Hinton, V. J., De Vivo, D. C., Fee, R., Goldstein, E., & Stern, Y. (2004). Investigation of poor academic achievement in children with Duchenne muscular dystrophy. *Learning Disabilities Research & Practice, 19,* 146–154.

Hinton, V. J., De Vivo, D. C., Nereo, N. E., Goldstein, E., & Stern, Y. (2000). Poor verbal working memory across intellectual level in boys with Duchenne dystrophy. *Neurology, 54,* 2127–2132.

Hutzler, Y., Flies, O., Chacham, A., & Van den Auweele, Y. (2002). Perspectives of children with physical disabilities on inclusion and empowerment: Supporting and limiting factors. *Adapted Physical Activity Quarterly, 19,* 300–317.

Johnson, E. R., Abresch, R. T., Carter, G. T., Kilmer, D. D., Fowler, W. M., Jr., Sigford, B. J., & Wanlass, R. L. (1995). Myotonic dystrophy. *American Journal of Physical Medicine and Rehabilitation, 74*(Suppl.), S104–S116.

Karpati, G., Hilton-Jones, D., & Griggs, R. C. (Eds.). (2001). *Disorders of voluntary muscle* (7th ed.). New York: Cambridge University Press.

Khurana, T. S., & Davies, K. E. (2003). Pharmacological strategies for muscular dystrophy. *Nature Reviews, 2,* 379–390.

Kilmer, D. D., Abresch, R. T., McCrory, M. A., Carter, G. T., Fowler, W. M., Jr., Johnson, E. R., et al. (1995). Facioscapulohumeral muscular dystrophy. *American Journal of Physical Medicine and Rehabilitation, 74*(Suppl.), S131–S139.

Kinnunen, E., Farkkila, M., Hovi, T., Juntunen, J., & Weckstrom, P. (1989). Incidence of Guillain–Barre syndrome during a nationwide oral poliovirus vaccine campaign. *Neurology, 39,* 1034–1036.

Kwon, J. M., Elliott, J. L., Yee, W. C., Ivanovich, J., Scavarda, N. J., Moolsintong, P. J., & Goodfellow, P. J. (1995). Assignment of a second Charcot–Marie–Tooth Type II locus to chromosome 3q. *American Journal of Human Genetics, 57,* 853–858.

Leiden, J. M. (1995). Gene therapy—promise, pitfalls, and prognosis. *New England Journal of Medicine, 333,* 871–873.

Livneh, H., & Antonak, R. F. (1994). Review of research on psychosocial adaptation to neuromuscular disorders: I. Cerebral palsy, muscular dystrophy, and Parkinson's disease. *Journal of Social Behavior and Personality, 9,* 201–230.

McDonald, C. M., Abresch, R. T., Carter, G. T., Fowler, W. M., Jr., Johnson, E. R., & Kilmer, D. D. (1995). Becker's muscular dystrophy. *American Journal of Physical Medicine and Rehabilitation, 74*(Suppl.), S93–S103.

McDonald, C. M., Abresch, R. T., Carter, G. T., Fowler, W. M., Jr., Johnson, E. R., Kilmer, D. D., & Sigford, B. J. (1995). Duchenne muscular dystrophy. *American Journal of Physical Medicine and Rehabilitation, 74*(Suppl.), S70–S92.

McDonald, C. M., Johnson, E. R., Abresch, R. T., Carter, G. T., & Fowler, W. M., Jr. (1995). Limb–Girdle Syndromes. *Journal of Physical Medicine and Rehabilitation, 74*(Suppl.), S117–S130.

Mercuri, E., & Muntoni, F. (2001). Congenital muscular dystrophies. In A. E. H. Emery (Ed.), *The muscular dystrophies* (pp. 10–38). Oxford, England: Oxford University Press.

Moxley, R. T., Chinnery, P., & Turnbull, D. (2001). The metabolic myopathies. In G. Karpati, D. Hilton-Jones, & R. C. Griggs (Eds.), *Disorders of voluntary muscle* (7th ed., pp. 560–579). New York: Cambridge University Press.

Newsom-Davis, J., & Beeson, D. (2001). Myasthenia gravis and myasthenic syndromes: Autoimmune and genetic disorders. In G. Karpati, D. Hilton-Jones, & R. C. Griggs (Eds.), *Disorders of voluntary muscle* (7th ed., pp. 660–675). New York: Cambridge University Press.

Odom, S. L., Peterson, C., McConnell, S., & Ostrosky, M. (1990). Ecobehavioral analysis of early education/specialized classroom settings and peer social interaction. *Education and Treatment of Children, 13,* 316–330.

Roberts, R. G., Bobrow, M., & Bentley, D. R. (1992). Point mutations in the dystrophin gene. *Proceedings of the National Academy of Sciences of the United States of America, 89*, 2331–2335.

Ropper, A. H., Wijdicks, E. F. M., & Truax, B. T. (1991). *Guillain–Barre syndrome.* Philadelphia: F. A. Davis.

Schaumburg, H. H., Berger, A. R., & Thomas, P. K. (1992). *Disorders of peripheral nerves* (2nd ed.). Philadelphia: F. A. Davis.

Strong, K. E. (1998). Peer group entry and social adaptation of children with a neuromuscular disease (Doctoral dissertation, University of California, Davis, 1998). *Dissertation Abstracts International Section A: Humanities and Social Sciences, 59*, 1911.

Strong, K., & Sandoval, J. (1999). Mainstreaming children with a neuromuscular disease: A map of concerns. *Exceptional Children, 65*, 353–366.

Thompson, T. G., DiDonato, C. J., Simard, L. R., Ingraham, S. E., Burges, A. H., Crawford, T. O., et al. (1995). A novel cDNA detects homozygous microdeletions in greater than 50% of type I spinal muscular atrophy patients. *Nature Genetics, 9*, 56–62.

Toniolo, D. (2001). Emery–Dreifuss muscular dystrophy. In A. E. H. Emery (Ed.), *The muscular dystrophies* (pp. 95–108). Oxford, England: Oxford University Press.

Topaloglu, H., Brockington, M., Yuva, Y., Talim, B., Haliloglu, G., Blake, D., et al. (2003). FKRP gene mutations cause congenital muscular dystrophy, mental retardation, and cerebellar cysts. *Neurology, 60*, 988–992.

Upadhyaya, M., & Cooper, D. N. (2001). Facioscapulohumeral muscular dystrophy. In A. E. H. Emery (Ed.), *The muscular dystrophies* (pp. 137–172). Oxford, England: Oxford University Press.

Wallander, J. L., & Varni, J. W. (1989). Social support and adjustment in chronically ill and handicapped children. *American Journal of Community Psychology, 17*, 185–201.

Wollmann, T., Barroso, J., Monton, F. I., & Nieto, A. (2002). Neuropsychological test performance of patients with Friedreich's Ataxia. *Journal of Clinical and Experimental Neuropsychology, 24*, 677–686.

Worton, R. (1995, November 3). Muscular dystrophies: Diseases of the dystrophin-glycoprotein complex. *Science, 270*, 755–756.

13

PERVASIVE DEVELOPMENTAL DISORDERS

DEBORAH KING KUNDERT AND CARRIE L. TRIMARCHI

OVERVIEW

The term *pervasive developmental disorders* (PDDs) was first introduced in 1980 to describe a class of conditions that encompass a wide range of delays of different magnitude in different domains (Tsai, 1998). The term *pervasive* indicates that these developmental disorders affect or pervade all domains of the individual's life; that is, multiple developmental and behavioral problems are associated with these conditions (Tidmarsh & Volkmar, 2003). At present, included under this broad category are autistic disorder, Asperger's disorder, childhood disintegrative disorder, Rett's disorder, and pervasive developmental disorder—not otherwise specified (NOS; American Psychiatric Association, 2000).

This chapter provides a description of autistic disorder, Asperger's disorder, and Rett's disorder, the three PDDs most documented in the available literature. In addition, medical, behavioral, and educational consequences of these disorders are outlined. The chapter concludes with an overview of current medical and psychoeducational treatment options for these PDDs. In reviewing the literature, readers encounter the term *autism spectrum disorders*

(ASDs) used synonymously for PDDs (e.g., National Institute of Mental Health, 2004). Other authors reserve the use of *ASDs* in reference to autistic disorder, Asperger's disorder, and PDD-NOS only (Towbin, Mauk, & Batshaw, 2002).

All PDDs involve impairments in social interaction, communication, and behavioral abnormalities; they differ in the extent of these symptoms and in developmental course (Rodier, 2000). The estimated incidence rate for all forms of PDDs is at least 27.5/10,000 (Fombonne, 2003), indicating that PDDs are more common in childhood than cancer, Down syndrome, or cystic fibrosis (Kabot, Masai, & Segal, 2003). These disorders are seen across cultures, socioeconomic status, and ethnic groups (Ozonoff & Rogers, 2003). In general, PDDs are more frequent in boys than girls (male:female ratio, 3–4:1; Pennington, 2002).

It has been established in the literature that the PDDs are neurodevelopmental conditions with biological bases. These disorders are neurologic in nature with predominantly behavioral manifestations (Ozonoff & Rogers, 2003). Definitive neurodevelopmental genetic disorders (e.g., tuberous sclerosis, fragile X) have been identified in 10% to 20% of children diagnosed with PDDs (Ozonoff & Rogers, 2003). It has been estimated that 5 to 10 genes are involved in PDDs (Klinger, Dawson, & Renner, 2003).

Autistic Disorder

Autistic disorder is the most clearly defined of the PDDs (Tidmarsh & Volkmar, 2003). It involves significant disturbances in three domains—social, communication, and restricted behaviors and activities—with onset by age 3 years. These pathognomonic features were initially described by Kanner in 1943 and have been incorporated into the current definition and diagnostic criteria in the *Diagnostic and Statistical Manual of Mental Disorders* (4th ed., text rev.; American Psychiatric Association, 2000) and *International Statistical Classification of Diseases* (10th rev., World Health Organization [WHO], 1993).

In the social domain, impairments are noted in the use of nonverbal behaviors used in regulating social interaction (e.g., eye contact, facial expression, gestures) and developing age-appropriate peer relationships. In addition, children with autism rarely seek to share enjoyment or interests with others, and deficits in social reciprocity are observed. As Volkmar, Klin, Marans, and McDougle (1996) noted, social dysfunction in autism is fundamentally continuous over the life span, although its manifestations change with age and developmental level.

Disturbances in communication are a key feature in autism. Impaired expressive and receptive language is noted. Specifically, delays in the development of spoken language are common, with approximately 50% of children with autism largely or entirely mute (Pennington, 2002). Marked disability is typically apparent in the pragmatic aspects of language among speaking children with autism. They have difficulty initiating or sustaining conversations, as well as taking conversational turns. Their speech tends to be monotonic, and they fail to use appropriate inflection in conversations. Failure to listen, extreme literalness, irrelevant comments, and peculiar uses of speech are common (Klinger et al., 2003). In addition, they do not engage in pretend or social play. Likewise, children with minimal speech typically display immediate and delayed echolalia. The repetition of an expression of another person may be within a few seconds (immediate) or may occur hours, days, or weeks after the original exposure (delayed). Echolalic children frequently demonstrate pronoun reversal, although this may reflect echoing of the last pronoun heard (Newsom & Hovanitz, 1997).

Various remarkable behaviors are observed in individuals with autism. These behaviors are subsumed under the terms *insistence on sameness* or *restricted range of interests* in the available definitions. Turner (1999) suggested that these can be categorized into lower level behaviors characterized by repetitive motor movements and higher level or more complex behaviors that are characterized by insistence on routines and circumscribed interests. Common repetitive motor movements include rocking; toe walking; arm, hand, or finger flapping; and whirling (Towbin et al., 2002). These repetitive motor movements are more often observed in younger children and lower functioning children with autism (Turner, 1999). Attachment to moving objects is seen in their fascination with spinning tops or fans, washing machines, and windshield wipers (Newsom & Hovanitz, 1997). The more complex behaviors are seen in individuals with mild mental retardation and those with high-functioning autism (Klinger et al., 2003). Individuals with autism exhibit an inflexible adherence to routines (e.g., dressing, food) and demonstrate significant difficulty tolerating even trivial changes in their routines or environments. The routines may be nonfunctional rituals. Intense preoccupation with idiosyncratic interests or objects is common. They may obsess about numbers, letters, time, dinosaurs, or the solar system, or they may collect simple objects (e.g., paper, pieces of string).

A variety of other features are often seen in individuals with autism. These most commonly include self-injurious behaviors, sleep disturbances, eating disturbances, and oversensitivity to sensory stimulation. Self-injurious behaviors, such as head banging, finger biting, or hair pulling, have been commonly reported in individuals diagnosed with autism. Furthermore, these behaviors occur more often in individuals with autism than in children with mental retardation (Lord, Rutter, & Le Couteur, 1994). It has been hypothesized that when children with autism become frustrated, they often have no means for verbally expressing their feelings or needs and as a result engage in self-injury as a means for expressing their frustration (Carr & Durand, 1985). Finally, available research (e.g., Richdale, 1999) has indicated that 44% to 83% of children with autism experience sleep problems, particularly before age 8. These problems typically include difficulty falling and staying asleep, shortened sleep, and early waking.

Parents frequently report eating disturbances in children with autism; however, little research is available (Klinger et al., 2003). Klinger et al. indicated that food preferences may be based on texture, color, or specific taste. Apparently, eating problems may not resolve in adulthood. Frequently adults with autism must be supervised to ensure that they eat a well-balanced diet (Klinger et al., 2003).

It has been noted that individuals with autism may fail to respond to common sounds (e.g., their names) and overreact to environmental sounds (e.g., panic in response to vacuum cleaner sounds; Volkmar et al., 1996). Because of the lack of response to some sounds, many parents may initially believe their child has impaired hearing. Similar response variation has been noted for tactile stimulation. They often seem insensitive to pain although at the same time hypersensitive to clothing touching their skin (Klinger et al., 2003).

Prevalence estimates for autism range from .7 in 10,000 to 72.6 in 10,000 (Fombonne, 2003). On the basis of extensive examination of multiple studies, Fombonne adopted the rate of 10 in 10,000 for autism prevalence. Furthermore, as noted earlier, autism occurs more frequently in males than females, approximately 3 to 4:1 (Fombonne, 1999). When females are affected, they are more likely to be severely mentally retarded; high-functioning females with autism are rare (American Academy of Child and Adolescent Psychiatry [AACAP], 1999).

The research to date clearly indicates that autism is the product of developmental brain abnormalities with significant genetic effect (e.g., Towbin et al., 2002). Current evidence directly contradicts the early conventional thought that the disorder was due to social learning, parenting, and adverse environmental conditions (Towbin et al., 2002). Furthermore, recent data indicate that it is unlikely autism is the result of infections, poor nutrition, or immunizations (Towbin et al., 2002). Evidence for genetic influences is based on twin studies and extensive family studies. Specifically, the rate of autism is much higher among identical twins (70%–91%) than among fraternal twins (0%–10%; Bailey et al., 1995). In addition, rates of autism are increased among siblings (2%–6%) of children with autism compared with the general population (<0.1%; Towbin et al., 2002). It is estimated that 5% to 18% of individuals with autism have identifiable genetic anomalies (Bailey, Phillips, & Rutter, 1996; Pennington, 2002).

A number of neurological abnormalities associated with autism have been identified in the literature. The most consistently reported finding is macrocephaly (large head size) in about 20% of cases (Piven et al., 1995). Other structural differences include hydrocephalus and lateral ventricle enlargement (Bailey et al., 1996), as well as hypoplasia in the cerebellar vermis, and brain-stem abnormalities (Courchesne, 1995). In addition, abnormal electroencephalograms (EEGs) and hyperserotonemia have been identified (Trottier, Srivastava, & Walker, 1999).

Asperger's Disorder

First described by Asperger (1944/1991) and later expanded on by Wing (1981), Asperger's disorder (AD) was not recognized as a developmental condition by the American Psychiatric Association until 1994. In general, the diagnosis of AD typically involves intact intellectual and language functioning, with impairments in reciprocal social interaction, restricted behaviors and interests, and odd patterns of verbal and nonverbal communication (Klinger et al., 2003). Considerable debate exists as to whether AD is a distinct diagnostic entity (McLaughlin-Cheng, 1998), a disorder falling along the autism spectrum (e.g., Attwood, 1998), or merely a higher functioning form of autism (e.g., Gillberg, 1998). Further complicating the issue is the fact that the available studies have not used consistent diagnostic criteria for AD, thus producing difficulties in making definitive statements about the disorder (Klinger et al., 2003).

Clinically, the degree and severity of social impairment is the most striking feature in AD (Szatmari, 1996). According to Myles and Simpson (1998), children with AD lack developmentally appropriate social skills, display poor social relatedness, fail to appreciate the give-and-take of social relationships, and have difficulty empathizing with others. They relate differently with others, either ignoring or invading, and are therefore thought of as annoying. Other researchers have described individuals with AD as socially isolated, naive, prone to teasing, immature, odd, and socially obtuse (e.g., Attwood, 1998). When engaged in joint play, children with AD tend to impose or dictate the activity and insist that other children play by their rules (Attwood, 1998). In addition, children with AD have particular difficulties acting spontaneously in social interactions that require quick and intuitive judgment (Volkmar & Klin, 2000). As a result of their social difficulties, these children show a strong preference to interact with adults, who are more interesting, knowledgeable, and tolerant than other children (Attwood, 1998), with younger children, or with girls (Szatmari, 1996). Szatmari stated that the essential feature of AD is the qualitative impairment in social relationships "that cannot be explained by other factors such as shyness, short attention span, aggressive behavior, or lack of experience" (p. 196). Individuals with AD appear to lack the skill to modulate their social behavior to the demands of the social context or the environment (Szatmari, 1996).

Many authors (e.g., Attwood, 1998; Klin & Volkmar, 1997) have described the language impairments that individuals with AD commonly demonstrate. In terms of pragmatics, these individuals may make irrelevant comments, follow conventional scripts, and appear oblivious to the reactions of the listener. They tend to interpret conversation literally and are less aware of hidden, implied, or multiple meanings. The prosody or melody of their speech lacks variation in pitch, stress, and rhythm. Their tone sounds flat, monotonous, and overprecise. Overly formal, pedantic speech and idiosyncratic use of words have been noted.

The degree and nature of the social impairments demonstrated by individuals with AD may vary as a function of their limited repertoire of interests and behaviors. Researchers have suggested that the patterns of behavior characteristic of AD tend to entail collecting vast amounts of factual information about a circumscribed area of interest (e.g., Klin, Volkmar, & Sparrow, 2000). Children and adolescents with AD are often described as "little professors" because of their intense absorption in certain subjects and the extraordinary amount of information they can consume and reiterate on a given topic (e.g., Attwood, 1998; Myles & Simpson, 1998). Intense fascination with a topic may dominate their thoughts, time, and conversations. The topic of interest may change over time, typically becoming more unusual and narrowly focused (Klin & Volkmar, 1997). Their interests may seem idiosyncratic to others and usually involve order (e.g., cataloging information, creating tables). Individuals with AD will read avidly, ask incessant questions, and obsessively collect objects to build on their encyclopedic knowledge of a topic. They may exhibit exceptional concentration and memory for their interest, but this may hinder their motivation for and attention to other activities (Klin, Carter, & Sparrow, 1997).

Children and adolescents with AD also follow and enforce strict, repetitive routines. These routines usually develop in early childhood (Attwood, 1998). The rigid behavior that individuals with AD demonstrate is often characterized by insistence on a set of events, compulsion to finish what has been started, difficulty accepting deviation from routine, insistence on rules, and difficulty predicting the future (Barnhill, 2001). They may become distressed over changes in small details in their environment (Klin, Sparrow, Volkmar, Cicchetti, & Rourke, 1995). Finally, children and adolescents with AD may display either oversensitivity or blatant insensitivity to sensory stimulation. It has been suggested that as many as 40% of individuals diagnosed with AD may have some abnormality of sensory sensitivity (Attwood, 1998).

Given the wide use of different diagnostic definitions and the scarcity of studies that have attempted to explore epidemiological issues related to AD, prevalence rates are speculative. The estimates range from as low as 2.5 in 10,000 (Fombonne, 2003), to 8.4 in 10,000 (Ozonoff & Rogers, 2003), to as high as 10 to 26 in 10,000 (Szatmari, 1996). Furthermore, AD is more common in boys (male:female ratio, 4:1; Gillberg, 1998). Yet much of what is known about the cause of AD has emerged from the broader literature on the etiology of autism. The causal factors appear to be variable and complex. No one factor can account for the heterogeneous presentation of symptoms that are specific to a diagnosis of AD. Both genetic and environmental factors are hypothesized to play a role.

Rett's Disorder

Rett's Disorder (RD) is a rare, neurodevelopmental disorder characterized by a brief period (6–12 months) of normal development followed by regression resulting in significant cognitive and physical impairment. Although the disorder was first reported in 1966, it was not until a series of papers were published in English in 1983 (Hagberg, Aicardi, Dias, & Ramos) that awareness of this condition in the United States was noted (Volkmar, 1996). The estimated prevalence of RD is 1 in 15,000 (Volkmar, 1996). This behavioral syndrome has typically been diagnosed in girls only, although recently it has been suggested that RD can occur in boys (Kerr, 2002). Although the clinical features and course of RD are distinctive, there may be some confusion with autism in the preschool years (Volkmar, 1996).

Four stages in RD have been identified (Hagberg et al., 1983): early onset (Stage I), regression (Stage II), essentially stable, pseudo-stationary (Stage III), and late motor impairment (Stage IV). Prenatal and perinatal development is relatively normal. Head circumference at birth is within normal limits, and psychomotor development initially proceeds appropriately. Subtle neurodevelopmental abnormalities (mild hypotonia, tremulous neck movements, abnormal hand movements [excess hand waving, twisting of the wrists and arms], and abnormal language development) may present in infancy (Klinger et al., 2003). These early symptoms are often mild and are not sufficient to alert the pediatrician or caregiver. This period of "apparently normal" but subtly abnormal development typically ends between 6 and 18 months of age (Kerr, 2002).

Most commonly between the ages of 1 and 4 years, a period of stagnation in the acquisition of new skills (for some months) is observed, which is followed by a period of developmental regression (Kerr, 2002). Regression may be rapid or gradual and typically lasts for several months. During this stage, a reduction in head growth is noted, indicating interrupted brain development. Overall growth delays are also noted (i.e., the child is abnormally small and thin). In addition, losses are noted in social interaction (loss of face-to-face contact) and communication (loss of spoken language; Kerr, 2002). Repeated small movements of the hands may be observed, along with declines in voluntary hand use. Sleep disturbances and breathing irregularities commonly occur during regression (Kerr et al., 2001).

As Percy (1992) noted, during Stage III (ages 2–10), most cases show an improvement in mood, attention, and communication. They are described as more aware socially; they reestablish interpersonal contact, and head growth often resumes. Hand skills may recover to some extent. Locomotor skills may continue to develop, and occasional further development of speech and limited learning may occur (Kerr, 2002). During this period, the onset of seizures and scoliosis is commonly noted.

During the final stage (age 10+), increasing motor difficulties are observed. No decline in cognition and communication is noted. Decreased mobility in adolescence and wheelchair dependence in adulthood have been reported (Tidmarsh & Volkmar, 2003). Scoliosis is most prominent. Increasing muscle rigidity, dystonia (i.e., altered muscle tone leading to contorted body positioning), and contractures (i.e., irreversible shortening of muscle fibers that cause decreased joint mobility) are noted. Breathing abnormalities and seizures may become less pronounced with age. Continued improvement in attention and eye contact may be seen. Some purposeful hand movements may be recovered during this period.

Classic characteristics of RD are noted in the areas of posture and growth, involuntary movement disorder and voluntary hand use, autonomic control, epilepsy, and feeding and gastrointestinal function (Kerr, 2002). Muscle tone is always disturbed in RD. During regression, hypotonia is typical. Both during and after regression, a tendency for increased muscle tone, especially in the lower limbs, becomes apparent (Kerr, 2002). Joint contractures, often in ankles, knees, and hips, may occur. Scoliosis develops and tends to worsen with growth and age (Kerr, 2002). Short stature is often noted (Kerr, 2002). RD is a rare disorder, so little is known about the long-term prognosis and life expectancy. Barring complications and severe illnesses, survival into adulthood is likely. Girls with RD have a 95% chance of surviving to the age of 20 to 25, and after age 35 the survival rate drops to 70% (Naidu, 1997). For those with profound mental retardation, the survival rate is 27%, likely due to an abnormality in the autonomic nervous system (Naidu, 1997).

A number of involuntary movements are observed in RD. The most prominent feature is the stereotyped hand movements (repetitive wringing, twisting, clapping, or rubbing of hands in the midline). In contrast, voluntary hand use is absent or significantly impaired (dyspraxia). Kerr (2002) noted that some spontaneous hand movements are not affected (swimming, moving to music, grasping when a fall is imminent). Other involuntary movements include grimacing and bruxism (teeth grinding). Likewise, irregular waking respiratory rhythm, resulting in panting, shallow or deep breathing, breath holding, and hyperventilation is another classic symptom of RD (Kerr, 2002). In contrast, the sleeping respiratory rhythm is normal (Kerr, 2002). Among individuals with the most severe hypotonia, inadequate, shallow breathing resulting in increased carbon dioxide levels has been noted (Kerr, 2002). Additional autonomic symptoms include poor heart and blood pressure regulation (Kerr, 2002). Finally, feeding difficulties are commonly noted in RD (Kerr, 2002). Increased muscle tone of the tongue, as well as involuntary movements of the tongue and jaws, poor mouth closure and movement of food in the mouth, and irregular breathing all affect feeding (Kerr, 2002). Loss of appetite in adolescence and adulthood has been noted in British studies (Kerr, 2002). Also common in RD are gastroesophageal reflux and constipation.

RD is an X-linked dominant chromosome disorder caused by mutations in the gene MECP2 at Xq28 (Amir et al., 1999). This gene codes for the methyl-CpG-binding protein 2, which is important in early brain development (Amir et al., 1999). The mutation interferes with maturation of specific parts of the brain involved in cognition and movement. Amir et al. identified more than 100 mutations at this site. As Volkmar (1996) indicated, higher rates of RD in monozygotic twins have been noted, as well as cases in extended family members, although familial cases account for only a small proportion of affected individuals; most cases appear to be sporadic in nature.

OUTCOMES

A number of disorders have been observed to co-occur with PDDs. These include mental retardation, internalizing and externalizing disorders, seizure disorders, tic disorders, other medical disorders, and social difficulties. Cognitively, mental retardation is always reported among those diagnosed with RD. Level of cognitive functioning has been found to range from mentally retarded (approximately 75%) to average in individuals with autism. Typically, intelligence in AD is within normal limits, although the few studies that have directly investigated the cognitive profiles in this group have presented inconsistent results (Barnhill, Hagiwara, Myles, & Simpson, 2000). In terms of overall IQ, reports range from below normal intelligence (Carpentieri & Morgan, 1994) to average to above average scores (American Psychiatric Association, 2000; Barnhill et al., 2000; WHO, 1993). Despite their apparent intelligence, however, children and adolescents with AD may experience various cognitive difficulties. They display weaknesses on tasks that require social knowledge and problem solving, abstract reasoning, and concept formation. They may be unable to cope with novelty and tend to have difficulties with auditory input (Attwood, 1998). In addition, a relative weakness in cognitive flexibility has been noted. Individuals with AD tend to have "one-track minds" (Attwood, 1998). They display rigid thinking and have difficulties with change or failure. As a result, they typically have only one approach to solving a problem and are often unable to produce alternative solutions. This cognitive inflexibility makes it difficult for them to generalize information that they have learned (Attwood, 1998).

Research suggests that individuals with PDDs may experience significant levels of emotional distress and behavioral problems (e.g., Kim, Szatmari, Bryson, Streiner, & Wilson, 2000; Tonge, Brereton, Gray, & Einfield, 1999). Children with PDDs display emotional vulnerability and stress, making them easy targets for bullies (Myles & Simpson, 2001). Both depression and anxiety have been identified as comorbid with PDDs, although these symptoms may not be verbalized because of impaired communication. Lainhart (1999) indicated that depression rates in individuals with PDDs range from 4% to 58%. Symptoms of comorbid depression may include a worsening in behaviors, agitation, social withdrawal, compulsions, and changes in sleep and appetite. It has been noted that depression tends to occur more often in higher functioning individuals during adolescence, when they develop greater insight into their differences from others or an increased desire to have friendships (Kim et al., 2000).

Anxiety and the PDDs co-occur in approximately 84% of patients, (Muris, Steerneman, Merckelbach, Holdrinet, & Meesters, 1998). Furthermore, anxiety is manifested at an early age in those with PDDs (Tidmarsh & Volkmar, 2003). The most common anxiety disorders observed include generalized anxiety disorder, agoraphobia, separation anxiety disorder, and simple–specific phobia (Lainhart, 1999). Symptoms of obsessive–compulsive disorder are reportedly common (16%–81%) in individuals with PDDs, with the rate of comorbid diagnosis of a PDD and OCD ranging from 1.5% to 29% (Lainhart, 1999). As Klinger et al. (2003) noted, it is often difficult to determine whether anxiety and obsessive–compulsive symptoms represent separate conditions or are part of the PDD. Furthermore, there is a greater incidence of anxiety disorders in adolescents with high functioning autism and AD. In addition, fear of loud noises and worry over changes in routines have been noted, although children with PDDs also demonstrate common childhood fears (e.g., dogs, snakes; Matson & Love, 1991). Furthermore, in response to increased stress, some researchers report an increase in behavior problems, marked by defiance, noncompliance, manipulation, obsessive–compulsive rituals, and extremely rigid behavior (e.g., Tonge et al., 1999).

One of the common neurological disorders observed across individuals with PDDs is seizures; 11% to 39% of patients diagnosed with PDDs have seizures. Seizures are most frequently noted in individuals with autism and RD (25%–90%) and are less common in those diagnosed with AD (Tidmarsh & Volkmar, 2003). Moreover, seizure disorders are more common among individuals with comorbid mental retardation and in girls and women (Klinger et al., 2003). Two peak periods are noted for the onset of seizures: before age 3 or during puberty (ages 11–14; Towbin et al., 2002). Abnormal EEGs without clinical seizures have been found in 21% of individuals with autism (Tuchman & Rapin, 1997). No specific type of epilepsy has been consistently associated with PDDs.

Tic disorders are observed more frequently in individuals with PDDs (4%–30% incidence), than in the general population (Stern & Robertson, 1997). As Klinger et al. (2003) noted, it is difficult to distinguish complex motor tics from the stereotypies and volitional vocal outbursts that are commonly observed in some individuals diagnosed with PDDs. Family histories strongly suggest a genetic component to the observed tics; 78% of children diagnosed with comorbid Tourette syndrome had a family history of tics or obsessive–compulsive disorder (Klinger et al., 2003).

PDDs have been found in association with a variety of medical disorders with some frequency (5%–30% of individuals; Dykens & Volkmar, 1997). Common issues include physical anomalies, genetic syndromes, chromosome anomalies, and seizures (as discussed previously). In a review of Danish data, Lauritsen, Mors, Mortensen, and Ewald (2002) found congenital anomalies in 5.3% of their sample with autism. These included disorders of the eyes (coloboma [i.e., congenital cleft in the retina, iris, or other structure of the eye], eyelid anomalies, glaucoma), ears (cochlear disease, hearing impairment), central nervous system (spina bifida, cerebral atrophy, neurofibromatosis), heart (patent ductus arteriosus), extremities (polydactyly, pelvic girdle anomaly), and urinary system (accessory kidney, medullary sponge kidney). Shevell, Majnemer, Rosenbaum, and Abrahamowicz (2001) noted that approximately 10% to 20% of children with PDDs have a definable neurodevelopmental genetic syndrome (e.g., fragile X, Angelman syndrome, 15q duplication, Down syndrome, tuberous sclerosis). Medical services for individuals with RD typically include physical therapy and occupational therapy for orthopedic issues (e.g., scoliosis, contractures) and respiratory therapy (for breathing issues). For those with seizures, ongoing medical intervention is warranted to maintain optimal functioning.

A variety of residual social difficulties are noted in individuals with PDDs (Ozonoff & Rogers, 2003). The results of a follow-up study by Kobayashi, Murata, and Yoshinaga (1992) of individuals who received early intervention indicated that 27% of their sample had achieved social independence (i.e., they were employed) or had a good chance for social independence (i.e., they were students in college or trade school). The remaining individuals in their sample continued to need considerable supervision and were not employed. The social deficits associated with autism affect attempts at integration (Klin & Cohen, 1994). Individuals diagnosed with RD typically require high-level support and supervision (Volkmar, 1996). Perseverative, circumscribed interests are common among older and higher functioning individuals with PDDs (South, Ozonoff, & McMahon, 2001), and these may limit their social interactions.

IMPLICATIONS

At this time, much controversy exists over which treatment approach is most effective for individuals with PDDs. The available treatments have not been well evaluated. Few comparative studies that directly contrast different approaches have been conducted, so it is difficult to firmly claim superiority for any one intervention for individuals with PDDs (Ozonoff & Rogers, 2003). Most of the investigations have examined behavioral approaches (applied behavior analysis) for individuals with autism to date. At present, the focus is on identification and use of empirically supported treatments. Features that are seen across the efficacious treatments, regardless of model, philosophy, or type, have been consistently identified: Effective treatments begin early, are intensive in nature (= 25 hours/week), are individualized and developmentally appropriate, and are family centered (Rogers, 1998).

Given this, three challenges in the treatment of those diagnosed with PDDs have been identified in the literature: (a) The complexity of the disorders requires input of multiple professionals and of the parents, (b) there is a pressing need to train personnel about PDDs and using evidenced-based interventions for teaching and treating and managing behavioral issues, and (c) increased attention should be paid to the social and emotional well-being of individuals with PDDs (Bryson, Rogers, & Fombonne, 2003). Current research suggests that people with PDDs can improve when provided with certain kinds of interventions (Ozonoff & Rogers, 2003). Interventions for those with PDDs are typically aimed at improving overall functioning by promoting the development of communication, social, adaptive, behavioral, and academic skills; lessening maladaptive and repetitive behaviors; and helping the family manage the stress associated with raising a child with a disability (American Academy of Pediatrics, Committee on Children With Disabilities, 2001b). These approaches include medical and psychoeducational interventions.

Medical

Medications typically play a more modest role in the treatment of individuals with PDDs. As Volkmar et al. (1996) noted, drug therapy can be a useful adjunctive treatment in reducing many of the behavioral disturbances associated with PDDs (e.g., anxiety, aggression, agitation) with resultant improvements in the quality of life for the individual and family. Few controlled clinical trials of psychopharmacologic agents for the treatment of children with PDDs have been conducted, however (des Portes, Hagerman, & Hendren, 2003). Harden and Lubetsky (2005) described data suggesting that patients with autism respond to many psychotropic medications similarly to typically developing individuals, although response rates tend to be poorer and more variable, with the occurrence of more side effects. Despite this, 55% of individuals with PDDs are prescribed one medication, and 29.3% are prescribed two or more medications (des Portes et al., 2003). For those patients with associated neurologic disorders, seizures, or tics, medications may be of benefit. Currently, selective serotonin reuptake inhibitors (SSRIs) and atypical antipsychotics are believed to provide the greatest benefit in reducing behavioral issues (des Portes et al., 2003), and these medications are frequently prescribed: 21.7% and 16.8%, respectively (Harden & Lubetsky, 2005). Atypical neuroleptics, such as haloperidol (Haldol), risperidone (Risperdal), clozapine (Clozaril), and olanzapine (Zyprexa), have been extensively studied in individuals with autism; only risperidone has been proven efficacious in controlled clinical trials (AACAP, 1999). The use of these medications suggests benefit in terms of reduced stereotypies, aggression, motor tics, inattention, overactivity agitation, self-injurious behaviors, and withdrawal (Arnold et al., 2000). Other drugs used in treating behavior symptoms (e.g., aggression, self-injury, depression), as well as anticonvulsants (carbamazepine [Tegretol], valproic acid [Depakote], levetiracetam [Keppra]) and mood stabilizers (lithium), have also been prescribed for individuals with PDDs. SSRIs (fluoxetine [Prozac], paroxetine [Paxil], sertraline [Zoloft]) have been prescribed to decrease ritualistic behaviors, stereotyped movements, anxiety, and difficulties making transitions (McDougle et al., 2000). Although psychostimulants are prescribed for 11% to 13.9% of individuals with autism, mixed responses have been noted with the use of these medications (e.g., methylphenidate [Ritalin, Concerta], dextroamphetamine/amphetamine [Adderall]); in some cases psychostimulants have been observed to increase self-stimulatory behavior, irritability, and social withdrawal (Aman, Lam, & Collier-Crespin, 2003; Aman & Langworthy, 2000). Clonidine, an antihypertensive agent, has shown some short-term success in controlling hyperactivity and sleep problems (Riddle et al., 1999).

For individuals with RD, treatments from a number of medical specialties are routinely indicated to maintain physical functioning. Given the motor characteristics, ongoing orthopedic consultation and treatment are warranted to maintain optimal motor functioning and reduce contractures. Gastroenterology and nutrition address issues related to feeding, fluid intake, and gastrointestinal concerns. For heart and breathing issues, cardiology and ear–nose–throat specialists are indicated. Medications more specific to individuals with RD include levodopa (L-dopa) to alleviate muscle stiffness, naltrexone (ReVia) to stabilize breathing irregularities, and busperidone (Buspar) to improve breathing rhythm (International Rett Syndrome Association, 2005).

Psychoeducational

As noted by Towbin et al. (2002), the mainstay of treatment for PDDs is education. Individuals with PDDs present a number of challenges to educators because of the nature and severity of their disabilities across the cognitive, behavioral, social, and language domains (Simpson, deBoer-Ott, & Smith-Myles, 2003). All children with PDDs require individualized planning to experience educational success. Irregular patterns of cognitive and educational strengths and deficits, including splinter skills and isolated discontinuous abilities, have often been observed in individuals with PDDs (Simpson et al., 2003). As Simpson et al. noted, there is significant, ongoing debate over the efficacy and appropriateness of recommending students with PDDs for placement in general education settings in inclusion programs. Although students with special needs are increasingly being served in general education programs, few models and procedures have been advanced to facilitate the successful placement and maintenance of students with PDDs in these settings (Simpson et al., 2003). It appears that intensive special education interventions are associated with better outcomes than less structured approaches (Volkmar et al., 1996). Furthermore, early intervention leads to better prognosis, including increased likelihood of developing language, being placed in regular education classes, and higher intelligence scores (Klinger et al., 2003). At this time, adaptive behavior, intelligence, and language have been identified as the best indicators of outcome in adulthood (Bryson et al., 2003). It has been noted that most individuals with PDDs improve with time and age (Ozonoff & Rogers, 2003). Furthermore, it seems that AD has a better outcome than autism, whereas the outcome seems significantly worse for those with RD than for those with autism (Volkmar, 1996).

Education typically begins with enrollment in an early intervention program during the preschool years. All successful early intervention programs (e.g., Princeton Child Development Institute, Douglass Developmental Disabilities Center, LEAP Program, and TEACCH) for children with PDDs consider the influence of environmental stimulation, highly structure the teaching, and present materials in a systematic and well-planned manner (Kabot et al., 2003). Diverse approaches have been determined to be effective in providing educational services. These include discrete trial training (e.g., Lovaas, 1987), naturalistic behavioral interventions (e.g., Koegel, Koegel, & Carter, 1998), and developmental–pragmatic interventions (e.g., Prizant & Wetherby, 1998).

For school-age students with PDDs, special education and behavioral interventions often facilitate learning and adjustment. Significant debate exists over the efficacy and appropriateness of recommending students with PDDs for placement in general educational settings (Simpson et al., 2003). Actual placement and services must be determined on an individual basis. Prevocational and vocational training is important for adolescents with PDDs. Depending on the skills and behaviors of the individual, the goal may be for independent or supported employment that provides opportunities for continued social development (Gerhardt & Holmes, 1997).

Language interventions are often provided to children with PDDs to develop expressive and receptive language skills, as well as pragmatics. Approximately 50% of all children with autism acquire language and learn to communicate with useful speech (Howlin, 1997). For those who are nonverbal or speak minimally, augmentative and alternative communication strategies can be effective. For example, the Picture Exchange Communication System (PECS) teaches children to exchange a picture of the desired item with the teacher, who immediately honors the request (Frost & Bondy, 1994). Verbal prompts are not used, thereby allowing the child to initiate an interaction and avoiding prompt dependency.

Social competency interventions vary along important dimensions: who is initiating the social exchange (adult vs. peer), the context (individual vs.

group), and the social goal being taught (initiations vs. play; Mastergeorge, Rogers, Corbett, & Solomon, 2003). Adult-delivered interventions include social skills groups, social stories, visual cueing, social games, and video modeling. Most of the available literature has focused on peer-mediated social interventions (Mastergeorge et al., 2003). Rather than teaching specific verbal responses (e.g., individual words), pivotal response training teaches "pivotal" communication behaviors that can have broad effects on language (e.g., requesting; Koegel et al., 1998). Furthermore, typical peers in inclusive classes can be taught to use these techniques to enhance peer interactions of children with PDDs (Pierce & Schreibman, 1997).

Behavioral features of PDDs can interfere with learning and social success. As discussed previously, these maladaptive behaviors may carry meaning and should not be presumed to be random. Applied behavior analysis (ABA), functional behavioral assessment, and functional analysis procedures consider the origin of the behavior, teach effective ways to achieve the desired result, and increase social adaptability (Towbin et al., 2002). Behavioral supports have been effective in establishing daily routines; extinguishing self-injurious, aggressive, or destructive behaviors; and responding to tantrums (Howlin, 1998). In addition, individuals with PDDs can be taught to self-monitor their behavior and reinforce appropriate or desirable behaviors (Koegel, Koegel, Hurley, & Frea, 1992).

Beginning in the 1990s, positive behavioral support (PBS) approaches have emerged. These approaches attempt to increase positive behaviors and decrease problem behavior while improving the individual's lifestyle. Interventions are based on individual growth and development, motivation and learning, and preferences and choices (Parrish, 2002). Outcomes that are acceptable to the participants (individual, parents) are the major goal of PBS (Haring & DeVault, 1996).

Family involvement and support have been identified as key factors in any intervention with individuals with PDDs. Parents are an important source of information, and they are critical partners in implementing appropriate interventions. They are advocates for appropriate services for their children. Parents and siblings may have special needs (Marcus, Kunce, & Schopler, 1997). Parents have been found to be at increased risk for depression as a result of the unique challenges of living with a child with a disability (Marcus et al., 1997). In addition, siblings may have a difficult time comprehending the disorder and often do not understand the explanations their parents provide (Glasberg, 2000).

Alternative Treatments

Significant attention is being paid to alternative approaches for the treatment of PDDs (American Academy of Pediatrics, Committee on Children With Disabilities, 2001a). These nontraditional approaches have rarely been studied in a scientific manner. Most often testimonials are offered, although it is unknown whether the intervention or some unknown was instrumental in the improvement (Towbin et al., 2002). As Nickel (1996) noted, 50% of children with autism use alternative treatments, and in many cases the physicians are unaware of their use. These alternative treatments fall into various categories: (a) unproven, benign biological treatments (e.g., megavitamins and nutritional supplements); (b) unproven, benign biological treatments that have some basis in theory (use of secretin [i.e., a pancreatic hormone that mediates digestion]; gluten-free diets); (c) unproven, potentially harmful biological treatments (Nystatin or Diflucan, chelation therapy [i.e., a synthetic amino acid that binds with heavy metals which are then eliminated from the body]); and (d) nonbiological treatments (e.g., sensory integration training, brushing, weighted vests, facilitated communication, holding therapy, patterning, auditory training; AACAP, 1999; Hyman & Levy, 2000). In an evaluation of sensory and motor interventions (e.g., sensory integration therapy, weighted vests, brushing, Irlen lenses) for children with autism, Baranek (2002) indicated that "at least some positive findings are noted . . . and future research must move from the current level small-scale, poorly controlled, unsystematic studies of effectiveness to . . . well-controlled large-scale designs" (p. 418). For example, occupational therapists report using weighted vests with young children with autism to improve on-task behavior and attention span (Olson & Moulton, 2004). Baranek identified two studies that examined this type of treatment. These studies (McClure & Holtz-Yotz, 1990; Zisserman, 1991) provided case reports using weighted garments (gloves and vests) to reduce self-stimulatory behaviors. In her evaluation, Baranek (2002) noted that these were weak case reports (e.g., no functional analysis of the behaviors prior to treatment). Zisserman (1991) noted improvements using gloves, although not for the weighted vest; no carryover effects were demonstrated once the gloves were removed. McClure and Holtz-Yotz (1990) used elastic wraps with a 13-year-old boy, although investigator biases, medication, and poor reliability and validity for the measures used significantly restrict any conclusions that might be made. In general, Baranek (2002) noted that studies of sensory and motor interventions yield "some positive, albeit modest outcomes," although methodological constraints (small sample sizes, uncontrolled designs, observer bias) severely limit conclusions that can be drawn and the "generalizability of much of the work" (p. 415).

Given that these treatments are used, the following guidelines have been proposed: (a) the therapy should not compromise the child's attendance at program or delay entry into a program, (b) it should not be too expensive, and (c) it should be safe and noninvasive (Towbin et al., 2002). Maintaining the health and safety of the child and ensuring that families do not forgo treatments of proven effectiveness in favor of alternative treatments of undetermined efficacy is of paramount importance (des Portes et al., 2003). Further research needs to evaluate the scientific merits of each therapeutic approach, ensure that treatments are implemented with integrity and consistency, identify the risks or potential harmful effects, determine which treatments are effective for which children (American Academy of Pediatrics, Committee on Children With Disabilities, 2001a).

CONCLUSION

Autism, AD, and RD are neurodevelopmental disorders with a genetic basis that present in infancy and young childhood. They share impairments in social reciprocity and communication, as well as behavior abnormalities, although they may differ in the level of severity. In addition to the characteristics of each disorder, a number of associated conditions may be present. At this time, there is no consensus treatment to address the multiple aspects of these PDDs. Individualized, multidimensional intervention is the standard of care and can lead to improvements.

REFERENCES

Aman, M. G., Lam, K. S., & Collier-Crespin, A. (2003). Prevalence and patterns of use of psychoactive medicines among individuals with autism in the Autism Society of Ohio. *Journal of Autism and Developmental Disorders, 33*, 527–534.

Aman, M. G., & Langworthy, K. S. (2000). Pharmacotherapy for hyperactivity in children with autism and other pervasive developmental disorders. *Journal of Autism and Developmental Disorders, 30*, 451–459.

American Academy of Child and Adolescent Psychiatry. (1999). Practice parameters for the assessment and treatment of children, adolescents, and adults with autism and other pervasive developmental disorders. *Journal of the American Academy of Child and Adolescent Psychiatry, 38*(Suppl. 12), 32S–54S.

American Academy of Pediatrics, Committee on Children With Disabilities. (2001a). Counseling families who choose complementary and alternative medicine for their child with chronic illness or disability. *Pediatrics, 107*, 598–601.

American Academy of Pediatrics, Committee on Children With Disabilities. (2001b). *Technical report: The pediatrician's role in the diagnosis and management of autistic spectrum disorder in children.* Retrieved June 29, 2005, from http://www.pediatrics.org/cg/content/full/107/5/e85

American Psychiatric Association. (2000). *Diagnostic and statistical manual of mental disorders* (4th ed., text rev.). Washington, DC: Author.

Amir, R. E., Van den Veyver, I. B., Wan, M., Tran, C. Q., Francke, U., & Zoghbi, H. (1999). Rett syndrome is caused by mutations in X-linked MECP2, encoding methyl CpG binding protein 2. *Nature Genetics, 23*, 185–188.

Arnold, L. E., Aman, M. G., Martin, A., Collier-Crespin, A., Vitiello, B., Tierney, E., et al. (2000). Assessment in multisite randomized clinical trials of patients with autistic disorder: The Autism RUPP Network. Research Units on Pediatric Psychopharmacology. *Journal of Autism and Developmental Disorders, 30,* 99–111.

Asperger, H. (1991). "Autistic psychopathy" in childhood. In U. Frith (Ed. & Trans.), *Autism and Asperger syndrome* (pp. 37–92). Cambridge, England: Cambridge University Press. (Original work published 1944)

Attwood, T. (1998). *Asperger's syndrome: A guide for parents and professionals.* London: Kingsley.

Bailey, A., LeCouteur, A., Gottesman, I., Bolton, P., Simonoff, E., Yuzda, F. Y., et al. (1995). Autism as a strongly genetic disorder: Evidence from a British twin study. *Psychological Medicine, 25,* 63–77.

Bailey, A., Phillips, W., & Rutter, M. (1996). Autism: Towards an integration of clinical, genetic, neuropsychological, and neurobiological perspectives. *Journal of Child Psychology and Psychiatry, 37,* 369–392.

Baranek, G. T. (2002). Efficacy of sensory and motor interventions for children with autism. *Journal of Autism and Developmental Disorders, 32,* 397–422.

Barnhill, G. (2001). What is Asperger's syndrome? *Intervention in School and Clinic, 36,* 258–265.

Barnhill, G., Hagiwara, T., Myles, B. S., & Simpson, R. L. (2000). Asperger syndrome: A study of the cognitive profiles of 37 children and adolescents. *Focus on Autism and Other Developmental Disabilities, 15,* 146–153.

Bryson, S. E., Rogers, S. J., & Fombonne, E. (2003). Autism spectrum disorders: Early detection, intervention, education, and psychopharmacological management. *Canadian Journal of Psychiatry, 48,* 506–516.

Carpentieri, S. C., & Morgan, S. B. (1994). A comparison of patterns of cognitive functioning of autistic and nonautistic retarded children on the Stanford–Binet—fourth edition. *Journal of Autism and Developmental Disorders, 24,* 215–223.

Carr, E. G., & Durand, V. M. (1985). The social–communicative basis of severe behavior problems in children. In S. Reiss & R. Bootzin (Eds.), *Theoretical issues in behavior therapy* (pp. 219–254). New York: Academic Press.

Courchesne, E. (1995). New evidence of cerebellar and brainstem hypoplasia in autistic infants, children, and adolescents. The MR imaging study by Hashimoto and colleagues. *Journal of Autism and Developmental Disorders, 25,* 19–22.

des Portes, V., Hagerman, R. J., & Hendren, R. L. (2003). Pharmacotherapy. In S. Ozonoff, S. J. Rogers, & R. L. Hendren (Eds.), *Autism spectrum disorders: A research review for practitioners* (pp. 161–186). Washington, DC: American Psychiatric Publishing.

Dykens, E. M., & Volkmar, F. R. (1997). Medical conditions associated with autism. In D. J. Cohen & F. R. Volkmar (Eds.), *Handbook of autism and pervasive developmental disorders* (pp. 388–407). New York: Wiley.

Fombonne, E. (1999). The epidemiology of autism: A review. *Psychological Medicine*, *29*, 769–786.

Fombonne, E. (2003). Epidemiological surveys of autism and other pervasive developmental disorders: An update. *Journal of Autism and Developmental Disorders*, *33*, 365–382.

Frost, L., & Bondy, A. (1994). *PECS: The Picture Exchange Communication System training manual*. Cherry Hill, NJ: Pyramid Educational Consultants.

Gerhardt, P. F., & Holmes, D. L. (1997). Employment: Options for adolescents and adults with autism. In D. J. Cohen & F. R. Volkmar (Eds.), *Handbook of autism and pervasive developmental disorders* (pp. 650–664). New York: Wiley.

Gillberg, C. (1998). Asperger syndrome and high-functioning autism. *British Journal of Psychiatry*, *172*, 200–209.

Glasberg, B. A. (2000). Development of siblings' understanding of autism spectrum disorders. *Journal of Autism and Developmental Disorders*, *30*, 143–156.

Hagberg, B., Aicardi, J., Dias, K., & Ramos, O. (1983). A progressive syndrome of autism, dementia, ataxia, and loss of purposeful hand use in girls: Rett's syndrome. Report of 35 cases. *Annals of Neurology*, *14*, 471–479.

Harden, B. L., & Lubetsky, M. (2005). Pharmacotherapy in autism and related disorders. *School Psychology Quarterly*, *20*, 155–171.

Haring, N. G., & DeVault, G. (1996). Discussion: Family issues and family support. In L. K. Koegel, R. L. Koegel, & G. Dunlap (Eds.), *Positive behavior support: Including people with difficult behavior in the community* (pp. 115–120). Baltimore: Brookes Publishing.

Howlin, P. (1997). *Autism: Preparing for adulthood*. London: Routledge.

Howlin, P. (1998). Practitioner review: Psychological and educational treatments for autism. *Journal of Child Psychology and Psychiatry and Allied Disciplines*, *39*, 307–322.

Hyman, S. L., & Levy, S. E. (2000). Autistic spectrum disorders: When traditional medicine is not enough. *Contemporary Pediatrics*, *17*, 101–116.

International Rett Syndrome Association. (2005, June 17). *Treatments and therapies*. Retrieved June 27, 2005, from http://www.rettsyndrome.org/main/general.htm

Kabot, S., Masai, W., & Segal, M. (2003). Advances in the diagnosis and treatment of autism spectrum disorders. *Professional Psychology: Research and Practice*, *34*, 26–33.

Kanner, L. (1943). Autistic disturbances of affective contact. *Nervous Child*, *2*, 217–250.

Kerr, A. (2002). Annotation: Rett syndrome: Recent progress and implications for research and clinical practice. *Journal of Child Psychology and Psychiatry*, *43*, 277–287.

Kerr, A. M., Nomura, Y., Armstrong, D., Anvret, M., Belichenko, P. V., Budden, S., et al. (2001). Guidelines for reporting clinical features in cases with MECP2 mutations. *Brain and Development*, *23*, 208–211.

Kim, J. A., Szatmari, P., Bryson, S. E., Streiner, D. L., & Wilson, F. J. (2000). The prevalence of anxiety and mood disorders among children with autism and Asperger syndrome. *Autism, 4,* 117–132.

Klin, A., Carter, A., & Sparrow, S. S. (1997). Psychological assessment of children with autism. In D. J. Cohen & F. R. Volkmar (Eds.), *Handbook of autism and pervasive developmental disorders* (2nd ed., pp. 418–427). New York: Wiley.

Klin, A., & Cohen, D. J. (1994). The immorality of not-knowing: The ethical imperative to conduct research in child and adolescent psychiatry. In J. Hattab (Ed.), *Ethics in child psychiatry* (pp. 217–242). Jerusalem: Gefan.

Klin, A., Sparrow, S. S., Volkmar, F. R., Cicchetti, D. V., & Rourke, B. P. (1995). Asperger syndrome. In B. P. Rourke (Ed.), *Syndrome of nonverbal learning disabilities: Neuropsychological manifestations* (pp. 93–118). New York: Guilford Press.

Klin, A., & Volkmar, F. R. (1997). Asperger's syndrome. In D. J. Cohen & F. R. Volkmar (Eds.), *Handbook of autism and pervasive developmental disorders* (2nd ed., pp. 94–122). New York: Wiley.

Klin, A., Volkmar, F. R., & Sparrow, S. (Eds.). (2000). *Asperger syndrome.* New York: Guilford Press.

Klinger, L. G., Dawson, G., & Renner, P. (2003). Autistic disorder. In E. J. Mash & R. A. Barkley (Eds.), *Child psychopathology* (2nd ed., pp. 409–454). New York: Guilford Press.

Kobayashi, R., Murata, T., & Yoshinaga, K. (1992). A follow-up study of 201 children with autism in Kyushu and Yamaguchi areas, Japan. *Journal of Autism and Developmental Disorders, 22,* 395–411.

Koegel, L. K., Koegel, R. L., & Carter, C. M. (1998). Pivotal responses and the natural language teaching paradigm. *Seminars in Speech and Language, 19,* 355–371.

Koegel, L. K., Koegel, R. L., Hurley, C., & Frea, W. D. (1992). Improving social skills and disruptive behavior in children with autism through self-management. *Journal of Applied Behavior Analysis, 25,* 341–353.

Lainhart, J. (1999). Psychiatric problems in individuals with autism, their parents and siblings. *International Review of Psychiatry, 11,* 278–298.

Lauritsen, M. B., Mors, O., Mortensen, P. B., & Ewald, H. (2002). Medical disorders among inpatients with autism in Denmark according to ICD-8: A nationwide register-based study. *Journal of Autism and Developmental Disorders, 32,* 115–119.

Lord, C., Rutter, M., & Le Couteur, A. (1994). Autism Diagnostic Interview— Revised: A revised version of a diagnostic interview for caregivers of individuals with possible pervasive developmental disorders. *Journal of Autism and Developmental Disorders, 24,* 659–685.

Lovaas, O. I. (1987). Behavioral treatment and normal education and intellectual functioning in young autistic children. *Journal of Consulting and Clinical Psychology, 55,* 3–9.

Marcus, L. M., Kunce, L. J., & Schopler, E. (1997). Working with families. In D. J. Cohen & F. R. Volkmar (Eds.), *Handbook of autism and pervasive developmental disorders* (pp. 631–649). New York: Wiley.

Mastergeorge, A. M., Rogers, S. J., Corbett, B. A., & Solomon, M. (2003). Non-medical interventions for autism spectrum disorders. In S. Ozonoff, S. J. Rogers, & R. L. Hendren (Eds.), *Autism spectrum disorders: A research review for practitioners* (pp. 133–160). Washington, DC: American Psychiatric Publishing.

Matson, J. L., & Love, S. R. (1991). A comparison of parent-report fear for autistic and normal age-matched children and youth. *Australian and New Zealand Journal of Developmental Disabilities, 16*, 349–358.

McClure, M. K., & Holtz-Yotz, M. (1990). The effects of sensory stimulatory treatment on an autistic child. *American Journal of Occupational Therapy, 45*, 1138–1145.

McDougle, C. J., Scahill, L., McCracken, J. T., Aman, M. G., Tierney, E., Arnold, L. E., et al. (2000). Research Units on Pediatric Psychopharmacology (RUPP) Autism Network. Background and rationale for an initial controlled study of risperidone. *Child and Adolescent Psychiatric Clinics of North America, 9*, 201–224.

McLaughlin-Cheng, E. (1998). Asperger syndrome and autism: A literature review and meta-analysis. *Focus on Autism and Other Developmental Disabilities, 13*, 234–245.

Muris, P., Steerneman, F., Merckelbach, H., Holdrinet, I., & Meesters, C. (1998). Comorbid anxiety symptoms in children with pervasive developmental disorders. *Journal of Anxiety Disorders, 12*, 387–393.

Myles, B. S., & Simpson, R. L. (1998). *Asperger syndrome: A guide for educators and practitioners*. Austin, TX: PRO-ED.

Myles, B. S., & Simpson, R. L. (2001). Effective practices for students with Asperger syndrome. *Focus on Exceptional Children, 34*, 1–14.

Naidu, S. (1997). Rett syndrome: A disorder affecting early brain growth. *Annals of Neurology, 42*, 3–10.

National Institute of Mental Health. (2004). *Autism spectrum disorders (pervasive developmental disorders)*. Retrieved January 13, 2005, from http://www.nimh.nih.gov/publicat/autism.cfm

Newsom, C., & Hovanitz, C. (1997). Autistic disorder. In L. G. Terdal & E. J. Mash (Eds.), *Assessment of childhood disorders* (3rd ed., pp. 408–452). New York: Guilford Press.

Nickel, R. (1996). Controversial therapies for young children with developmental disabilities. *Infants and Young Children, 8*, 29–40.

Olson, L. J., & Moulton, H. J. (2004). Use of weighted vests in pediatric occupational therapy practice. *Physical and Occupational Therapy in Pediatrics, 24*, 45–60.

Ozonoff, S., & Rogers, S. J. (2003). From Kanner to the millennium: Scientific advances that have shaped clinical practice. In S. Ozonoff, S. J. Rogers, & R. L. Hendren (Eds.), *Autism spectrum disorders: A research review for practitioners* (pp. 3–33). Washington, DC: American Psychiatric Publishing.

Parrish, J. M. (2002). Promoting adaptive behavior while addressing challenging behavior. In M. L. Batshaw, *Children with disabilities* (5th ed., pp. 607–628). Baltimore: Brookes Publishing.

Pennington, B. F. (2002). *The development of psychopathology*. New York: Guilford Press.

Percy, A. K. (1992). The Rett syndrome: Recent advances in genetic studies in the USA. *Brain Development, 14*(Suppl.), 104–105.

Pierce, K., & Schreibman, L. (1997). Multiple peer use of pivotal response training to increase social behaviors of classmates with autism: Results from trained and untrained peers. *Journal of Applied Behavior Analysis, 30,* 157–160.

Piven, J., Arndt, S., Bailey, J., Havercamp, S., Andreasen, N. C., & Palmer, P. (1995). An MRI study of brain size in autism. *American Journal of Psychiatry, 152,* 1145–1149.

Prizant, B. M., & Wetherby, A. M. (1998). Understanding the continuum of discrete-trial traditional behavioral to social-pragmatic developmental approaches in communication enhancement for young children with autism/PDD. *Seminars in Speech and Language, 19,* 329–352.

Richdale, A. (1999). Sleep problems in autism: Prevalence, cause, and intervention. *Developmental Medicine and Child Neurology, 41,* 60–66.

Riddle, M. A., Bernstein, G. A., Cook, E. H., Leonard, H. L., March, J. S., & Swanson, J. M. (1999). Anxiolytics, adrenergic agents, and naltrexone. *Journal of the American Academy of Child and Adolescent Psychiatry, 38,* 546–556.

Rodier, P. M. (2000, February). The early origins of autism. *Scientific American, 282,* 56–63.

Rogers, S. J. (1998). Empirically supported comprehensive treatments for young children with autism. *Journal of Clinical Child Psychology, 27,* 167–178.

Shevell, M. I., Majnemer, A., Rosenbaum, P., & Abrahamowicz, M. (2001). Etiological yield of autistic spectrum disorders: A prospective study. *Journal of Child Neurology, 16,* 509–512.

Simpson, R. L., de Boer-Ott, S. R., & Smith-Myles, B. (2003). Inclusion of learners with autism spectrum disorders in general education settings. *Topics in Language Disorders, 23,* 116–134.

South, M., Ozonoff, S., & McMahon, W. M. (2001, April). *Repetitive behavior and cognitive functioning in high-functioning autism and Asperger's syndrome*. Paper presented at the biennial meeting of the Society for Research and Child Development, Minneapolis, MN.

Stern, J. S., & Robertson, M. M. (1997). Tics associated with autistic and pervasive developmental disorders. *Neurologic Clinics, 15,* 345–355.

Szatmari, P. (1991). Asperger's syndrome: Diagnosis, treatment, and outcome. *Psychiatric Clinics of North America, 14,* 81–93.

Szatmari, P. (1996). Asperger's disorder and atypical pervasive developmental disorder. In F. R. Volkmar (Ed.), *Psychoses and pervasive developmental disorders in childhood and adolescence* (pp. 191–221). Washington, DC: American Psychiatric Publishing.

Tidmarsh, L., & Volkmar, F. R. (2003). Diagnosis and epidemiology of autism spectrum disorders. *Canadian Journal of Psychiatry, 48,* 517–525.

Tonge, B. J., Brereton, A. V., Gray, K. M., & Einfield, S. I. (1999). Behavioral and emotional disturbance in high-functioning autism and Asperger syndrome. *Autism, 3,* 117–130.

Towbin, K. E., Mauk, J. E., & Batshaw, M. L. (2002). Pervasive developmental disorders. In M. L. Batshaw (Ed.), *Children with disabilities* (5th ed., pp. 365–387). Baltimore: Brookes Publishing.

Trottier, G., Srivastava, L., & Walker, C. D. (1999). Etiology of infantile autism: A review of recent advances in genetic and neurobiological research. *Journal of Psychiatry and Neuroscience, 24,* 103–115.

Tsai, L. Y. (1998). *Briefing paper: Pervasive developmental disorders.* Washington, DC: National Dissemination Center for Children With Disabilities.

Tuchman, R. F., & Rapin, I. (1997). Regression in pervasive developmental disorders: Seizures and epileptiform electroencephalogram correlates. *Pediatrics, 88,* 1211–1218.

Turner, M. (1999). Annotation: Repetitive behavior in autism: A review of psychological research. *Journal of Child Psychology and Psychiatry, 40,* 839–849.

Volkmar, F. R. (1996). The disintegrative disorders: Childhood disintegrative disorder and Rett's disorder. In F. R. Volkmar (Ed.), *Psychoses and pervasive developmental disorders in childhood and adolescence* (pp. 223–248). Washington, DC: American Psychiatric Publishing.

Volkmar, F. R., & Klin, A. (2000). Diagnostic issues in Asperger syndrome. In A. Klin, F. R. Volkmar, & S. S. Sparrow (Eds.), *Asperger syndrome* (pp. 25–71). New York: Guilford Press.

Volkmar, F. R., Klin, A., Marans, W. D., & McDougle, C. J. (1996). Autistic disorder. In F. R. Volkmar (Ed.), *Psychoses and pervasive developmental disorders in childhood and adolescence* (pp. 129–190). Washington, DC: American Psychiatric Publishing.

Wing, L. (1981). Asperger's syndrome: A clinical account. *Psychological Medicine, 11,* 115–129.

World Health Organization. (1993). *International classification of diseases* (10th rev.). Geneva, Switzerland: Author.

Zisserman, L. (1991). The effects of deep pressure on self-stimulating behaviors in a child with autism and other disabilities. *American Journal of Occupational Therapy, 46,* 547–551.

14

RESPIRATORY IMPAIRMENTS

MELISSA A. BRAY, THOMAS J. KEHLE,
LEA A. THEODORE, AND HEATHER L. PECK

This chapter provides an overview of asthma, bronchitis, pneumonia, pneumococcal pneumonia, croup, cystic fibrosis, tonsillitis, and the common cold. Medical, behavioral, and educational consequences are outlined. Medical and psychoeducational preventative measures and treatment options are also provided for the disorders.

OVERVIEW

Respiratory disorders minimally include asthma, bronchitis, pneumonia, croup, cystic fibrosis, tonsillitis, and common colds. Agrawal, David, and Harris (2003) noted that approximately 50% of symptomatic infants could be classified in accordance with textbook criteria for the diagnoses of varied respiratory disorders. Among the major disease groups, chronic respiratory impairments rank fifth in prevalence (Ward, Javitz, Smith, & Whan, 2002). Although heritability estimates are associated with most chronic respiratory impairments, lung development is also particularly susceptible to numerous insults during pregnancy and the first few years of life. Therefore, environmental insults are likely to exacerbate genetic predisposition for respiratory impairments, and together they may be the etiology of a substantial proportion of later respiratory impairments and diseases (Merkus, 2003).

Asthma is a chronic respiratory disease characterized by obstruction of the airways, tissue inflammation, congestion, muscle constriction, and airway irritability that results in coughing, wheezing, and shortness of breath (National Heart, Lung, & Blood Institute, 1997). Persistent asthma is defined as one of the following occurring during a 1-year period: (a) the need for asthmatic medication on four or more occasions, (b) one or more emergency room visits for which asthma was the primary problem, (c) one or more hospital admissions for asthma, and (d) at least one or more ambulatory visits for asthma and two occasions requiring medication (Fuhlbrigge et al., 2005). The causes of asthmatic attacks include viral infections, allergies, airborne irritants, strenuous exercise, weather and temperature fluctuations, and emotional reactions. Particularly noteworthy is that since the early 1980s, asthma rates in children have steadily increased and currently may affect as many as 7% of American children (Mingroni, 2004). Furthermore, asthma, AIDS, and tuberculosis are the only chronic illnesses that have been recently associated with increasing death rates.

Bronchitis is a swelling of the bronchi or bronchial tubes that causes reduced air flow to the lungs and severe mucous. Chronic bronchitis includes a mucous-laden cough most every day for at least 3 months of the year in 2 consecutive years in the absence of another cause for the cough. Chronic bronchitis, which may be accompanied with emphysema, can reoccur for 2 years or more (Haas, 2000). Acute bronchitis is typically a brief episode caused by a virus that attacks the bronchial tubes that carry air through the trachea (windpipe) to the lungs. Bacterial infections that cause bronchitis are rare. The tubes become inflamed and mucous builds up, leading to coughing, difficult breathing, and often an accompanying cold. Individuals with heart disease experience relatively more severe bronchitis that can develop into pneumonia. Interestingly, fever is not a usual symptom of this disorder. It can last from 3 days to several months. Children younger than 2 years may be more susceptible to this disorder (usually acute in nature) in the late winter and early spring, and it usually lasts approximately 2 weeks. Typically, children will begin with a dry cough, runny nose, wheezing, and rapid breathing. These symptoms often occur after the child has had a cold. The incidence rate of acute bronchitis in the United States within any particular year is approximately 5%; however, it is diagnosed most often in preschool children. The incidence rate in children younger than 5 years is approximately 11%. Individuals with recurrent episodes of acute bronchitis often are eventually diagnosed as having asthma. A physician should be contacted immediately if the child is breathing very fast (i.e., more than 40 breaths in 1 minute), cannot talk or swallow, looks blue, is visibly moving his or her ribs when breathing, is coughing with a barking noise, has chest pain, is vomiting, is 3 months or younger, or has a preexisting heart disease.

Pneumonia is an inflammation of the lungs that can be caused by viruses, bacteria, and, at times, fungi. The swelling is the immune system's response to an infection. Lung tissue can fill with pus or mucous. Cough, fever, and difficult breathing are the main symptoms. The most common causes of pneumonia are viruses including influenza and adenovirus. With regard to young children, respiratory syncytial virus is a common cause. Less common, but more serious, than viral pneumonia is that caused by the *Streptococcus pneumoniae* bacteria (AlonsoDeVelasco, Verheul, Verhoef, & Snippe, 1995). The term *double pneumonia* refers to both lungs being affected and *walking pneumonia* refers to a mild case. Furthermore, pneumonia combined with influenza is the fifth leading cause of death in the United States. With respect to ethnic minorities, Native American children are particularly susceptible to the disease with an incidence rate 5 to 10 times that of Caucasians. Also, African Americans have an incidence rate 3 times higher than that of Caucasians.

Pneumococcal pneumonia is a lung infection caused by the *S. pneumoniae* bacterium, which typically affects children under age 2 years and adults over age 65. The infection can affect the blood (i.e., bacteremia), lungs, middle ear (i.e., otitis media), eyes ("pink eye"—bacterial conjunctivitis), and the nervous system (i.e., meningitis). It is contagious, and the mechanism of contacting the disease is similar to that of the common cold in that it initially invades the upper respiratory tract (i.e., pharynx, larynx, and nasal passages) through physical contact or inhalation of infected droplets. Approximately one third of individuals who are infected with *S. pneumoniae* eventually develop the serious health threat of bacteremia, which is the fifth leading cause of death in the United States. Symptoms include high fever, cough, shortness of breath, rapid breathing, and chest pains. Following antibiotic treatment, symptoms usually decrease or become nonexistent within 12 to 36 hours. Overuse of antibiotics increases the probability of the bacteria becoming resistant to treatment, however (AlonsoDeVelasco et al., 1995). Symptoms of viral pneumonia are similar to pneumococcal pneumonia and include fever, coughing, rapid and difficult breathing, chest or abdominal pain, loss of appetite, vomiting, and physical exhaustion. The symptoms associated with viral pneumonia typically appear more gradually, however, and are less severe than those associated with bacteria-based pneumococcal pneumonia.

Croup is a term that encompasses several illnesses (i.e., laryngotracheobronchitis, laryngotracheobronchopneumonia, and spasmodic croup) that infect the larynx, trachea, and bronchi (Knutson & Aring, 2004). This upper airway obstruction is usually preceded by low-grade fever progressing to the characteristic barking cough often accompanied by other symptoms such as hoarseness, dyspnea, stridor, and wheezing (Knutson & Aring, 2004). These symptoms tend to become more pronounced during the night and peak within 1 or 2 days. Typically the duration of croup is less than a week (Knutson & Aring, 2004). Croup is most common between ages 6 months and 4 years. The causes of croup are infection, trauma, or aspiration. Children with croup should receive prompt attention and appropriate management because certain symptoms can quickly progress to a life-threatening level (Hammer, 2004). Croup is one of the most common respiratory impairments in infants and young children. The annual incidence rate is approximately 6% in children younger than 6 years (Ausejo et al., 1999), and approximately 2% to 6% of these children require hospitalization. As such, croup is the leading cause of hospitalizations of preschool children (Knutson & Aring, 2004). Severe croup is marked by extreme difficulty in breathing, high-pitched vocal noises, rapid breathing, and pale or bluish skin tone. If there is a probability for respiratory failure, the definitive diagnostic procedure that should have priority involves airway protection and endoscopy (Hammer, 2004).

Cystic fibrosis is a genetic condition that causes thick mucous to be formed in the lungs. This can cause lung infections and pancreas obstruction. The condition requires a recessive gene for the disorder from each parent, in which case there is a 25% chance in each pregnancy that the child will have the disease. It occurs in approximately 1 in 3,200 live births. Cystic fibrosis is most common in people of northern and western European descent. Symptoms can vary, but most typically include salty skin, coughing, shortness of breath, poor weight gain, and greasy bowl movements. The condition is diagnosed via a sweat test looking for high salt levels.

The tonsils are tissue clusters at the back of the throat. Tonsillitis is inflammation of the tonsils, usually because of an infection (bacterial or viral). Whether an infection is bacterial or viral can be determined with a throat culture. The tonsils become large, red, and coated with mucous. In children, the condition usually starts with a sore throat, pain while swallowing, swollen glands, and lack of appetite. In infants, difficulty feeding, fever, and runny nose are more common. It is contagious; if caused by the common Group A streptococci, incubation is from 2 to 7 days. Parents should take precautions to prevent spreading the condition. Keep glasses and towels separate, wash hands frequently, and keep the child somewhat isolated from others in the home. Typically, tonsillitis will last for 1 week with treatment but may take many weeks for the swelling of glands and tonsils to subside.

Common colds are the most frequent respiratory infection in humans (Wat, 2004). Although there are more than 200 viruses that can infect the nasal cells, rhinovirus is most common (Wat, 2004). The body reacts with inflammation, which results in sneezing and coughing. Furthermore, fever, nasal discharge, stuffiness, swelling of the sinuses, sore throat, and headache typically accompany the cold. As indicated by Wat, diagnosis of the common cold is not straightforward because it is based on assessment of clinical symptoms that are similar to those associated with pharyngitis and bronchitis. In addition, allergen insults of the upper airways also have symptoms similar to that of the common cold. Finally, young children have difficulty expressing their symptoms to the physician, making it difficult to distinguish between relatively benign viral infections and severe invasive bacterial infections. The duration of the cold is typically 1 to 2 weeks. Because of their underdeveloped immune systems, children are more susceptible to colds and typically have 6 to 10 episodes per year. Regardless of their benign nature, the common cold is a major cause of mortality throughout the world (Wat, 2004). Several myths surround the causes of contacting a cold, such as being exposed to cold weather, overheating, exercising, inappropriate diet, or enlarged tonsils and adenoids.

OUTCOMES

In addition to absences from school and restriction of physical activities, asthma is also associated with relatively poor social relationships (de Mesquita & Fiorello, 1998), higher incidences of behavioral problems, lower self-esteem (Vila, Nollet-Clemencon, deBlic, Mouren-Simeoni, & Scheinmann, 2000), depression, and mood disorders (Chaney et al., 1999; Miller & Wood, 1994). Children with asthma also tend to be more fatigued, feel relatively more hopeless and worthless (Lehrer, Feldman, Giardino, Song, & Schmaling, 2002), and express a diminished sense of well-being in contrast to their peers (Bray et al., 2003). Furthermore, approximately 40% of children with asthma evidence both anxiety disorders and clinically significant psychological stressors (Vila et al., 2000). In addition to exacerbating asthmatic symptoms and triggering attacks, anxiety and stress may also function to increase their susceptibility to other respiratory illnesses (Cohen, Tyrell, & Smith, 1991).

Children with other respiratory impairments such as bronchitis, pneumonia, croup, tonsillitis, and common colds may evidence similar psychological problems as children with asthma. Because of the relatively brief duration of these respiratory illnesses, the psychological problems would most probably be less severe. For example, children with bronchitis, colds, and croup will probably be sick for a week; children with pneumonia typically are on antibiotic therapy for 3 to 5 days; and children with tonsillitis will most likely be ill for at least 1 to 2 weeks. Generally, any restriction of physical activities, together with the physical symptoms associated with the respiratory illness, may also increase the probability of depression accompanied with abridgement of peer and social interactions, threats to self-esteem, feelings of incompetence, and sense of loss of personal control (Kehle & Bray, 2004).

MEDICAL AND PSYCHOEDUCATIONAL IMPLICATIONS

Preventative Measures

There are preventative interventions that, to varying degrees, reduce the severity or probability of contacting respiratory impairments. One such intervention involves the reduction of indoor home and school-based air pollutants. It is obvious that tobacco smoke should not be allowed in any closed setting. It is also widely known that dust, aerosol products, inhalation of dusting powder or talc, household chemical cleaners, and fireplace smoke can all be particularly irritating to children with respiratory impairments. Less obvious pollutants are bathroom fumes, molds, and mildew, along with the chemical substances used to clean bathrooms. These are particularly problematic in settings that do not have exhaust fans, a common situation in school restrooms. These fumes can be the source of considerable irritation to children with respiratory problems. Another less obvious source of pollution is household plants that can be a major source of mold, a common irritant.

Transmission and spread of respiratory viruses and bacteria can be attenuated primarily by controlling contact with noninfected individuals. For example, rhinovirus, the virus most associated with the common cold, is spread primarily by touching contaminated skin or surface areas. Depending on the length of time of exposure, rhinovirus can also be transmitted by infected children through the air and by infected respiratory secretions (Wat, 2004). In both cases, close contact with an infected classmate would greatly increase the probability of transmission. The mechanism of contacting pneumococcal pneumonia is similar to that of the common cold in that it initially invades, through physical contact or inhaling infected droplets, the upper respiratory tract (i.e., pharynx, larynx, and nasal passages).

Wat (2004) suggested that knowledge of some broad generalizations regarding seasonal variation in incidence of various viral and bacterial infections may be helpful in planning control strategies. For example, it is apparent that common cold epidemics tend to occur during the early autumn and late spring months. "The reservoir for rhinovirus is school children, who transmit rhinovirus infections among their peers and infect other family members at home" (Wat, 2004, p. 80). In autumn, the rhinovirus is responsible for approximately 80% of all upper respiratory illness (Arruda, Pitkaranta, Witek, Doyle, & Hayden, 1997). Nevertheless, we are unaware of any alternation of the school academic year calendar as a specific strategy to attenuate the relatively high rate of transmission during these months.

Treatment Alternatives

Treatment of respiratory impairments should include not only pharmacological and medical interventions but also sensitivity to the beneficial effects of psychological interventions.

Medical Treatments

Generally, two categories of medications are used to treat asthma. These include "controllers," or antiinflammatory drugs (corticosteroids), and "relievers," or bronchodilators (beta-adrenergic receptor agonists). The antiinflammatory drugs are typically used for prevention of asthmatic attacks and maintenance of normal lung functioning, whereas bronchodilators are used as a rescue medication for sudden attacks (Berkow, 1997). The most common reliever is albuterol, which dilates the airways.

The controllers function as preventive medications designed to attenuate symptoms and are typically taken on a daily basis. Therefore, regardless of the presence of any symptoms, children with asthma are generally required to inhale corticosteroids twice daily. Preventative controllers can also be ingested in the form of a tablet. Because the controllers tend not to have an immediate effect on sudden episodes, fidelity to the twice-daily treatment regimen is often compromised. The treatment regimen should be associated with other daily tasks such as morning and evening teeth brushing to help the child remember the routine. Regimented corticosteroid treatment is vital in that it is the only known medication that actually heals the existing airway inflammation. Inflammation causes swelling, mucus, and potential thickening of the airway linings, resulting in possible permanent deleterious effects on pulmonary function (Adams, Fuhlbrigge, & Finkelstein, 2001).

The appropriate treatment or management of acute bronchitis continues to be controversial; however, addressing the symptoms remains the most common therapeutic intervention (Gwynne & Newton, 2004). The majority of cases of acute bronchitis are caused by viruses, and consequently antibiotics are not an informed choice of treatment. Although antibiotics have not been shown to be efficacious in the treatment of acute bronchitis, survey results indicate that approximately 80% of adults continue to be treated with such medication. According to Nash, Harman, Wald, and Kelleher (2002), antibiotic prescribing for children with bronchitis is also still common but is slowly declining. In addition to not being efficacious, overuse of antibiotic medication may contribute to the development of drug-resistant organisms.

The use of infant or children's acetaminophen (e.g., Tylenol) is recommended if the child has a fever. Pain relievers can be used for sore throats, and cough suppressants are available to reduce coughing.

A recent study reported by Gwynne and Newton (2004) suggested that an extract derived from *Pelargonium sidoides* (geranium root) had a substantial effect on the reduction of severity and duration of symptoms associated with acute bronchitis. The extract resulted in few, if any, side effects. Additionally, encouraging the child to drink liquids to prevent dehydration, use a cool mist vaporizer, take a fever-reducing medication (not aspirin), or inhale hot steam helps to improve breathing. Exposure to secondhand smoke should be reduced as much as possible because it can exacerbate the bronchitis. Bronchodilators (e.g., inhalers) may also be prescribed in an attempt to open the airways. Because bronchitis and the common cold are spread in like ways, similar precautions should be taken to prevent bronchitis from spreading (e.g., washing hands, keeping towels separate, isolation of the ill child from other children).

Treatment recommendations for less severe cases of acute pneumonia include a 3-day course of amoxicillin or trimethoprim-sulfamethoxazole oral antibiotics. This finding is based on a large sample double-blind experimental study conducted by Walling (2002) that examined children aged 2 to 5 years with nonsevere pneumonia who took 15 mg/kg of oral amoxicillin every 8 hours for 3 days. For the last 2 of the 5 days, the control group was given a placebo, and the experimental group continued taking amoxicillin. The authors concluded that 3-day treatment was as effective as 5-day treatment with respect to respiratory rate, wheezing, and chest radiography results.

A pneumococcal conjugate vaccine (PCV7, Prevnar) is also available. It is recommended for individuals over age 65, children under 2 years, and for those with lowered immune systems (American Academy of Pediatrics, 2000). Because many of the *S. pneumoniae* bacteria are resistant to some antibiotics, the disease is becoming more difficult to treat (American Academy of Pediatrics, 2000).

In mild cases of croup, home-based treatments consisting of the use of a cool mist vaporizer, sleeping in cool night air, taking a hot steam shower, and drinking plenty of cold liquids have long been popular and effective treatments. Cough suppressants can be of some aid as well. For children 1 year and older, use of cold fluids such as water, juice, Jell-O water, 7-Up, Sprite, ginger ale, lemonade, or Kool-Aid and frozen popsicles may help as well. Children with croup tend to want to sit, or to be held, in an upright position. Agitation and crying, not uncommon with ill children, may exacerbate the symptoms (Knutson & Aring, 2004).

Generally, croup has an excellent prognosis in that the disease is usually self-limiting (Knutson & Aring, 2004); however, children with a history of croup may have an increased risk for developing asthma (Castro-Rodriguez et al., 2001). A physician should be consulted if the child's symptoms are not reduced after treatment or if he or she has difficulty swallowing, is drooling, has throat pain, has a fever 102° or above, has rapid breathing (> 40 breaths/minute for a child younger than 3 months old, > 30 breaths/minute over 3 months old), wheezing, difficulty breathing, looks blue around mouth or fingernails, or is restless or exhausted.

The use of corticosteroids has been the preferred treatment in moderate to severe cases of croup. Corticosteroid treatment, compared with placebo, typically reduces hospitalizations, duration of the illness, and subsequent need for treatments (Rittichier, 2004). According to Rittichier, although nebulized budesonide is effective, it is often not used in place of oral corticosteroids. Although controversy exists as to whether mild cases of croup should be treated with corticosteroids, some clinicians use it to treat all cases of croup, regardless of the degree of severity. Corticosteroids have gained universal acceptance because they are effective, well tolerated, and inexpensive (Rittichier, 2004).

Cystic fibrosis is not curable, but it is treatable. Lung symptoms are most commonly treated with physical or respiratory therapy. This treatment primarily includes clearing the lungs of the mucus. Antibiotics are used to fight lung infections. Individuals with cystic fibrosis may enjoy relatively normal and productive adult lives. As they age, however, other problems may occur, such as osteoporosis and reproductive disorders.

Antibiotics are the treatment of choice for bacterial tonsillitis. In addition, altering the child's diet to include foods that are easily swallowed (e.g., soups, ice cream, etc.), drinking plenty of fluids, encouraging gargling with salty water, use of cool mist vaporizer for sore throat, wearing a warm towel about the neck to reduce the swelling of glands, and monitoring fever all tend to reduce the symptoms and facilitate recovery.

If a child has several episodes of tonsillitis, approximately seven in 1 year or five in 2 years, a tonsillectomy may be advised. This is a common procedure, but recently medical professionals are questioning its worth because of the observation that there is little or no therapeutic impact for the procedures. For example, there are no differences in the recurrence of fever and infections between children who have the surgery and those who do not. Several fiction books describe the condition and treatment to children (e.g., Leigh & Fox, 2002).

The common cold, particularly for school children, is a debilitating and contagious disease that interferes with students' social and academic functioning. Prevention in the home setting includes frequent hand washing, avoidance of individuals with colds, and structuring the home environment to ensure that each child has his or her own towels and drinking glasses. The obvious preventative school-based strategy would be not to allow an infected child to attend school for the duration of the cold. The majority of school systems have no policy on preventing children with colds from attending school, however. Furthermore, working parents, and particularly working single parents, often are unwilling to have their children stay out of school given the difficulty and expense associated with requesting a week's leave from their jobs.

The most irritating symptoms of a cold are nasal discharge and stuffiness (Wat, 2004). The irritation is somewhat exacerbated in young children who have not yet developed effective "nose blowing" techniques. With younger infected children who continue to attend school, some school systems have attempted to teach them to sneeze or cough into the crevice of their bent arms in a relatively ineffective attempt to reduce the possibility of transmission of the cold to their classmates.

The development of a vaccine for rhinovirus is unlikely in that it has more than 100 serotypes (Wat, 2004). Using interferon in the nose appears to have some preventative value, however, reducing the probability of contracting a cold by approximately 40% (Wat, 2004). A relatively new finding with respect to prevention of the common cold involves the daily ingestion of vitamin E. Although the research is limited, it appears that vitamin E may strengthen the immune system (Meydani et al., 2004).

To facilitate recovery, parents should encourage bed rest, drinking of fluids, gargling with warm salt water, and the use of non-aspirin-based fever reducers. Antiviral treatment alone may not be sufficient to address successfully the inflammation of the pathways. According to Wat (2004), because reliable and effective treatments are not yet available, the only remaining treatment strategy is to focus on alleviating the symptoms. Wat noted, however, that further research on host inflammatory response along with the use of combination therapies may prove to be efficacious in long-term treatment.

Although unnecessary antibiotic treatment should be avoided, occasionally the common cold can result in a secondary sinus or middle ear infection. In these cases, which can result in high fevers, glandular swelling, facial pain, and a severe cough, antibiotic treatment may be warranted. Treatment myths include the use of vitamin C and inhalation of steam, which have not been shown to ease the common cold.

Psychoeducational Treatments

The field of psychoneuroimmunology (PNI) examines the multidirectional relationships among the psychological, neurological, and immune systems. Although the precise mechanisms are not known, it appears that an individual's perceived stress or anxiety is communicated biochemically to his or her immune cells via neuropeptides (Dunn, 1996). Therefore, stressors with accompanying psychopathologies such as depression or anxiety directly affect biological processes and increase disease risk. As Pert (1986) explained, "indeed, the more we know about neuropeptides, the harder it is to think in the traditional terms of a mind and a body. It makes more and more sense to speak of a single integrated entity, a bodymind" (p. 9).

In accord with PNI, interventions that promote mental health simultaneously promote physical health. The definition of mental health, according to Kehle and Bray (2004) and as expressed in Bertrand Russell's (1930) *Conquest of Happiness*, is synonymous with a sense of well-being or happiness and encompasses a realization of competence, intimacy or friendship formation, autonomy or a sense of independence, and physical health. It is increasingly clear that a sense of well-being or happiness that includes components of independence, intimacy, and competence are protective of both psychological and physical health. According to Kehle and Bray, the definition of each is derived from the other three. These components have also been shown to be inversely related to anxiety and depression (Kehle & Bray, 2004). Furthermore, interventions designed to promote any one of these four components also enhance the remaining three, and the converse is also true. Simply stated, a happy individual is more likely to be physically healthier, and this relationship is bidirectional (Kehle & Bray, 2004; Seligman, Steen, Park, & Peterson, 2005).

Based on this reasoning, although the research is limited, asthma, bron-chitis, pneumonia, croup, cystic fibrosis, tonsillitis, and the common cold are all medical conditions that may benefit from interventions designed to pro-mote psychological wellness. The following example of asthma was selected to illustrate the mind–body connection because of its ample research base.

Psychologically based treatments for asthma have included family therapy, biofeedback, yoga, hypnosis, stress management, relaxation tech-niques, relaxation techniques combined with guided imagery (RGI), and written-emotional expression (WEE; Bray, Kehle, Theodore, Zhou, & Peck, 2004). Most of these treatments use strategies that are either directly or indirectly related to Kehle and Bray's (2004) definition of psychological well-being or happiness. For example, Peck, Bray, and Kehle's (2003) treat-ment focused on helping middle school children with asthma establish a sense of control over their lung functioning (forced expiratory volume in 1 second [FEV_1] and forced expiratory flow 25–75 [FEF_{25-75}]) through the use of RGI. RGI required the children to engage in relaxation exercises while simultaneously imagining internal healing specific to improving lung func-tion. The results of Peck et al.'s (2003) investigation indicated that the ef-fect of RGI on lung functioning and anxiety was substantial with most of the children. It was found that FEV_1 improved and anxiety decreased in all stu-dents, whereas, FEF_{25-75} improved in 3 of 4 participants. The effect sizes were impressive and ranged from –0.98 to –1.88 for FEV_1, 0.20 to –1.93 for FEF_{25-75} (negative effects demonstrated improved lung function), and 2.19 to 4.06 for anxiety.

Correspondingly, Castes et al. (1999) reported the results of a multicom-ponent intervention for children with asthma that combined RGI, education about asthma, and self-esteem workshops. The experimental group children indicated significant improvement in lung function, immunological function-ing, reduced asthmatic episodes, and decreased need for medication.

As would be predicted by Kehle and Bray (2004), improvement in the children's general health as evidenced by improved lung functioning also was accompanied by positive effects on their sense of well-being or happi-ness. In the Peck et al. (2003) study, the children's anxiety was also substan-tially diminished. Similarly, Slater (1993) found that RGI improved lung function and also reduced anxiety. Furthermore, Freeman's (1998) use of RGI resulted not only in better lung function but also a decrease in the sever-ity of symptoms, decreased anxiety, increased self-efficacy, and a trend to-ward improved peak flow outcomes.

It has also been suggested that writing about past emotionally trau-matic episodes can not only change cognitions but may also result in improv-ing physical health (Klein & Boals, 2001; Smyth, 1998; Smyth, Stone, Hurewitz, & Kaell, 1999). Using WEE, the individual spends 10 to 20 min-utes daily writing about upsetting, stressful, or distressing past experiences. With respect to improving general physical health, Smyth (1998) and Smyth et al. (1999) noted the WEE resulted in decreased medical visits, improvement of the immune system, and increased feelings of subjective well-being.

Interventions based on WEE have been shown to improve lung function in adults (Smyth et al., 1999), adolescents and college students (Bray et al., 2003), and elementary school children (Bray et al., 2004). The results of the Bray et al. (2004) study indicated that the WEE intervention improved both the children's lung functioning and perceptions of quality of life. With respect to lung functioning, the effect sizes were large, ranging from −1.14 to −1.44 (negative effects demonstrated improved lung function) and, with one exception, were maintained at follow-up. Furthermore, the intervention is well suited for use in schools because it is relatively easy to implement, in addition to being time- and cost-efficient.

Children with cystic fibrosis typically have difficulty initiating and maintaining friendship because of their relative small stature, immature development, and lack of participation in physical activities. Pyschoeducational treatments designed for children with cystic fibrosis focus primarily on friendship formation through techniques such as social skills training, peer counseling, and anxiety reduction (Clark, Striefel, Bedlington, & Naimon, 1989).

CONCLUSION

Children with respiratory impairments, in addition to experiencing debilitating physical symptoms, absences from school, and restrictions of physical activities, may also evidence psychological problems. In addition to pharmacological and medical interventions, prevention and treatment of respiratory impairments should include psychological interventions that promote happiness or well-being. These include strategies to promote children's sense of independence or personal control, feelings of competence, and intimacy or friendship formation. Happiness is postulated to be defined by these characteristics and is synonymous with psychological health, which in turn is protective of physical health.

REFERENCES

Adams, R., Fuhlbrigge, A., & Finkelstein, J. (2001). Use of inhaled anti-inflammatory medication in children with asthma in managed care settings. *Archives of Pediatric Adolescent Medicine, 155,* 501–507.

Agrawal, V., David, R. J., & Harris, V. J. (2003). Classification of acute respiratory disorders of all newborns in a tertiary care center. *Journal of the National Medical Association, 95,* 585–595.

AlonsoDeVelasco, E., Verheul, A., Verhoef, J., & Snippe, H. (1995). *Streptococcus pneumoniae:* Virulence factors, pathogenesis, and vaccines. *Microbiology, 59,* 591–603.

American Academy of Pediatrics, Committee on Infectious Diseases. (2000). Policy statement: Recommendation for the prevention of pneumococcal infections, including the use of Prevnar, pneumococcal polysaccharide vaccine, and antibiotic prophylaxis. *Journal of Pediatrics, 106*, 362–366.

Arruda, E., Pitkaranta, A., Witek, T. J., Doyle, C. A., & Hayden, F. G. (1997). Frequency and natural history of rhinovirus infections in adults during autumn. *Journal of Clinical Microbiology, 11*, 2864–2868.

Ausejo, M., Saenz, A., Pham, B., Kellner, J. D., Johnson, D. W., & Moher, D. (1999). The effectiveness of glucocorticoids in treating croup: Meta-analysis. *British Medical Journal, 319*, 595–600.

Berkow, R., (Ed.). (1997). *Merck manual of medical information.* New York: Pocket Books.

Bray, M. A., Kehle, T. J., Theodore, L. A., Zhou, Z., & Peck, H. L. (2004). Enhancing subjective well-being in individuals with asthma. *Psychology in the Schools, 41*, 95–100.

Bray, M. A., Theodore, L. A., Patwa, S. S., Margiano, S., Alric, J., & Peck, H. (2003). Written emotional expression as an intervention for asthma. *Psychology in the Schools, 40*, 193–207.

Castes, M., Hagel, I., Palenque, M., Canelones, P., Corao, A., & Lynch, N. R. (1999). Immunological changes associated with clinical improvement of asthmatic children subjected to psychosocial intervention. *Brain, Behavior, and Immunity, 13*, 1–13.

Castro-Rodriguez, J. A., Holberg, C. J., Morgan, W. J., Wright, A. L., Holonen, M., Taussig, L. M., et al. (2001). Relation of two different sub-types of croup before age three to wheezing, atopy, and pulmonary function during childhood: A prospective study. *Pediatrics, 107*, 512–518.

Chaney, J., Mullins, L., Uretsky, D., Pace, T., Werden, D., & Hartman, V. (1999). An experimental examination of learned helplessness in older adolescents and young adults with long-standing asthma. *Journal of Pediatric Psychology, 24*, 259–270.

Clark, H., Striefel, S., Bedlington, M., & Naimon, D. (1989). A social skills developmental model: Coping strategies for children with chronic illnesses. *Children's Health Care, 18*, 19–29.

Cohen, S., Tyrell, D., & Smith, A. (1991). Psychological stress in humans in susceptibility to the common cold. *New England Journal of Medicine, 325*, 606–612.

de Mesquita, P. B., & Fiorello, C. A. (1998). Asthma (childhood). In L. Phelps (Ed.), *Health-related disorders in children and adolescents* (pp. 74–81). Washington, DC: American Psychological Association.

Dunn, A. (1996). Psychoneuroimmunology, stress, and infection. In H. Friedman, T. W. Klein, & A. Friedman (Eds.), *Psychoneuroimmunology and infection* (pp. 25–46). Boca Raton, FL: CRC Press.

Freeman, L. W. (1998). Effects of a comprehensive psychoneuroimmunological program on asthma symptoms and mood states in adult asthmatic patients (Doctoral dissertation, Saybrook Institute, 1997). *Dissertation Abstracts International,* 58(11-B), 6221.

Fuhlbrigge, A. L., Carey, V. J., Finkelstein, J. A., Lozano, P., Inui, T. S., Weiss, S., & Weiss, K. B. (2005). Validity of the HEDIS criteria to identify children with persistent asthma and sustained high utilization. *American Journal of Managed Care, 11,* 325–330.

Gwynne, M., & Newton, W. (2004). Geranium extract reduces bronchitis symptoms. *Journal of Family Practice, 53,* 180–181.

Haas, F. (2000). *The chronic bronchitis and emphysema handbook.* New York: Wiley.

Hammer, J. (2004). Acquired upper airway obstruction. *Pediatric Respiratory Review, 5,* 25–33.

Kehle, T. J., & Bray, M. A. (2004). RICH Theory: The promotion of happiness. *Psychology in the Schools, 41,* 43–49.

Klein, K., & Boals, A. (2001). Expressive writing can increase working memory capacity. *Journal of Experimental Psychology, 130,* 520–533.

Knutson, D., & Aring, A. (2004). Viral croup (Practical Therapeutics). *American Family Physician, 69,* 535–540.

Lehrer, P., Feldman, J., Giardino, H., Song, H., & Schmaling, K. (2002). Psychological aspects of asthma. *Journal of Consulting and Clinical Psychology, 70,* 691–711.

Leigh, J., & Fox, W. (2002). *Harriet has tonsillitis.* New York: Red Kite Books.

Merkus, P. J. (2003). Effects of childhood respiratory diseases on the anatomical and functional development of the respiratory system. *Pediatric Respiratory Review, 4,* 28–39.

Meydani, S. N., Leka, L. S., Fine, B. C., Dallal, G. E., Keusch, G. T., Singh, M. F., & Hamer, D. H. (2004). Vitamin E and respiratory tract infections in elderly nursing home residents. *Journal of the American Medical Association, 292,* 828–836.

Miller, B. D., & Wood, B. L. (1994). Psychophysiologic reactivity in asthmatic children: A cholinergically mediated confluence of pathways. *Journal of the American Academy of Adolescent Psychiatry, 33,* 1236–1245.

Mingroni, M. A. (2004). The secular rise in IQ: Giving heterosis a closer look. *Intelligence, 32,* 65–83.

Nash, D. R., Harman, J., Wald, E. R., & Kelleher, K. J. (2002). Antibiotic prescribing by primary care physicians for children with upper respiratory tract infections. *Archives of Pediatrics & Adolescent Medicine, 156,* 1114–1119.

National Heart, Lung, and Blood Institute. (1997). *Guidelines for the diagnosis and management of asthma: Expert panel report 2* (NIH Publication No. 97-4051). Bethesda, MD: Author.

Peck, H. L., Bray, M. A., & Kehle, T. J. (2003). Relaxation and guided imagery: A school-based intervention for children with asthma. *Psychology in the Schools, 40,* 657–675.

Pert, C. B. (1986). The wisdom of the receptors: Neuropeptides, the emotions, and bodymind. *Advances, 3,* 8–16.

Rittichier, K. K. (2004). The role of corticosteroids in the treatment of croup. *Treatments in Respiratory Medicine, 3,* 139–145.

Russell, B. (1930). *The conquest of happiness.* New York: Liveright.

Seligman, M. E., Steen, T., Park, N., & Peterson, C. (2005). Positive psychology progress: Empirical validation of interventions. *American Psychologist, 60,* 410–421.

Slater, S. B. (1993). Relaxation training as an adjunctive treatment for asthma (Doctoral dissertation, Yeshiva University, 1992). *Dissertation Abstracts International, 54,* 3330.

Smyth, J. M. (1998). Written emotional expression: Effect sizes, outcome types, and moderating variables. *Journal of Consulting Clinical Psychology, 66,* 174–184.

Smyth, J. M., Stone, A. A., Hurewitz, A., & Kaell, A. (1999). Effects of writing about stressful experiences on symptom reduction in patients with asthma or rheumatoid arthritis. *Journal of the American Medical Association, 281,* 1304–1309.

Vila, G., Nollet-Clemencon, C., deBlic, J., Mouren-Simeoni, M., & Scheinmann, P. (2000). Prevalence of DSM-IV anxiety and affective disorders in a pediatric population of asthmatic children and adolescents. *Journal of Affective Disorders, 58,* 223–231.

Walling, A. D. (2002). Pakistan multicentre amoxicillin short course therapy pneumonia study group: Clinical trial efficacy of 3 days versus 5 days of oral amoxicillin for treatment of childhood pneumonia using a multicentre double-blind trial. *Lancet, 360,* 835–841.

Ward, M. M., Javitz, H. S., Smith, W. M., & Whan, M. A. (2002). Lost income and work limitations in persons with chronic respiratory disorders. *Journal of Clinical Epidemiology, 55,* 260–268.

Wat, D. (2004). The common cold: A review of the literature. *European Journal of Internal Medicine, 15,* 79–88.

15

SEX CHROMOSOME ANOMALIES

DAVID L. WODRICH

OVERVIEW

This chapter is an overview of selected syndromes caused by anomalies in the distribution or functioning of either the X or Y chromosome. Turner syndrome, Klinefelter syndrome, fragile X syndrome, Lesch–Nyhan disease, and Lowe syndrome are reviewed (see Table 15.1). The chapter includes a synopsis of sex chromosomes, a brief description of some of the ways in which malfunctions occur, and a review of each disorder mentioned. Medical, socioemotional, behavioral, and educational consequences are provided for each disorder. Also included are treatment options, with emphasis on those supported by empirical data or endorsement by disorder-specific professional groups.

Most individuals are born with 46 chromosomes. Of these, 44 are auto-somes and two are sex chromosomes. Two X chromosomes result in a female infant, and an X and Y result in a male infant. Rarely, an extra or missing sex

The author would like to thank Saunder Bernes, MD, Department of Neurology at Phoenix Children's Hospital, for reviewing this chapter.

TABLE 15.1
Sex Chromosome Disorders

Disorder	Anomaly	Prevalence	Gender distribution	Effects
Fragile X syndrome	Faulty repeat of CGG sequence on X chromosome	1:4,000 males; 1:8,000 females	Both males and females	Extremely variable: includes mental retardation, autism, and subtle learning or emotional problems
Turner syndrome	Absence of X chromosome	1:2,000 to 1:5,000 females	Females only	Variable: short stature, absence of secondary sex characteristics, visuospatial and math problems
Klinefelter syndrome	Presence of one or more extra X chromosomes	1:800 males	Males only	Tall stature, lack of secondary sex characteristics, social and learning problems
Lesch–Nyhan	Faculty gene on the X chromosome	1:380,000 live births	Males only	Kidney disease, movement disorders, self-mutilation
Lowe syndrome	Faulty gene on X chromosome	Up to 1:100,000 males	Males only	Visual defects, kidney disease, seizures, and mental retardation

chromosome occurs, which results in an individual with a type of sex chromosome disorder. When an X is missing (XO), a girl with Turner syndrome is born. When an extra X chromosome is present (XXY), a boy with Klinefelter syndrome results. Sometimes a defect at a specific site on the X chromosome occurs. Because females have two X chromosomes (XX) to males' one (XY), this produces more conspicuous outcomes in boys than girls. More than 200 genes on the X chromosome are estimated to cause learning disabilities (Hagerman & Hagerman, 2002).

Unlike many of the medical conditions reviewed in this book (e.g., kidney disease, neurological impairment), genetic disorders may present with relatively subtle signs and symptoms. Accordingly, psychologists, not physicians, may first recognize the prospect of a syndrome, and their alert response may prompt a referral for a definitive medical diagnosis. Furthermore, because many interventions are behavioral and educational, psychologists may assume planning, advocacy, and psychotherapeutic roles as important as medical treatment. That is, psychologists may help assess neurocognitive, academic, and socioemotional dimensions and devise programs based on patterns of strengths and weaknesses. As various genetic disorders become better understood in coming years, programming will increasingly consider the particular vulnerabilities associated with each. Likewise, disorder-specific interventions at school and sensitivity to the challenges of parenting will be needed. Psychologists, as health care providers and behavioral scientists, may be uniquely qualified to help (Wodrich, 2004).

Turner Syndrome

Turner syndrome, a condition affecting 1 in 2,000 to 1 in 5,000 females, appears when a single X chromosome, rather than the normal two X complement denoting a female, is present (the genotype is 45,XO). The father's X chromosome is almost always the missing one; risk of recurrence in subsequent pregnancies is low (Gardner & Sutherland, 2004). In the absence of a second X chromosome, approximately 99% of fetuses abort spontaneously; survivors are phenotypically female (Batshaw, 2002). As with many sex chromosome disorders, variations exist, with approximately 30% of females with Turner syndrome showing a deletion (XO) in only some of the cells with the rest being genetically normal (46,XX). Those with the most common form of Turner (45,XO) have short stature, webbed neck, risk of hearing impairments, structural heart problems, and neurocognitive deficits. In Turner variations, more subtle physical stigmata and associated problems may exist. Turner syndrome is confirmed by karyotyping (a standard arrangement of the chromosomes in the laboratory so that they can be studied under a microscope). Girls may be well into their school career before short stature, absence of secondary sex characteristics, or academic problems prompt a conclusive medical evaluation (Berch & Bender, 2000).

Outcomes

Turner syndrome may not limit life expectancy, although obesity, diabetes, hypothyroidism, heart disease, hypertension, stroke, liver cirrhosis, and osteoporosis are more common than in the general population (Gardner & Sutherland, 2004). Interestingly, one of Turner's original child patients from 1937 reportedly was still thriving at age 75 (Smith, 1999). Turner syndrome appears to be associated with several interrelated neurocognitive problems, such as deficits in spatial processing, mathematics, attention, and social interaction. Fortunately, affected girls do not appear particularly vulnerable to mental retardation as was once thought (Ross, Zinn, & McCauley, 2000), but spatial deficits abound and these can be detected on tests such as the Wechsler Intelligence Scale for Children—III (WISC–III). For example, Rovet (1993) found Wechsler performance IQ to be about 15 points lower than verbal IQ, and this pattern has been replicated in subsequent studies (see Nijhuis van der Sanden, Eling, & Otten, 2003).

Mathematics deficits are prevalent. Problems often appear early, with girls as young as 5 years nearly twice as likely to encounter arithmetic problems as classmates with other genetic syndromes and similar IQ scores (Mazzocco, 2001). Math problems continue to be present into the middle school years and may actually intensify at that time (Mazzocco, 2001). Studies have documented deficits in math at rates of 43% and 55%, far exceeding those of the general population. Perhaps surprisingly, a direct link between math failure and visuospatial processing may not exist. Limited understanding of concepts and restricted knowledge of arithmetic facts can be as pronounced as computational skill deficits, which presumably require managing complex spatial arrays (e.g., columns when adding). Working memory and executive deficits, as discussed later, may be responsible, as are failures of rote memory and limited retention of basic arithmetic rules (Bruandet, Molko, Cohen, & Dehaene, 2004). The ability to divide and shift attention, track one's progress through a series of operations, or retain numbers in working memory are all required during math tasks. Somewhat surprisingly, Rovet (1993) also established problems in reading decoding (although these were less severe than those in math), even though many girls with Turner syndrome profess a love of reading. It may be that hyperactivity and impulsivity play a role in academic problems, including those in math. Rovet (1993) found attention-deficit/hyperactivity disorder (ADHD) symptoms to be prevalent in a group of girls with Turner syndrome. Temple, Carney, and Mullarkey (1996) and Temple (2002) also documented executive dysfunction, often associated with ADHD-spectrum problems.

Social problems, not surprisingly, are common among girls with Turner syndrome. The combination of math, visuospatial, and social difficulties is reminiscent of nonverbal learning disability (NLD; Rourke, 2000). NLD is, in fact, characterized in part by visuospatial, math, and social deficits. It is still unclear, however, whether the social problems of girls with Turner syndrome share underlying causes with NLD (e.g., right hemisphere dysfunction). Alternatively, they might arise from social stigma associated with short stature or other, yet unknown neurocognitive impairments. Nonetheless, social withdrawal and anxiety are more common among girls with Turner syndrome, leading some researchers to speculate that difficulty understanding social cues may be responsible (Downey, Ehrhardt, Gruen, Bell, & Morishima, 1989; Lawrence et al., 2003). Social problems might also be attributable to impairments in facial expression (Lesniak-Karpiak, Mazzocco, & Ross, 2003).

The outcome for those with Turner syndrome during womanhood awaits systematic research, but many girls continue to be referred for evaluation and receive services (e.g., school accommodations, psychotherapy) through the high school and into the college years. Nonetheless, a cross-sectional study of 240 affected adults found no differences in educational achievement, occupational status, or personal happiness compared with genetically normal peers (Orten & Orten, 1992), although sampling bias may have been present in this and most other studies of those identified by means other than genetic screenings. Magnetic resonance imaging (MRI) and related techniques do not currently play a role in routine clinical diagnosis or treatment of the disorder (although neuroimaging studies suggest the presence of reduced size of various brain structures; Reiss et al., 1993).

Medical and Psychoeducational Implications

Turner syndrome requires appropriate referral for medical diagnosis with direct referral to a geneticist or endocrinologist appropriate. Many girls with Turner syndrome are candidates for growth hormone replacement, typically managed by an endocrinologist. Almost all remain infertile, however. Nonetheless, treatment may increase growth, with one trial finding final height about 5 cm better for a treated than an untreated control group (Cave, Bryant, & Milne, 2003).

Equivalent empirical trials of psychosocial interventions for females with Turner syndrome do not yet appear to exist. Nonetheless, regarding school, Rovet (1993) recommended the following: (a) early psychoeducational evaluation and required learning disability services, (b) classroom modifications and consideration of pharmacotherapy if ADHD is present, (c) reliance on verbal strengths and circumvention of spatial problems (e.g., copying from the board), (d) support of self-esteem through positive feedback, (e) steps to prevent teasing about stature, and (f) vocational guidance that directs them away from areas where their deficiencies would limit success. Some evidence suggests that academic interventions teaching strategies through reliance on well-developed verbal skills provide strategies for solving nonverbal tasks (Williams, Richman, & Yarbrough, 1992). Psychosocial services may be required to deal with short stature and disclosing diagnostic information to friends and potential mates, as well as to address the grieving process over potential life-limiting factors, such as infertility, and to promote long-term adjustment (Powell & Schulte, 1999). Individual counseling or participation in support groups may be needed. Social skills training, typically performed in groups of same-age girls, may also help.

Klinefelter Syndrome

Klinefelter syndrome is caused by the presence of one (or, rarely, several) extra X chromosomes (e.g., 47, XXY), which can be inherited from either parent. It occurs exclusively among male phenotypes and is characterized by tall stature, obesity, lack of facial hair, and enlarged breasts (gynecomastia) but no distinctive facial dysmorphology. Klinefelter is estimated to affect between 1 in 400 to 800 individuals, making it relatively common (Geschwind, Boone, Miller, & Swerdloff, 2000). Klinefelter syndrome is often unrecognized until puberty when secondary sex characteristics fail to emerge, with many individuals going through life without detection of the disorder. Psychologists can sometimes promote detection.

Outcomes

The presence of an extra X chromosome is associated with diminished testosterone levels, typically arising in late adolescence, which results in a lack of secondary sex characteristics. Affected boys frequently appear tall (with especially long limbs) and thin until puberty, but tend toward obesity later (Jones, 1997). Even before puberty, genital abnormalities (e.g., small testes) may exist. Nearly all are infertile.

In general, the neurocognitive effects of Klinefelter syndrome are less debilitating than those associated with some genetic disorders, with variable impact in school and social settings. Verbal deficits are most frequently reported, with verbal IQs about 20 points lower than those of siblings and clearly inferior to their own nonverbal scores (Rovet, Netley, Keenan, Bailey, & Stewart, 1996). Impairments often include delayed linguistic milestones, as well as problems with articulation, word finding, phonemic processing, verbal memory, language comprehension, expressive problems and diminished speed of processing of linguistic material (Geschwind et al., 2000). Many of these deficits are reminiscent of those underlying developmental dyslexia in genetically normal children. Indeed, 92% of individuals with Klinefelter syndrome admitted difficulty learning to read, and 70% demonstrated objective evidence of a reading disability on standardized psychometrics (e.g., ability–achievement discrepancy or absolute reading deficit; Geschwind et al., 2000). In contrast, nonverbal and visuospatial skills are typically average. Global IQ impairments are not common, although Klinefelter was recently found to be present in eight boys with mental retardation who underwent genetic screening (Khalifa & Struthers, 2002). Written language problems and arithmetic deficits are also fairly common (Rovet et al., 1996). Between 40% and 80% of these boys required special education services. Whether academic problems derive from core linguistic problems or are related to other underlying problems is unclear. Boys with Klinefelter have deficits in manual dexterity (e.g., as indicated by the Grooved Pegboard Test) and are often cited as clumsy and averse to sports (Geschwind et al., 2000). Nonetheless, actual outcomes include many individuals who complete high school successfully, and even a few who pursue postsecondary education.

There is some evidence that left hemisphere dysfunction (perhaps related to diminished gray matter, lack of expected hemispheric asymmetry, or both) cause the predominate linguistic and reading problems described here. Executive and frontal deficits may also be present. These have not been reported reliably in a childhood cohort, but among adults with Klinefelter, more than half have difficulties with establishing and maintaining a response set (Wisconsin Card Sorting Test), inhibition (Stroop Test), and mental flexibility (Trailmaking B; Geschwind et al., 2000).

There are enduring myths that Klinefelter syndrome is associated with sociopathy and criminal behavior, but most of these are now debunked. In fact, psychiatric problems are reportedly rare among individuals with Klinefelter syndrome (Geschwind et al., 2000). Nonetheless, introversion, unassertiveness, and a paucity of ambition may be present, in addition to impulsivity and social inappropriateness. Such difficulties further indicate that frontal–executive functions, which subsume motivation, inhibition, judgment, and flexibility, may be at fault.

Medical and Psychoeducational Implications

Learning and language problems, poor adjustment, or social and body image issues may bring boys with Klinefelter syndrome into contact with psychologists. Referral to the child's primary care physician, endocrinologist, medical geneticist, or neurologist is indicated. A diagnosis can be established by karyotyping. Maternal age is a risk factor, but errors may arise from either parent; recurrence of the disorder in children born to the same parents is low (Gardner & Sutherland, 2004). Some individuals receive exogenous testosterone at puberty, which may ameliorate left hemisphere gray matter impairments and concomitantly improve verbal skills (Patwardhan, Eliez, Bender, Linden, & Reiss, 2000). Some researchers question the evidence supporting testosterone-linked language improvements (Kates & Singer, 2000), whereas others suggest improvements occur in attention–executive functions but not language (Geschwind et al., 2000).

No psychological or educational interventions, however, appear to have been validated for children having Klinefelter syndrome. Careful evaluation of language, executive, and motor function is essential in understanding the full scope of problems that these individuals encounter. Early speech/language services have been advocated (Rovet et al., 1996). Accommodations for deficits in motor output, language reception and expression, and processing speed are all logical as well, although each particular deficit needs to be established through individual evaluation. The combined presence of Klinefelter and struggling school status should prompt special education services rather than hoping that the child will outgrow his problem.

Fragile X

Fragile X syndrome is due to an anomaly in an X chromosome and is estimated to be present in 1 in 4,000 males and 1 in 8,000 females (Crawford et al., 1999). A trinucleotide repeat expansion in a specific gene located near the end of the long arm of the X chromosome was discovered in 1991, and the gene came to be called the fragile X mental retardation 1 gene. When advanced diagnostic techniques (microscopic DNA analysis) became available, moderate repeats (called premutations) in the CGC sequence were discovered to signify a carrier with normal IQ (but at risk for emotional problems). DNA studies also can detect full mutations, involving many more repeats concurrent with a gene responsible for inhibiting production of a specific protein (FMRP), in a process called methylation. Deficient FMRP causes physical stigmata, intellectual impairments, and behavioral disturbance that characterize fragile X syndrome (Hagerman & Lampe, 1999). Mothers with premutation in a certain range always produce a full mutation in one of their two X chromosomes; hence, there is a 50% chance the fully mutated X chromosome is passed to a son. Fathers with premutations always pass on the premutation, but not the full mutation, to their daughters (the fathers' sperm has only the premutation). The next generation of boys born to these daughters is likely to have the full mutation, however. Because the X chromosome is never transmitted from father to son, men with fragile X premutation or full mutation never have affected sons.

Outcomes

Individuals with fragile X have high rates of mental retardation, with FMRP playing a crucial role. A mean IQ of 41 has been reported among those with full mutation plus an abnormal FMR1 gene, a mean IQ of 60 among those with mosaic (affected and unaffected cell lines existing in the same individual), and a mean IQ of 88 among those with fragile X but no or only partially abnormal FMR1 gene (Tassone et al., 1999). Accordingly, a precise DNA analysis allows general insight into the future of a particular child. Besides IQ, WISC–III verbal working memory (Digit Span) scores appear to be most directly affected in boys and girls, whereas in girls alone attention, speediness, and sequential ability (i.e., as measured by WISC–III Picture Arrangement and Symbol Search subtests) are also affected (Loesch et al., 2002). Extra-IQ deficits, such as poor motor planning, diminished inhibition, and deficits in sequential processing, also typify the disorder, and some of these impairments also appear linked to variations in the FMR1 gene (Loesch et al., 2003; Powell, Houghton, & Douglas, 1997).

Clinical lore contains numerous references to the peculiar behavior and social awkwardness of children with fragile X. Language problems are common, with speech characterized as tangential, perseverative, and repetitive (Sudhalter & Belser, 2004) and devoid of pragmatics, such as the ability to sustain conversation, even though most children with fragile X are socially motivated. Social skills accordingly are often deficient, and frankly odd behavior is present. In fact, nearly 50% of children with fragile X have clinical levels of autism on rating scales (Demark, Feldman, & Holden, 2003). A variation of pervasive developmental disorder, however, rather than full syndrome autism, may best describe these children. Although the behavior of many children with fragile X improves with time, hallmark shyness, aversion to eye contact, and speech peculiarities typically continue, the latter two commonly persisting into adulthood (Einfeld, Tonge, & Turner, 1999).

Girls appear to be less cognitively impaired than boys (Bromham & Jupp, 1991) but may still express schizotypal features and communication disorders, such as those mentioned earlier (Feinstein & Reiss, 1998; Freund, Reiss, Hagerman, & Vinogradov, 1992). Although often less affected than boys, girls with fragile X may still be slow to initiate social interaction, even when they are not obviously anxious (Lesniak-Karpiak et al., 2003). Neuroimaging studies have identified differences in the brains of male and female individuals with fragile X (e.g., decreased size in portions of the cerebellum and increased size of ventricles; Reiss, Freund, Tseng, & Joshi, 1991), although MRI and related techniques are not currently used for clinical diagnostic purposes.

All of this means that children with fragile X are prevalent in clinical populations; 6 boys per 100 with autism may have fragile X syndrome (Brown et al., 1986), although epidemiological studies suggest fewer (Fombonne, DuMazaubrun, Cans, & Grandjean, 1997). Between 2% and 3% of boys with mental retardation of unknown etiology may have fragile X (Slaney et al., 1995). Roughly 1 in 400 children in special education have the fragile X mutation (Crawford et al., 1999). Accordingly, the Academy of Neurology's practice guidelines suggest that karyotyping and DNA analysis should be preformed under any of the following conditions: (a) mental retardation, (b) developmental or emotional problems concurrent with a family history of autism, and (c) dysmorphic features (compatible with fragile X; Filipek et al., 2000).

Medical and Psychoeducational Implications

The first task when psychologists are involved is to make sure that biomedical syndromes (including fragile X) are identified rather than focusing on administrative labels alone (e.g., mild mental retardation, autism). Because the signs of fragile X may not be recognized until adolescence, psychologists should be alert to family history of mental retardation, long jaw or high forehead, large or protuberant ears, hyperextensible joints, soft and velvety palmar skin, enlargement of testes (reported by family or checked by physician), initial shyness, lack of eye contact followed by friendliness, and verbosity (Shevell et al., 2003). Use of these signs to determine who should undergo more detailed studies leads to effective use of genetic testing. Prompt detection of fragile X permits genetic counseling and family planning. Carriers can be identified by DNA analysis; prenatal testing is also available (Gardner & Sutherland, 2004). There is some empirical evidence that sensitizing individuals, including prospective referring professionals, promotes ascertainment of families with the fragile X chromosome (Keenan et al., 1992), which sets the stage for family planning.

Informing teachers of the features of fragile X and disorder-specific classroom behavior has been suggested (Braden, 2004; York, von Fraunhofer, Turk, & Sedgwick, 1999). Etiology-based interventions (Hodapp & Fidler, 1999) have been advocated for disorders with uniform representation, possibly including fragile X. Because many children with fragile X have language, attention, interpersonal, sequential processing, and mathematics problems, intervention plans often need to consider these dimensions. Instruction may need to incorporate sequential processing (via direct instruction and organization of life routines). Similarly, these children often require training in social and communication skills (especially pragmatics), as well as external structure and guidance, but any such plan should spring from a comprehensive evaluation (including assessment of memory, attention–executive functioning, social skills, and language). Test batteries comprising only IQ and achievement tests are incomplete. Highly structured classroom settings sometimes diminish odd behavior and attention problems. A study of boys with fragile X and coexisting mental retardation found that a structured special education classroom promoted fairly high levels of academic engagement and relatively low levels of stereotypic and self-injurious behavior (Symons, Clark, Roberts, & Bailey, 2001).

After confirmation of fragile X, medical treatment involves monitoring for possible epilepsy, which occurs in 10% to 30% of cases (Turk, 2004). Psychopharmacotherapy may be warranted as well for ADHD, aggression and violent outbursts, self-injurious behavior, sleep problems, and mood disturbances (Turk, 2004). Most pharmacotherapy is symptomatic, addressing presenting symptoms, rather than the underlying biochemical pathology of fragile X. Thus, empirical support exists for general medication effects only.

Lesch–Nyhan

Lesch–Nyhan disease is a rare (1 in 380,000 live births) congenital error of metabolism. It occurs when purine is improperly metabolized, resulting in its elevation to toxic levels. This arises because of a mutation of a specific gene located on the X chromosome. Various pernicious physiologic outcomes result, including chronic kidney disease and central nervous system (CNS) impairments (Nyhan & Wong, 1996). Rather than structural lesions, neurotransmitter deficiencies (i.e., in dopamine) appear to underlie CNS disease. The dopamine pathways are known to involve basal ganglia (symmetrical masses composed of gray matter) and connected structures (e.g., frontal lobes) and to subserve movement, reward, planning, and response inhibition. Dopamine and dopaminergic pathways are involved in various movement disorders that include elements of compulsion and dysregulation, such as Tourette syndrome. Thus, some of the impairments that characterize Lesch–Nyhan are understandable.

Lesch–Nyhan is an X-linked recessive disorder that expresses almost exclusively in males. Because a second X chromosome (XX) in females results in sufficient production of deficient enzyme (HPRT), normal brain development occurs in girls. Mothers of affected boys, however, are always the carriers. Diagnosis is made by DNA analysis of the index child. Mothers can be tested for carrier status, and prenatal (fetal) testing is also available (Morales, 1999).

Outcomes

These children have such severe impairments that most (perhaps all) are identified very early. Severe spasticity and involuntary movements typically begin in the first year. So may the appearance of orange crystals in diapers, indicating renal insufficiency; gout may arise later. As motor deficits intensify, most babies lose the ability to sit or stand, with ambulation rarely developing. Increased muscle tone, spasticity, rigidity, and spasms of flexor muscles ensue, as do severe involuntary movements characterized by slow, irregular twisting of upper extremities (athetosis) or muscle-contraction-induced inclining of the head to one side (torticollis; Morales, 1999). Confinement to a wheelchair with supports at the chest is almost universal, as is nearly complete dependency for activities of daily living. Related speech problems are present, which slows expression and limits intelligibility. Eating problems are common, which can compromise caloric intake and may result in aspiration and subsequent pneumonia.

Self-injurious behavior, especially biting off fingers, end of the tongue, and hunks of flesh is the most troubling aspect of the disorder (Robey, Reck, Giacomini, Barabas, & Eddey, 2003). Individuals may hit or poke themselves, bang their head, or rub themselves raw. Some form of self-mutilation is nearly unanimously present, although these children remain sensitive to pain. For many, aggressive actions are also aimed at caregivers. Both self-mutilation and aggression, however, are distinctly compulsive in nature; afterward children almost always report feeling powerless to refrain and communicate regret (Morales, 1999).

As might be expected, cognitive assessment is hard to accomplish because of speech and motor limitations and self-abusive actions. Practitioners must use instruments that can be fairly administered and validly interpreted based on each youngster's particular physical and behavior impairments. Group data have been collected using standardized IQ instruments that provide general cognitive parameters. Matthews, Solan, Barabas, and Robey (1999) assessed a group of boys three times over approximately 4 years. As a group, these boys' skills reached a plateau between ages 13 and 17 years in abstract visual reasoning and aspects of short-term memory, ostensibly because older boys had decreased attentiveness and diminished flexibility of thinking. Many of these teenage boys enjoyed continued growth in some areas, however (e.g., vocabulary and memory for objects). The latter findings are consistent with observations of keen awareness of their environment and facility at incidental learning. Parents report that their sons have quite variable mental abilities, and some boys appear to possess surprisingly well-preserved skills and diverse interests (Anderson, Ernst, & Davis, 1992).

Medical and Psychoeducational Implications

No medical treatment is available to correct the fundamental HPRT enzyme deficiency, but allopurinol, an oral medication, can manage excessive uric acid in the blood. This treatment fails to improve CNS functioning, however, and most individuals die before age 20 (Morales, 1999). Medications to reduce self-mutilation and aggression have been attempted without obvious success, but they may still be tried on individual bases.

Mechanical restraints (e.g., gloves, masks, and helmets) are needed to reduce self-mutilation. Interestingly, most children with Lesch–Nyhan welcome these restraints, as they apparently harbor no wish to harm but simply cannot resist self-abusive or aggressive compulsions. Behavioral techniques may reduce aggressive acts against caregivers. Stress sometimes triggers self-abuse, and thus managing anxiety can represent an effective strategy. Because these children represent enormous management and basic care burdens, institutional living is often necessary. For those who remain at home, family support is required. Outcomes associated with various placement options or with providing parents with supports, however, do not to appear have been systematically examined.

Lowe Syndrome

Lowe syndrome is a low-incidence genetic disorder (probably fewer than 1 individual in 100,000) characterized by physical handicaps, medical problems, and mental retardation. It is sometimes called oculocerebrorenal (OCRL) syndrome because of eye, brain, and kidney involvement (see the Lowe Syndrome Association Web page at http://www.lowesyndrome.org, 2003). Lowe syndrome is an X-linked recessive disorder with only boys expressing symptoms; mothers are carriers. The gene has now been mapped (Nussbaum, Orrison, Janne, Charnas, & Chinault, 1997) and the resultant deficient enzyme identified (Suchy & Nussbaum, 2002). Diagnosis is made by detecting a missing enzyme (phosphatidylinositol 4,5-biphosphate 5 phosphatase) in a culture grown from a small skin sample or by DNA analysis.

Outcomes

Congenital cataracts are present that typically require surgical repair during the first months of life. Glasses or contact lenses are required, but corrected vision is rarely better than 20/100. About half of boys with the syndrome develop glaucoma during their first years. In addition, elevated intraocular pressure is often present, necessitating surgery or routine use of eye-drops. Likewise, kidney damage (Fanconi-type renal tubular dysfunction) begins for most boys around age 1 year. This includes abnormal excretion of various substances (e.g., bicarbonate, sodium, potassium) in the urine. Fanconi-type dysfunction is of variable severity. Seizures arise in about half of affected boys. Hypotonia and choreathetoid movements (involving frequent, spastic movements of the limbs), some bizarre appearing, may be present (Magalini & Magalini, 1997). Overall motor coordination is poor. Global cognitive impairment is typically present, with IQs often in the moderate range of mental retardation, although one quarter of children may score above the mental retardation cutoff (Kenworthy, Park, & Charnas, 1993). White matter destruction surrounding the ventricles may represent part of the underlying CNS pathology (Pueschel, Brem, & Nittoli, 1992). Behavior problems, especially stubbornness, temper tantrums, and stereotypic movements or screaming are common (Kenworthy et al., 1993).

Other physical problems are also present. Facial stigmata include deeply set eyes, frontal bossing, and sparse hair in temporal regions (Gropman et al., 2000). These boys have short stature and orthopedic impairments, which may include rickets, bone fractures, scoliosis, and joint problems. Life expectancy is typically limited to 30 to 40 years, if complications do not exist.

Medical and Psychoeducational Implications

Antiepileptic drugs are sometimes necessary to control seizures. Despite identification of the deficient enzyme, no treatment of the underlying malfunction exists. Prevention is a treatment option. When Lowe's syndrome is identified, mother's carrier status can be confirmed by karyotyping, and other women in the family who may be carriers can be tested. Prenatal testing is also possible (Suchy, Lin, Horwitz, O'Brien, & Nussbaum, 1998), which extends genetic counseling and family planning options for some couples.

Most boys with Lowe syndrome require special education and related services throughout school. Self-contained placements are often necessary because of the array of mobility, vision, and cognitive problems that many of these boys endure. Nonetheless, many boys with Lowe syndrome are affectionate and sociable, enjoy humor, and love music. These attributes are sometimes used to help place boys with Lowe syndrome in mainstream settings.

CONCLUSION

Numerous sex chromosome anomalies are currently known to exist or will be discovered in the foreseeable future. Five such anomalies with implications for psychologists were reviewed here. Although much is currently known about the diagnosis, medical and psychological management, and education of individuals with these disorders, disorder-specific investigations continue. As advances in molecular biology, clinical genetics, and psychology are brought to bear on each distinctive genetic disorder, their treatment will benefit from increasing guidance from empirical research.

REFERENCES

Anderson, L. T., Ernst, M., & Davis, S. V. (1992). Cognitive abilities of patients with Lesch–Nyhan disease. *Journal of Autism and Developmental Disorders, 22,* 189–203.

Batshaw, M. L. (2002). *Children with disabilities* (5th ed.). Washington, DC: Brookes Publishing.

Berch, D. B., & Bender, B. G. (2000). Turner syndrome. In K. O. Yeates, M. D. Ris, & H. G. Taylor (Eds.), *Pediatric neuropsychology: Research, theory, and practice* (pp. 252–275). New York: Guilford Press.

Braden, M. (2004). The effects of fragile X syndrome on learning. In D. Dew-Hughes (Ed.), *Educating children with fragile X syndrome* (pp. 43–47). London: RoutledgeFalmer.

Bromham, S., & Jupp, J. (1991). Intellectual functioning in fragile X syndrome school children. *Australia and New Zealand Journal of Developmental Disabilities, 17*, 49–57.

Brown, W. T., Jenkins, E. C., Cohen, I. L., Fisch, G. S., Wolf-Schein, E. G., Gross, A., et al. (1986). Fragile X and autism: A multicenter study. *American Journal of Medical Genetics, 23*, 341–352.

Bruandet, M., Molko, N., Cohen, L., & Dehaene, S. (2004). Cognitive characterization of dyscalculia in Turner syndrome. *Neuropsychologia, 42*, 288–298.

Cave, C. B., Bryant, J., & Milne, R. (2003). Recombinant growth hormone in children and adolescents with Turner syndrome. *The Cochrane Database of Systematic Reviews, 1*, CD003887. Available from The Cochrane Library Web site, http://www.cochrane.org

Crawford, D. C., Meadows, I. L., Newman, J. L., Taft, L. F., Pettay, D. L., Gold, L. B., et al. (1999). Prevalence and phenotypic consequence of FRAXA and FRAXE alleles in a large, ethnically diverse, special-needs population. *American Journal of Human Genetics, 64*, 495–507.

Demark, J. L., Feldman, M. A., & Holden, J. J. A. (2003). Behavioral relationship between autism and fragile X syndrome. *American Journal on Mental Retardation, 108*, 314–426.

Downey, J. I., Ehrhardt, E. A., Gruen, R., Bell, J. J., & Morishima, A. (1989). Psychopathology and social functioning in women with Turner syndrome. *Journal of Nervous and Mental Disease, 177*, 191–196.

Einfeld, S., Tonge, B., & Turner, G. (1999). Longitudinal course of behavioral and emotional problems in fragile X syndrome. *American Journal of Medical Genetics, 87*, 436–439.

Feinstein, C., & Reiss, A. L. (1998). Autism: The point of view from fragile X studies. *Journal of Autism and Developmental Disorders, 28*, 393–405.

Filipek, P. A., Accardo, P. J., Ashwal, S., Baranek, G. T., Cook, E. H., Jr., Dawson, G., et al. (2000). Practice parameter: Screening and diagnosis of autism. *Neurology, 55*, 468–479.

Fombonne, E., DuMazaubrun, C., Cans, C., & Grandjean, H. (1997). Autism and associated medical disorders in a French epidemiological survey. *Journal of the American Academy of Child and Adolescent Psychiatry, 36*, 1561–1569.

Freund, L. S., Reiss, A. L., Hagerman, R., & Vinogradov, S. (1992). Chromosome fragility and psychopathology in obligate female carriers of the fragile X chromosome. *Archives of General Psychiatry, 49*, 54–60.

Gardner, R. J. M., & Sutherland, G. R. (2004). *Chromosome abnormalities and genetic counseling* (3rd ed.). New York: Oxford University Press.

Geschwind, D. H., Boone, K. B., Miller, B. L., & Swerdloff, R. S. (2000). Neurobehavioral phenotype of Klinefelter syndrome. *Mental Retardation and Developmental Disabilities Research Reviews, 6,* 107–116.

Gropman, A., Levin, S., Yao, L., Lin, T., Suchy, S., Sabnis, S., et al. (2000). Unusual renal features of Lowe syndrome in a mildly affected boy. *American Journal of Medical Genetics, 95,* 461–466.

Hagerman, R. J., & Hagerman, P. J. (2002). Fragile X syndrome. In P. Howlin & O. Udwin (Eds.), *Outcomes in neurodevelopmental and genetic disorders* (pp. 198–219). New York: Cambridge University Press.

Hagerman, R. J., & Lampe, M. E. (1999). Fragile X syndrome. In S. Goldstein & C. R. Reynolds (Eds.), *Handbook of neurodevelopmental and genetic disorders in children* (pp. 298–316). New York: Guilford Press.

Hodapp, R. M., & Fidler, D. J. (1999). Special education and genetics: Connections for the 21st century. *Journal of Special Education, 33,* 130–137.

Jones, K. L. (1997). *Smith's Recognizable Patterns of Human Malformation* (5th ed.). Philadelphia: W. B. Saunders.

Kates, W., & Singer, H. S. (2000). Sex chromosomes, testosterone, and the brain. *Neurology, 54,* 2201–2202.

Keenan, J., Kastner, T., Nathanson, R., Richardson, N., Hinton, J., & Cress, D. A. (1992). A statewide public and professional education program on fragile X syndrome. *Mental Retardation, 30,* 355–361.

Kenworthy, L., Park, T., & Charnas, L. R. (1993). Cognitive and behavioral profile of the oculocerebrorenal syndrome of Lowe. *American Journal of Medical Genetics, 46,* 297–303.

Khalifa, M. M., & Struthers, J. L. (2002). Klinefelter syndrome is a common cause of mental retardation of unknown etiology among prepubertal males. *Clinical Genetics, 61,* 49–53.

Lawrence, K., Campbell, R., Swettenham, J., Terstegge, J., Akers, R., Coleman, M., et al. (2003). Interpreting gaze in Turner syndrome: Impaired sensitivity to intention and emotion, but preservation of social cueing. *Neuropsychologia, 41,* 894–905.

Lesniak-Karpiak, K., Mazzocco, M. M. M., & Ross, J. L. (2003). Behavioral assessment of social anxiety in females with Turner or fragile X syndrome. *Journal of Autism and Developmental Disorders, 33,* 55–67.

Loesch, D. Z., Bui, Q. M., Grigsby, J., Butler, E., Epstein, J., Huggins, R., et al. (2003). Effect of fragile X status categories and the fragile X mental retardation protein levels on executive functioning in males and females with fragile X. *Neuropsychology, 17,* 646–657.

Loesch, D. Z., Huggins, R. M., Bui, Q. M., Epstein, J. L., Taylor, A. K., & Hagerman, R. J. (2002). Effects of the deficits of fragile X mental retardation protein on cognitive status of fragile X males and females assessed by robust pedigree analysis. *Journal of Developmental and Behavioral Pediatrics, 23,* 416–423.

Magalini, S. I., & Magalini, S. C. (1997). *Dictionary of medical syndromes* (4th ed.). Philadelphia: Lippincott-Raven.

Matthews, W. S., Solan, A., Barabas, G., & Robey, K. (1999). Cognitive functioning in Lesch–Nyhan syndrome: A 4-year follow-up study. *Developmental Medicine and Child Neurology, 41,* 260–262.

Mazzocco, M. M. M. (2001). Math learning disability and math LD subtypes: Evidence from studies of Turner Syndrome, fragile X syndrome, and neurofibromatosis type 1. *Journal of Learning Disabilities, 34,* 520–533.

Morales, P. C. (1999). Lesch–Nyhan syndrome. In S. Goldstein & C. R. Reynolds (Eds.), *Handbook of neurodevelopmental and genetic disorders in children* (pp. 478–498). New York: Guilford Press.

Nijhuis van der Sanden, M. W., Eling, P. A., & Otten, B. J. (2003). A review of neuropsychological and motor studies in Turner syndrome. *Neuroscience and Biobehavioral Reviews, 27,* 329–338.

Nussbaum, R. L., Orrison, B. M., Janne, P. A., Charnas, L., & Chinault, A. C. (1997). Physical mapping and genomic structure of the Lowe syndrome gene OCRL-1. *Human Genetics, 99,* 145–150.

Nyhan, W. L., & Wong, D. F. (1996). New approaches to understanding Lesch–Nyhan disease. *New England Journal of Medicine, 334,* 1602–1604.

Orten, J. D., & Orten, J. L. (1992). Achievement among women with Turner's syndrome. *Families in Society, 73,* 424–431.

Patwardhan, A. J., Eliez, S., Bender, B., Linden, M. G., & Reiss, A. L. (2000). Brain morphology in Klinefelter syndrome: Extra X chromosome and testosterone supplementation. *Neurology, 54,* 2218–2223.

Powell, L., Houghton, S., & Douglas, G. (1997). Comparison of etiology-specific cognitive functioning profiles for individuals with fragile X and individuals with Down syndrome. *Journal of Special Education, 31,* 363–376.

Powell, M. P., & Schulte, T. (1999). Turner syndrome. In S. Goldstein & C. R. Reynolds (Eds.), *Handbook of neurodevelopmental and genetic disorders in children* (pp. 277–298). New York: Guilford Press.

Pueschel, S. M., Brem, A. S., & Nittoli, P. (1992). Central nervous system and renal investigations in patients with Lowe syndrome. *Child's Nervous System, 8,* 45–48.

Reiss, A. L., Freund, L., Plotnick, L., Baumgardner, T., Green, K., Sozer, A. C., et al. (1993). The effects of X monosomy on brain development: Monozygotic twins discordant for Turner's syndrome. *Annals of Neurology, 34,* 95–107.

Reiss, A. L., Freund, L., Tseng, J. E., & Joshi, P. K. (1991). Neuroanatomy in fragile X females: The posterior fossa. *American Journal of Human Genetics, 49,* 279–288.

Robey, K. L., Reck, J. F., Giacomini, K. D., Barabas, G., & Eddey, G. E. (2003). Modes and patterns of self-mutilation in persons with Lesch–Nyhan disease. *Developmental Medicine and Child Neurology, 45,* 167–171.

Ross, J., Zinn, A., & McCauley, E. (2000). Neurodevelopmental and psychosocial aspects of Turner syndrome. *Mental Retardation and Developmental Disabilities Reviews, 6*, 135–141.

Rourke, B. P. (2000). Neuropsychological and psychosocial subtyping: A review of investigations within the University of Windsor laboratory. *Canadian Psychology, 41*, 34–51.

Rovet, J. (1993). The psychoeducational characteristic of children with Turner syndrome. *Journal of Learning Disabilities, 26*, 333–341.

Rovet, J., Netley, C., Keenan, M., Bailey, J., & Stewart, D. (1996). The psychoeducational profile of boys with Klinefelter syndrome. *Journal of Learning Disabilities, 29*, 180–196.

Shevell, M., Ashwal, S., Donley, D., Flint, J., Gingold, M., Hirtz, D., et al. (2003). Practice parameter: Evaluation of the child with global developmental delay. *Neurology, 60*, 367–380.

Slaney, S. F., Wilkie, A. O. M., Hirst, M. C., Charlton, R., McKinley, M., Pointon, J., et al. (1995). DNA testing for fragile X syndrome in school for learning difficulties. *Archives of Disease in Childhood, 72*, 33–37.

Smith, J. O. (1999). Turner's syndrome: Continuing to thrive at 75. *Journal of Gerontological Social Work, 31*, 187–195.

Suchy, S. F., Lin, T., Horwitz, J. A., O'Brien, W. E., & Nussbaum, R. L. (1998). First report of prenatal biochemical diagnosis of Lowe syndrome. *Prenatal Diagnosis, 18*, 1117–1121.

Suchy, S. F., & Nussbaum, R. L. (2002). The deficiency of PIP2 5-phosphatase in Lowe syndrome affects actin polymerization. *American Journal of Human Genetics, 71*, 1420–1427.

Sudhalter, V., & Belser, R. C. (2004). Atypical language production of males with fragile X syndrome. In D. Dew-Hughes (Ed.), *Educating children with fragile X syndrome* (pp. 25–31). New York: RoutledgeFalmer.

Symons, F. J., Clark, R. D., Roberts, J. P., & Bailey, D. B., Jr. (2001). Classroom behavior of elementary school-age boys with fragile X syndrome. *Journal of Special Education, 34*, 194–202.

Tassone, F., Hagerman, R. J., Ikle, D., Dyer, P. N., Lampe, M., Willemsen, R., et al. (1999). FMRP expression as a potential prognostic indicator in fragile X syndrome. *American Journal of Medical Genetics, 84*, 250–261.

Temple, C. M. (2002). Oral fluency and narrative production in children with Turner's syndrome. *Neuropsychologia, 40*, 1419–1427.

Temple, C. M, Carney, R. A., & Mullarkey, S. (1996). Frontal lobe function and executive skills in children with Turner syndrome. *Developmental Neuropsychology, 12*, 343–363.

Turk, J. (2004). The importance of diagnosis. In D. Dew-Hughes (Ed.), *Educating children with fragile X syndrome*. London: RoutledgeFalmer.

Williams, J. K., Richman, L. C., & Yarbrough, D. B. (1992). Comparison of visual-spatial performance strategy training in children with Turner syndrome and learning disabilities. *Journal of Learning Disabilities, 25*, 658–664.

Wodrich, D. L. (2004). Professional beliefs related to the practice of pediatric medicine and school psychology. *Journal of School Psychology, 42,* 265–284.

York, A., von Fraunhofer, N., Turk, J., & Sedgwick, P. (1999). Fragile-X syndrome, Down's syndrome and autism: Awareness and knowledge amongst special educators. *Journal of Intellectual Disability Research, 43,* 314–324.

16

VISUAL IMPAIRMENTS

JAMES P. DONNELLY

OVERVIEW

Visual impairment is commonly thought of as a problem of older adulthood, but many children experience some form of visual disorder, ranging from relatively mild and treatable to permanent and disabling. The primary goal of this chapter is to provide an overview of the more frequently encountered childhood visual disorders, particularly those involving disturbances of ocular motility, and to orient the reader to etiology, epidemiology, diagnosis, treatment, and outcomes of these conditions. A general definition of visual impairment was suggested by Corn and Koenig (1996): "any degree of vision loss that affects an individual's ability to perform the tasks of daily life, caused by a visual system that is not working properly or not formed correctly" (p. 452). The Individuals With Disabilities in Education Act (IDEA; 2004) definition of visual impairment includes blindness and means an impairment in vision that, even with correction, adversely affects a child's educational performance.

Vision is commonly measured in terms of visual acuity, scaled in terms of a ratio of the child's visual accuracy relative to a normal standard as well as the range of the visual field. The well-known "20/20" standard means that a child is able to see at 20 feet what a person with normal vision can see at that same distance of 20 feet (Shore, 1998). A child is considered legally blind if vision cannot be improved to better than 20/200 or if the visual field is less than or equal to 20 degrees. Children are said to be partially sighted or to have low vision if impairment is present but the child is not totally blind (Shore, 1998).

Valid and reliable estimates of the number of children with visual impairments are difficult to obtain. It has been estimated that, overall, 12.1 million school-age children have some form of visual impairment when broadly defined to include all forms of abnormal vision (approximately one in every four children; Flanagan, Jackson, & Hill, 2003). Only 14% of children received comprehensive vision examinations before starting school and global delays or severe learning disabilities (or both) are found in 43% of children with visual impairments (Flanagan et al., 2003).

Causes of visual impairment include damage or trauma to any part of the visual system from the eye through the optic nerve to the cortex. Such physical and mechanical problems may result from accidents, disease, genetics, or developmental complications (Mets et al., 1997; Rudanko, Fellman, & Laatikainen, 2003; Shore, 1998). A prospective study examining survival and disability in a cohort of 192 extremely premature infants (23–25 weeks gestational age) showed that although survival significantly improved over a previous similar study, disability rates had increased as well, particularly the rates of blindness and visual impairment, which had tripled (Emsley, Wardle, Sims, Chiswick, & D'Souza, 1998). Similarly, Cooke, Foulder-Hughes, Newsham, and Clarke (2004) identified premature birth as a significant risk factor for visual impairment, particularly strabismus (inability of one eye to attain binocular vision with the other because of imbalance of the eye muscles of the eyeball), which was 10 times more likely to be seen in the preterm group as the control group. In addition, visual impairment was associated with deficits in motor skills and general IQ as measured by standardized tests (the Developmental Test of Visual-Motor Integration, the Movement Assessment Battery for Children, and the Wechsler Intelligence Scale for Children—III—UK). Among the inherited causes of visual impairment, albinism is particularly important (Biswas & Lloyd, 1999). In addition to the observable impact of altered melanin synthesis on skin and hair pigmentation, the condition may be associated with reduced visual acuity, photophobia, nystagmus (a rapid, involuntary oscillation of the eyes), and other visual system manifestations. The study of genetic mutations associated with conditions such as albinism that produce visual disorders has become an increasingly productive area of study (Young, 2003). Beyond the neonatal stage, developmental aspects of visual impairment present significant challenges to children, their families, and to those who treat them and study their conditions.

The visual system matures throughout childhood, and variability in visual ability within and across children is typical. Development of normal and abnormal vision reflects both structural and functional events as the child grows. Because various visual functions mature at different rates, it may be difficult to predict the outcome of a particular impairment (Johnson, Minassian, Weale, & West, 2003).

In general, up to 82% (Harley, Lawrence, Sanford, & Burnett, 2000) of the visual impairment that occurs in children is a function of a refractive error, meaning that a clear image cannot be formed on the retina. The global term for refractive error problems is *ametropia* (Harley et al., 2000). Some optic problems, such as microcornea (very small corneal diameter) and microphthalmia (the eye itself is very small), are genetic deficiencies resulting in extreme hyperopia. These conditions may not be effectively treated with corrective lenses and require the provision of special education services. Beyond such optical problems, the largest area of concern in visual impairment is related to ocular motility, or the ability to coordinate both eyes so that the image received on the retina is identical. These conditions include amblyopia, strabismus, and nystagmus (Harley et al., 2000).

Amblyopia is commonly known as "lazy eye." As the colloquial term suggests, the condition involves an imbalance in the functioning of the eyes. It is caused by disuse of one eye during the developmental period, resulting in a reduction of visual acuity without overt signs of pathology (Thomas, 1995). Amblyopia is the most common childhood visual disorder, affecting approximately 2% to 3% of children (National Eye Institute [NEI], n.d.). Without successful early treatment, the condition persists into adulthood. It is the most common cause of monocular vision problems among young and middle-aged adults as well as children (NEI, n.d.). Untreated or permanent amblyopia may have long-term impact on vocation as well as binocular vision and will become a major problem in adulthood should the normal eye incur injury or disease (Hrisos, Clarke, & Wright, 2004).

Amblyopia may occur as a result of any problem that affects normal visual development, including strabismus, cataracts, and ptosis (drooping eyelids; Thompson, 2004). Childhood cataracts alone are considered the largest single cause of childhood blindness and, in those cases in which vision is not completely occluded, will often result in amblyopia (Long & Chen, 2004). The condition can also result from an inequity in another visual problem such that one eye is more nearsighted, farsighted, or astigmatic. Amblyopia may develop during sensitive periods of development, especially during the child's first year (Thompson, 2004). Although the exact mechanism has not been documented, the condition arises as a result of the failure of the visual cortex to process information from one or both eyes (Johnson et al., 2003).

A recent brain imaging study using functional magnetic resonance imaging (fMRI) investigated the psychophysical correlates in a sample of children with strabismus and amblyopia (Barnes, Hess, Dumoulin, Achtman, & Pike, 2001). Their analysis focused on the visual area of the cortex, which had been identified in prior animal studies. Most of the cases showed no normal functioning in this area, and the authors concluded that, given the limited number of alternative explanations, this site may be central to producing the symptoms of amblyopia. Clinically, the possibility of amblyopia is suggested when refractive errors in vision in an anatomically normal eye are corrected, but visual impairment remains (Johnson et al., 2003; Thompson, 2004). The most severe expression of this condition occurs as a result of stimulus deprivation, as in cataracts (Thompson, 2004). Because the condition may be reversible in childhood but not adulthood, early assessment and treatment have been recommended as practice guidelines, but the practice of early screening has been questioned in a series of recent studies. This issue highlights the elevated importance of evidence-based practice in recent years, as well as challenges in research design, interpretation of results, and translation of findings into public policy and professional practice.

For a significant number of children, there may be a misalignment of the eyes related to an imbalance in the ocular muscles. This condition is known as strabismus and most often results in diplopia, or double vision. It is estimated that approximately 1 in 50 children have strabismus (Flanagan et al., 2003). The condition is extremely common in children with cerebral palsy with estimates of occurrence in 75% of cases (Harley et al., 2000). In a retrospective case review, Brodsky and Fray (1997) identified congenital strabismus in 53% of cases with albinism. Symptoms include observable misalignment of the eyes (one eye may be turned in, out, up, or down), amblyopia, fatigue, reading difficulties including problems maintaining place and loss of interest, as well as affective and social consequences of teasing as a result of appearance (Harley et al., 2000). There are several common forms of strabismus depending on the particular deviation in alignment.

The term *heterotropia* describes the tendency of the eyes to diverge, with one fixed on an object while the other is unable to focus on that same point. Specific forms of heterotropia include esotropia (commonly called "crossed eyes"), in which one of the eyes is turned inward, and exotropia (known in lay terms as "walled eyes"), in which the divergent eye turns outward. In addition to diplopia, children may have difficulty with depth perception (stereopsis), and untreated strabismus may result in amblyopia. The terms *comitant* and *incomitant* are used to further classify the condition, with comitant strabismus referring to the case in which the degree of misalignment is constant in all directions of gaze and an incomitant deviation indicates that the degree of misalignment varies. As Newman-Toker and Rizzo (2001) noted, this distinction has great medical implications because whereas comitant strabismus is typically benign, the incomitant presentation may be indicative of significant pathology, including cancer. A variety of causes have been identified, including genetics, structural problems such as cataracts, and underlying pathology in the central nervous system, including the previously mentioned cerebral palsy as well as brain tumors and inflammation related to diseases such as meningitis (Harley et al., 2000). The various forms of strabismus may occur at any age but are estimated to most likely occur in the preschool years (Harley et al., 2000).

Many children with low vision will also have a condition known as nystagmus, an involuntary movement of one or both eyes (Harley et al., 2000). A degree of normal nystagmus can be elicited in most people. Pathological nystagmus involves a failure of the neural mechanisms needed to maintain a fixed gaze and will impair visual acuity. It presents as "repetitive, rhythmic oscillations of one or both eyes in any or all fields of gaze" (Riordan-Eva & Whitcher, 2004, p. 295). Children often attempt to compensate for the visual disturbance that nystagmus causes by tilting their heads (Harley et al., 2000). The condition may be linked to genetic, disease-, or drug-related causes. Congenital nystagmus will be noticeable within the first half year of life.

OUTCOMES

The outcomes of treatment for visual disorders such as amblyopia include both objective and subjective components. The objective domains have typically included visual acuity and visual fields (Johnson et al., 2003). The measurement of visual acuity has included a variety of procedures and definitions, however. Recently, Stewart, Moseley, and Fielder (2003) proposed that standard outcome measures should include two parameters: (a) the final visual acuity achieved with an optimal outcome defined as equalization of acuity in both eyes and (b) the proportion of the amblyopic deficit corrected by treatment. They provided specific guidelines for recording and interpreting these outcomes, and their adoption may become standard practice. Johnson et al. (2003) noted that the objective measures do not provide an indication of functional impairment and that measures relevant to adaptation in regard to educational, social, and personal functioning would be excellent supplements in the assessment of outcomes.

The subjective aspects of visual disorders including amblyopia have been less studied and do not yet include recommendations for standardization. Nonetheless, a few important studies of quality of life (Holmes et al., 2003), emotional impact (Hrisos et al., 2004), and integrative cost-effectiveness have been published (Konig & Barry, 2004; Lempert, 2004). These studies have used generic measures of the outcome variables in the absence of vision-specific measures. Recently, however, the Children's Visual Function Questionnaire (CVFQ) became available (Felius et al., 2004). This measure follows the development of a similar scale for adults developed with the support of the NEI (Mangione et al., 2001).

The CVFQ was developed for two age groups: less than 3 years and 3 years or older. Factor analytic study of the two such age groups ($n = 397$ and $n = 376$, respectively) suggested that the following subscales represented the data well: (a) general health, (b) general vision, (c) competence (in daily functioning), (d) personality, (e) family impact, and (f) treatment. Felius et al. (2004) reported that their validation work would continue and that they intended to distribute the measures without cost. In addition, a variety of children's well-being measures that may be relevant to visual impairment in both the research and clinical context are available (Naar-King, Ellis, & Frey, 2004).

The nomologic network of variables related to visual disorders in children has indeed become more comprehensive. To enhance consideration of this network, the conceptual model in Figure 16.1 was developed. The model includes variables that are suggested to have direct causal influence, as well as those that are likely to play moderating and mediating roles in determining outcomes. It is hoped that the model will be well received critically and that it may stimulate theory and research to further the development of evidence based treatment.

The Evidence With Regard to Objective Outcomes

The evidence base in treatment for pediatric vision problems was significantly advanced in 1997 with the formation of the Pediatric Eye Disease Investigator Group (PEDIG). This multicenter collaborative group is funded by the NEI, a branch of the National Institutes of Health (NIH). The group currently includes more than 60 participating sites and has concluded a number of randomized clinical trials related to amblyopia as well as other major visual disorders found in children. The group maintains a Web site (http://public.pedig.jaeb.org/Index.html) that describes its mission and current and completed studies and lists all its publications.

The two most frequently studied treatments for amblyopia are patching (a removable piece of cloth or other material covering one eye) and atropine eyedrops of the nonamblyopic eye (Pediatric Eye Disease Investigator, 2002). Both interventions are aimed at stimulating the weaker eye. Moderating factors include age of diagnosis, initial severity, and compliance. These treatments and the variables that modify response to treatment have been intensively studied in recent years, with major findings resulting from PEDIG's large collaborative clinical trials.

In the past 3 years, PEDIG has published three reports from a large multicenter randomized clinical trial of atropine and patching for amblyopia. These studies have addressed the question of which treatment, patching or atropine drops, is more effective, as well as potential moderators of effectiveness, including age, cause of amblyopia, and severity of initial deficit. The study included 419 children between ages 3 and 7 years who were randomly assigned to either a patching regimen of at least 6 hours per day or one drop of atropine per day in the nonamblyopic eye. The children were reassessed at 5 weeks, 16 weeks, and 6 months, with the primary outcome mea-

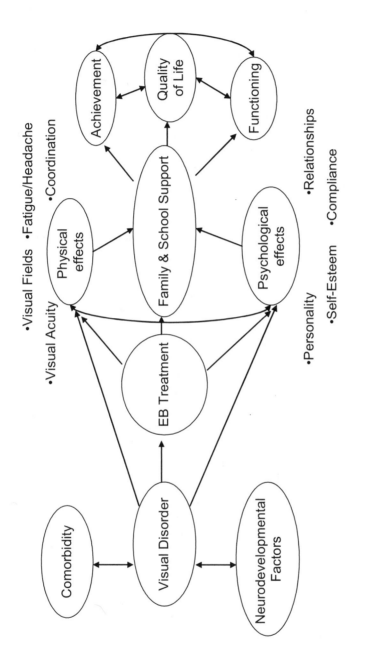

Figure 16.1. Conceptual model of the impact of childhood visual impairment. EB treatment = evidence-based treatment.

sure being visual acuity. The results showed that at 5 weeks, both groups had significantly improved vision, with a statistically significant advantage for the patching group relative to the atropine group ($p < .0001$). Interestingly, however, the patching advantage had disappeared by the time of the final assessment. The results were stable across the moderators included in the study: gender, age, initial severity, cause of amblyopia, and patching dosage (considered dichotomously as 6 to 8 vs. 10 or more hours of patching). The authors concluded that the choice of treatment may primarily be a function of child and parental preference. In an accompanying commentary, however, Kushner (2003) noted that although the final visual acuities were equivalent, the practical advantage of fewer trips to the doctor after only 5 weeks of treatment to reach normal vision in the patching group may be important and should be considered in consultation with families. In addition, the possibility of reaching the target outcome with a less intensive patching regimen opens the possibility that treatment can be effectively conducted after school, eliminating much of the social stigma and negative feedback that is likely to interfere with compliance.

Cobb, Russell, Cox, and MacEwen (2002) examined the predictive value of age of diagnosis and degree of anisometropia (unequal refractive power in the two eyes) in relation to visual outcomes. They tested regression models with a sample of 112 children who had been treated with spectacle correction and occlusion via patching, finding that both degree of refractive error and degree of anisometropia were significant predictors of visual acuity after treatment, but age of initial diagnosis was not related to acuity.

As noted previously, cataracts are a major cause of childhood blindness and may be comorbid with amblyopia and strabismus. The long-term visual outcome of early surgery for children with cataracts was investigated by Hosal, Biglan, and Elhan (2000). Their study of 171 children who had cataracts removed before age 8 suggested that visual acuity can be good following surgical treatment but that the presence of strabismus moderates this result in most cases. In addition, the most recent Cochrane review of surgical intervention for cataracts was consistent with the report of positive outcomes but noted that differential rates of side effects such as secondary opacification and compliance with follow-up care warrant further study of specific surgical procedures (Long & Chen, 2004)

The Evidence With Regard to Subjective Outcomes

In the largest such study to date, Hrisos et al. (2004) examined the subjective experiences of children and families during and after the course of treatment for amblyopia. Their initial cohort of 177 families was assessed via a mailed survey at three time points: during active treatment, at cessation of treatment, and 3 months after completion of treatment. Hrisos and colleagues examined both specific issues related to the child and family experience of the disorder and its treatment as well as the possible association with psychopathology. The latter was assessed with the Revised Rutter Parents Scale for Preschool Children.

The specific issues related to treatment were assessed via questionnaire items on compliance, emotional upset, and coping. Most parents reported that their children were coping "fairly or very well" (p. 1553), but there was significantly more emotional distress reported in children who were given occlusion (patching) treatment ($p = .03$). In addition, about half of the parents reported at least some difficulty with compliance with glasses, and three fourths reported similar experience with the patching regimen. In addition, teasing was reported by a significant number of children, was associated with wearing glasses, and persisted into the early school years. Despite these issues, the study also found that, overall, children were coping well and that there was no significant occurrence of psychopathology at any point in the treatment course or follow-up period. The study did suggest that increased difficulties in all domains might be expected with greater intensity treatments, a function of initial severity of amblyopia.

Reed, Kraft, and Buncic (2004) recently investigated academic and nonacademic outcomes in children with strabismus with a survey of parents. Their sample included the parents of 137 children between the ages of 6 and 16 as well as a comparison group of 50 parents of children without strabismus in a slightly younger cohort (aged 6–12 years). Reading difficulties were reported in 38% of cases with strabismus, but that proportion was not significantly greater than the comparison group, with 22% reporting that their child had trouble learning to read. Subsequent analyses of a variety of potential moderators, including type of strabismus, age of onset, and surgical treatment, were not associated with significant variance in the strabismic group. Higher rates of problems were reported in other school subject areas, including math, spelling, language and memory/attention, and physical education. The difference between the visually impaired and comparison groups in terms of the number of academic problems reported was statistically significant ($p < .025$). The study also reported that nonacademic problems such as stumbling, difficulty catching a ball, headaches, and eyestrain were more frequent in the group with strabismus ($p < .01$). They also noted that the presence of reading difficulties in the impaired group was predictive of other academic and nonacademic problems. They hypothesized that strabismus alone does not account for the observed differences and that further study should consider the possibility that additional perceptual problems (e.g., depth perception) as well as physical (e.g., headache) or affective (e.g., frustration) factors may be implicated in the learning problems of some children with strabismus.

Consideration of interactions between the functional and psychosocial aspects of strabismus has increased recently (Olitsky et al., 1999; Schworm & Rudolph, 2000). For example, Olitsky et al. (1999) studied the social perception of faces with strabismic eyes. Although the study was with adults, there were consistent negative ratings across 11 descriptive characteristics relevant to social acceptance and vocational functioning. A replication with a pediatric sample would be most interesting and important.

MEDICAL AND PSYCHOEDUCATIONAL IMPLICATIONS

The medical and psychoeducational implications of visual impairment range from the subtle to the more obvious and have been complicated by myths that continue to influence the treatment of children with visual impairment (Shore, 1998). These myths have particular relevance for the classroom. For example, there is no evidence that children will damage their eyes by holding a book close to the face or by reading in dim light. In fact, some children with albinism and cataracts may see better in dim light (Shore, 1998). In the long run, mistaken thinking about pediatric visual conditions can only be overcome with the dissemination of results of well-designed studies.

The impact of the evidence-based or best practices paradigm is apparent in the diagnosis and treatment of visual impairment in children despite the many challenges inherent in this area. The study of vision disorders and their correlates and consequences has been one of the more difficult areas of children's health research because they are relatively rare, and may be complicated by comorbidity, compliance problems, and the challenges of maintaining intact research cohorts in order to assess long-term outcomes (Rahi & Gilbert, 2004). In addition, the variability within and across children is due not only to the issues just cited, but also to the "moving target" that is the visual system of the developing young child. Yet the impact of visual disorders on important affective, social, educational, and vocational outcomes necessitates the sort of commitment, creativity, and collaboration seen in some of the large-scale trials to be reviewed herein.

In 1997, Snowdon and Stewart-Brown set off a major debate on the usefulness of screening for visual disorders with the publication of their comprehensive review. Following carefully described procedures, their systematic and critical review located an initial set of more than 5,000 studies, 85 of which were considered relevant to the question of efficacy of preschool screening. Snowdon and Stewart-Brown determined that, with regard to amblyopia, there were no trials that were sufficiently well designed to produce good evidence with regard to the benefits of screening (i.e., no trials included a no-treatment control group). The practical implication of the review, they suggested, was that the very existence of preschool vision screening should be reconsidered. This review sounded an alarm that was widely heard and resulted in serious reexamination of the issue in amblyopia and other conditions.

One of the subsequent studies used a longitudinal design in which children who had been initially screened and treated were reassessed up to 17 years after their initial examination (Ohlsson, Baumann, Sjostrand, & Abrahamsson, 2002). Of the initial sample of 44 children, 26 returned to the clinic for examination of their current visual acuity. The general pattern of results was characterized as one of stability, with most children (83%) either remaining stable or improving in the amblyopic eye. Four children declined in visual acuity, and the overall improvement was not statistically significant. Test results for the nonamblyotic eye were generally similar, with 92% remaining stable or improving in acuity and the mean improvement was significant ($p = .002$). The authors were encouraged by the pattern of results, yet their design again did not use a no-treatment control group.

A larger prospective study included a number of design improvements, including standardization of the time of assessment at 37 months, larger sample size with consideration of both statistical and clinical significance, and a randomized clinical trial embedded within the larger design (Williams et al., 2003). The study produced statistically significant evidence that early screening and treatment is likely to produce better visual acuity than no screening. The discussion of the study included important observations about the need for further consideration of clinical significance as well as cost–benefit analysis before the strongest possible recommendations about screening could be made.

Williams (2004) recently conducted a critical review of the evidence base in treatment. She located 11 randomized studies over the period 1968 to 1999 but none that included a no-treatment comparison. Considering the age of the trials and design limitations, Williams was reluctant to conclude that the evidence in favor of any treatment was compelling. In addition to the issue of inadequate control groups, treatment integrity related to non-compliance was cited as a limiting factor in interpretation of prior results (Williams, 2004). Williams regarded the evidence for screening and early intervention as slightly better but still not meeting national standards for evidence based ophthalmology. Thus, at this moment, debate and further study are likely to continue.

Hrisos et al. (2004) recommended that to maximize compliance, enhance visual and educational outcomes, and minimize distress, the following steps should be taken: (a) provide parents with detailed information about the condition and the recommended treatment; (b) use less intensive treatments whenever possible because these are associated with lower reports of distress and no difference in outcomes; (c) provide parents with as much choice as possible; and to (d) inform parents that although some distress may be observed, it is to be considered a normal reaction to treatment, that there is no risk of long-term psychological harm from treatment, and that, in fact, the goal of improved vision can be reached relatively quickly and permanently.

What expectations should children and school personnel have with regard to educational achievement in children with visual impairment? Layton and Lock (2001) suggested that children who receive appropriate intervention should be expected to perform in the normal range relative to their ability. Furthermore, the presence of a gap between performance and potential in such children suggests the possibility of a learning disability due to other problems in cognitive processing. That is, poor performance for visually impaired students should not be assumed to be consistent with visual processing deficits when other disabilities have not been ruled out.

The complexity of assessment of learning disabilities in children with visual impairment was thoroughly considered in the article by Layton and Lock (2001), which illustrates the usefulness of combined quantitative and qualitative assessment methods in tailoring an Individualized Education Plan (IEP) to the individual student and simultaneously enhancing the reliability and validity of the assessment. The quantitative assessment includes use of the Learning Disabilities Diagnostic Inventory, which produces scores in six performance areas and is considered valid for the assessment of children with low vision. Layton and Lock illustrated the interpretation of the inventory scores in the context of such qualitative data as work samples from the classroom, informal observation in academic and nonacademic settings, and the comments of other school personnel.

Special education personnel are obviously crucial to the successful assessment and implementation of IEPs for visually impaired students. Kirchner and Diament (1999) conducted a national survey to determine the kinds of specialists available to such children as well as their availability. They concluded that a significant shortage exists for students who are visually impaired as well as those with multiple disabilities in addition to vision.

LaVenture (2003) commented on the critical but frequently underappreciated role of parents in the success of IEPs for children with visual impairment. Her organization, the National Association for Parents of Children with Visual Impairments (NAPVI), has conducted parent education workshops to inform and empower parents to participate actively in educational planning and advocacy.

In addition to better use of human resources such as parents, evolving information technology will continue to develop with great implications for children with visual impairments. Recently, a special issue of the *Journal of Visual Impairment and Blindness* was devoted specifically to this topic (October, 2003). For example, Fruchterman (2003) described the evolution of multipurpose cell phones for children (and adults) with visual impairments, and Kurzweil (2003) reviewed the promise of lower costs and smaller designs for enhancing the functioning and quality of life of people with visual impairments.

CONCLUSION

In recent years significant progress has been made in strengthening the connection between research and practice in visual disorders of childhood.

The development of multicenter clinical trials as exemplified by PEDIG, the potential usefulness of technology in the scientist's lab, the doctor's office, the classroom, and the home, and recognition of the value of multidisciplinary teams working closely with parents should all be seen as promising signs in the future of children with visual impairments. In addition, subjective outcomes such as quality of life are becoming integral to conceptualization, assessment, and treatment of visual impairment. This broader and more integrative approach should be helpful to children and families on multiple levels, with long-term benefits not previously enjoyed in this population.

REFERENCES

Barnes, G. R., Hess, R. F., Dumoulin, S. O., Achtman, R. L., & Pike, G. B. (2001). The cortical deficit in humans with strabismic amblyopia. *Journal of Physiology, 533,* 281–297.

Biswas, S., & Lloyd, I. C. (1999). Oculocutaneous albinism. *Archives of Disease in Childhood, 80,* 565–569.

Brodsky, M. C., & Fray, K. J. (1997). The prevalence of strabismus in congenital nystagmus: The influence of anterior visual pathway disease. *Journal of AAPOS: American Association for Pediatric Ophthalmology and Strabismus, 1,* 16–19.

Cobb, C. J., Russell, K., Cox, A., & MacEwen, C. J. (2002). Factors influencing visual outcome in anisometropic amblyopes. *British Journal of Ophthalmology, 86,* 1278–1281.

Cooke, R. W., Foulder-Hughes, L., Newsham, D., & Clarke, D. (2004). Ophthalmic impairment at 7 years of age in children born very preterm. *Archives of Disease in Childhood: Fetal and Neonatal Edition, 89,* F249–F253.

Corn, A. L., & Koenig, A. J. (1996). *Foundations of low vision: Clinical and functional perspectives.* New York: American Foundation for the Blind.

Emsley, H. C., Wardle, S. P., Sims, D. G., Chiswick, M. L., & D'Souza, S. W. (1998). Increases survival and deteriorating developmental outcome in 23 to 25 week old gestation infants, 1990–4 compared with 1984–9. *Archives of Disease in Childhood: Fetal and Neonatal Edition, 78,* F99–F104.

Felius, J. D., Stager, D. R., Sr., Berry, P. M., Fawcett, S. L., Stager, D. R., Jr., Salomeo, S. R., et al. (2004). Development of an instrument to assess vision-related quality of life in young children. *American Journal of Ophthalmology, 138,* 362–372.

Flanagan, N. M., Jackson, A. J., & Hill, A. E. (2003). Visual impairment in childhood: Insights from a community-based survey. *Child Care, Health, and Development, 29,* 493–499.

Fruchterman, J. R. (2003). In the palm of your hand: A vision of the future of technology for people with visual impairments. *Journal of Visual Impairment and Blindness, 97,* 585–591.

Harley, R. K., Lawrence, G. A., Sanford, L., & Burnett, R. (2000). *Visual impairment in the schools.* Springfield, IL: Charles C Thomas.

Holmes, J. M., Beck, R. W., Kraker, R. T., Cole, S. R., Repka, M. X., Birch, E. E., et al., and the Pediatric Eye Disease Investigator Group. (2003). Impact of patching and atropine treatment on the child and family in the amblyopia treatment study. *Archives of Ophthalmology, 121,* 1625–1632.

Hosal, B. M., Biglan, A. W., & Elhan, A. H. (2000). High levels of binocular function are achievable after removal of monocular cataracts in children before 8 years of age. *Ophthalmology, 107,* 1647–1655.

Hrisos, S., Clarke, M. P., & Wright, C. M. (2004). The emotional impact of amblyopia treatment in preschool children: Randomized controlled trial. *Ophthalmology, 111,* 1550–1556.

Individuals With Disabilities in Education Act (IDEA). §300.7 *Child with a disability.* Retrieved August 27, 2004, from http://www.ideapractices.org/law/regulations/glossaryIndex.php

Johnson, G. J., Minassian, D. C., Weale, R. A., & West, S. K. (2003). *The epidemiology of eye disease.* London: Arnold.

Kirchner, C., & Diament, S. (1999). Estimates of the number of visually impaired students, their teachers, and orientation and mobility specialists: Part 1. *Journal of Visual Impairment and Blindness, 93,* 600–606.

Konig, H. H., & Barry, J. C. (2004). Cost-utility analysis of orthoptic screening in kindergarten: A Markov model based on data from Germany. *Pediatrics, 113,* e95–e108.

Kurzweil, R. (2003). The future of intelligent technology and its impact on disabilities. *Journal of Visual Impairment and Blindness, 97,* 582–584.

Kushner, B. J. (2003). Discussion. *Ophthalmology, 110,* 1632–1638.

LaVenture, S. (2003). The Individuals With Disabilities Act (IDEA): Past and present. *Journal of Visual Impairment and Blindness, 97,* 517–518.

Layton, C. A., & Lock, R. H. (2001). Determining learning disabilities in students with low vision. *Journal of Visual Impairment and Blindness, 95,* 288–299.

Lempert, P. (2004). A cost–benefit analysis of vision-screening methods for preschoolers and school-age children. *Journal of AAPOS: American Association for Pediatric Ophthalmology and Strabismus, 8,* 74–75.

Long, V., & Chen, S. (2004). Surgical interventions for bilateral congenital cataract. *Cochrane Database of Systematic Reviews, 3,* CD003171.

Mangione, C. M., Lee, P. P., Gutierrez, P. R., Spritzer, K., Berry, S., & Hays, R. D. (2001). Development of the 25-Item National Eye Institute Visual Function Questionnaire. *Archives of Ophthalmology, 119,* 1050–1058.

Mets, M. B., Holfels, E., Boyer, K. M., Swisher, C. N., Roizen, N., Stein, L., et al. (1997). Eye manifestations of congenital toxoplasmosis. *American Journal of Ophthalmology, 123,* 1–16.

Naar-King, S., Ellis, D. A., & Frey, M. A. (2004). *Assessing children's well-being: A handbook of measures.* Mahwah, NJ: Erlbaum.

National Eye Institute. (n.d.). *Amblyopia resource guide.* Retrieved August 24, 2004, from http://www.nei.nih.gov/health/amblyopia/index.asp

Newman-Toker, D. E., & Rizzo, J. F. (2001). Neuro-ophthalmic diseases masquerading as benign strabismus. *International Ophthalmology Clinics, 41,* 115–127.

Ohlsson, J., Baumann, M., Sjostrand, J., & Abrahamsson, M. (2002). Long term visual outcome in amblyopia treatment. *British Journal of Ophthalmology, 86,* 1148–1151.

Olitsky, S. E., Sudesh, S., Graziano, A., Hamblen, J., Brooks, S., & Shaha, S. H. (1999). The negative psychosocial impact of strabismus in adults. *Journal of American Association for Pediatric Ophthalmology and Strabismus, 3,* 209–211.

Pediatric Eye Disease Investigator. (2002). A randomized trial of atropine vs. patching for treatment of moderate amblyopia in children. *Archives of Ophthalmology, 120,* 268–278.

Rahi, J. S., & Gilbert, C. (2004). Paediatrics and ocular motility. In R. Wormald, L. Smeeth, & K. Henshaw (Eds.), *Evidence-based ophthalmology* (pp. 45–46). London: BMJ Publishing Group.

Reed, M. J., Kraft, S. P., & Buncic, R. (2004). Parents' observations of the academic and nonacademic performance of children with strabismus. *Journal of Visual Impairment and Blindness, 98,* 276–288.

Riordan-Eva, P., & Whitcher, J. P. (2004). *Vaughan and Asbury's general ophthalmology.* New York: McGraw-Hill.

Rudanko, S. L., Fellman, V., & Laatikainen, L. (2003). Visual impairment in children born prematurely from 1972 through 1989. *Ophthalmology, 110,* 1639–1645.

Schworm, H. D., & Rudolph, G. (2000). Comitant strabismus. *Current Opinion in Ophthalmology, 11,* 310–317.

Shore, K. (1998). *Special kids problem solver.* Paramus, NJ: Prentice Hall.

Snowdon, S. K., & Stewart-Brown, S. L. (1997). Preschool vision screening. *Health Technology Assessment, 1,* i–iv.

Stewart, C. E., Moseley, M. J., & Fielder, A. R. (2003). Defining and measuring treatment outcome in unilateral amblyopia. *British Journal of Ophthalmology, 87,* 1229–1231.

Thomas, C. L. (1995). *Taber's cyclopedic medical dictionary* (18th ed.). Philadelphia: F. A. Davis.

Thompson, G. (2004). Common childhood eye problems. *Practitioner, 248,* 46–52.

Williams, C. (2004). Unilateral amblyopia. In R. Wormald, L. Smeeth, & K. Henshaw (Eds.), *Evidence-based ophthalmology* (pp. 81–86). London: BMJ Publishing Group.

Williams, C., Northstone, K., Harrad, R. A., Sparrow, J. M., Harvey, I., & the ALSPAC Study Team. (2003). Amblyopia treatment outcomes after preschool screening v school entry screening: Observational data from a prospective cohort study. *British Journal of Ophthalmology, 87,* 988–993.

Young, T. L. (2003). Ophthalmic genetics/inherited eye disease. *Current Opinion in Ophthalmology, 14,* 296–303.

AUTHOR INDEX

Numbers in italics refer to listings in the references.

Fray, K. J., 274, *283*
Frea, W. D., 227, *232*
Freeman, J., *172*
Freeman, J. B., 103, *107*
Freeman, J. M., 103, 104, *107, 108*
Freeman, L. W., 247, *249*
French, J., 102, *107*
Freund, L., 261, *268*
Freund, L. S., 260, 261, *266, 268*
Frey, M. A., 276, *284*
Friedlander, A. H., 143, 145, *152*
Friedman, D., 9, *20*
Friedrich, W. N., 116, 119, *121*
Friesen, C. A., *122*
Friss, M. L., 101, *109*
Fritz, G., 119, *120*
Frost, L., 226, *231*
Fruchterman, J. R., 282, *283*
Fryer, A. E., 164, *173*
Fuggle, P. W., 77, *90*
Fuhlbrigge, A., 243, *248*
Fuhlbrigge, A. L., 238, *250*
Fujishiro, Y., 146, *153*
Fullerton, H. J., 185, *191*
Fung, C. M., 69, *89*
Furth, S. L., 125, 128, 129, 134, *136*

Gagnon, E. M., 51, *53*
Gaillard, W. D., 102, *107*
Gaily, E., 101, *107*
Garabedian, B., 139, *153*
Gardner, R. J. M., 255, 259, 261, *267*
Gardner, W. P., *21*
Gardner-Medwin, D., 195, *208*
Garstein, M. A., *22*
Gasche, C., 113, *121*
Gascon, G. G., *190*
Gauger, L. M., 140, *152*
Geisser, M., 97, *109*
Genel, M., 70, *86*
Genentech Inc. Cooperative Study Group, 70, *88*
Gennari, F. J., 132, *136*
George, R., 103, *108*
Gerhardt, C. A., *22*
Gerhardt, P. F., 226, *231*
Gerson, A. C., 125, 134, *136*
Geschwind, D. H., 257, 258, 259, *267*
Gettinger, M., 12, *21*
Ghafoor, A., *53*
Giacomini, K. D., 263, *268*
Giardino, H., 241, *250*

Gibb, A., 183, *192*
Gibikote, S. V., *171*
Gibson, R. J., 101, *106*
Gidal, B. E., 101, *109*
Gil, K. M., 50, 53, 188, *190*
Gilbert, C., 280, *285*
Gill, D. S., *171*
Gillberg, C., 164, *170*, 217, 218, *231*
Gillberg, I. C., 164, 165, *170*
Gilliam, F., 99, *108*
Gillon, G. T., 141, *152*
Gingold, M., *269*
Gionchetti, P., 112, *121*
Giraud, K., *152*
Glang, A., 189, *191*
Glasberg, B. A., 227, *231*
Gleason, M. M., 35, *38*
Goikhman, I., 98, *110*
Gold, L. B., *266*
Goldberg, R., 57, *66*
Goldfarb, L. P., 204, *209*
Goldman, M. B., *89*
Goldstein, E., 203, *209*
Gomez, M. R., 161, 162, 164, *170, 172, 173*
Gonzalez, R. C., 165, *170*
Goodfellow, P. J., *210*
Goodheart, C., 50, *55*
Goodman, M., 165, *170*
Gooskens, R. H. J. M., *190*
Gordon, A., *122*
Gorey-Ferguson, L., *191*
Gottesman, I., *230*
Goy, R. W., 83, *87*
Grandjean, H., 261, *266*
Granstrom, M. L., 101, *107*
Grant, D. B., 77, *90*
Gravel, J. S., 146, *153, 154*
Gray, K. M., 221, *235*
Graziano, A., *285*
Green, B., *137*
Green, K., *268*
Greenlee, J. D. W., 179, *191*
Greenley, R., 9, *20*
Greenwood, K. M., 203, *208*
Gres, C., *152*
Grew, R. S., 71, *87*
Griffin, P., 141, *154*
Griffiths, H., 181, *192*
Griggs, R. C., 193, 195, 196, 197, 198, 201, *209, 210*
Grigsby, J., *267*
Grimwood, K., 184, *189*

Livneh, H., 204, *210*
Lloyd, I. C., 272, *283*
Lobato, D., 45, *54*
Lock, R. H., 281, 282, *284*
Loesch, D. Z., 260, *267*
Loftus, E. F., 149, *151, 153*
Lombard, C., 168, *173*
Lombardino, L. J., 140, *152*
Long, V., 273, 278, *284*
Lopez, M. A., *23*
Lord, C., 215, *232*
Loucks, T., 143, *153*
Lovaas, O. I., 226, *232*
Love, S. R., 222, *233*
Loveland, K. A., 184, *191*
Lowe, P. A., 45, *54*
Lozano, P., *250*
Lubetsky, M., 224, *231*
Ludlow, C. L., 143, *153*
Luikkonen, E., 101, *107*
Lynch, M., 11, *20*
Lynch, N. R., *249*

Ma, K., *173*
MacEwen, C. J., 278, *283*
MacGillivray, M. H., 70, *88*
Mackie, E., 46, *54*
Maclean, R. E., 180, *190*
MacMillan, C., 184, *191*
Madan-Swain, A., 18, *21*, 26, 29, *38*
Madaus, M. M. R., 148, *153*
Maestrini, E., *208*
Mag, J. M., *155*
Magalini, S. C., 264, *268*
Magalini, S. I., 264, *268*
Magder, L. S., *191*
Mahoney, E. M., *191*
Mahr, G., 165, *170*
Mai, J., 101, *109*
Maixner, W. J., 180, *190*
Majnemer, A., 223, *234*
Mallick, M., *53*
Mancini, M., *208*
Mandel, E. M., 146, *151*
Mangione, C. M., 275, *284*
Manis, F., 140, *152*
Mann, L., 163, *172*
Manne, S., 45, *54*
Manolson, A., 142, *153*
Mansour, M. E., 145, *150*
Manz, P. H., 26, *39*
Marans, W. D., 214, *235*

March, J. S., *234*
Marchant, C. D., 146, *152*
Marcus, L. M., 227, *232*
Margiano, S., 149, *152, 249*
Marti, S., *90*
Martin, A., *230*
Martin, C. L., 83, *89*
Martin, M., 118, *121*
Martyn, C., *171*
Masai, W., 214, *231*
Mason, E. J., 58, *65*
Mastergeorge, A. M., 227, *233*
Matheson, P. B., 59, *64*
Matson, J. L., 222, *233*
Matthews, W. S., 263, *268*
Mauk, J. E., 214, *235*
Mauras, N., 70, *88*
Mautone, J. A., 19, *20*
Mazur, T., 80, 81, *88*
Mazzocco, M. M. M., 159, 160, *171*, 255, 256, *267, 268*
Mazzuca, L. B., 15, *22*
McAllister, T. W., 176, *192*
McCalla, J. L., *54*
McCartan, P., 142, *153*
McCauley, E., 255, *269*
McClean, T. W., 51, *54*
McClure, L. L., *54*
McClure, M. K., 228, *233*
McConnell, S., 205, *210*
McCracken, J. T., 148, *150, 233*
McCrory, M. A., *210*
McCurdy, B., 167, 168, *171*
McCurdy, E. A., 51, *54*
McDade, A., 142, *153*
McDaniel, J. S., *190*
McDonald, C. M., 194, 195, 197, 203, *208, 210*
McDougle, C. J., 214, 225, *233, 235*
McEwen, B. S., 83, *87*
McGoey, K. E., 19, *20*, 30, *38*
McGrath, N., 183, *192*
McGregor, A. L., 102, *109*
McGuire, D. E., 59, *65*
McInerney, T. K., *21*
McKee, J. R., 101, *108*
McKellop, J. M., 165, *173*
McKinlay, I. A., 164, *170*
McKinley, M., *269*
McLaughlin-Cheng, E., 217, *233*
McMahon, W. M., 223, *234*
McNally, R., 46, *54*

McQuaid, E. L., 48, *54*

Meador, K. J., 97, 104, *108, 109*

Meadows, A., *21, 53*

Meadows, I. L., *266*

Medley, L. P., 147, *153*

Medway, F. J., 189, *190*

Meeske, K., *21, 47, 53, 55*

Meesters, C., 222, *233*

Mehltretter, L., *192*

Mellits, E. D., 104, *108*

Melton, L., 82, *88*

Mendell, J. R., 195, 204, *208, 209*

Mendez, M. F., 143, *152*

Menezes, A. H., 179, *191*

Menna, R., *151*

Mensing, C., 74, 75, *88*

Merck, 115, 116, *121*

Merckelbach, H., 222, *233*

Mercuri, E., 197, *210*

Merkus, P. J., 238, *250*

Mets, M. B., 272, *284*

Meydani, S. N., 246, *250*

Meyer-Bahlburg, H. F. L., 69, 71, 84, 87, *88, 89*

Michael, P., 69, *90*

Mickelson, W., 14, *23*

Miehsler, W., 113, *121*

Mikati, M. A., *108*

Miller, B. D., 241, *250*

Miller, B. L., 257, *267*

Miller, C. K., 62, *65*

Miller, D., 45, *54*

Miller, M., 158, *171*

Miller, R. G., 195, *209*

Miller, S. L., 142, *155*

Milne, R., 257, *266*

Minassian, D. C., 273, *284*

Minchom, P. E., *190*

Miner, J., *23*

Mingroni, M. A., 238, *250*

Mings, E. L., *136*

Mirsky, A. F., 95, *108*

Mishra, A., *21*

Mody, M., 146, *153*

Moher, D., *249*

Molko, N., 256, *266*

Monobe, H., 146, *153*

Monton, F. I., 200, *211*

Moolsintong, P. J., *210*

Moore, B., *172*

Moore, B. D., 159, 160, *170, 171*

Moorman, A. S., *191*

Morales, P. C., 262, 263, *268*

Morgan, C. L., 96, *108*

Morgan, S. B., 221, *230*

Morgan, V., 59, *65*

Morgan, W. J., *249*

Morishima, A., 88, 256, *266*

Moro, M. R., 46, *55*

Morrison, M., *122*

Mors, O., 223, *232*

Morse, R., 134, *136*

Morselli, C., *121*

Mortensen, P. B., 223, *232*

Moseley, M. J., 275, *285*

Moulton, H. J., 228, *233*

Mouradian, W. E., 59, *66*

Mouren-Simeoni, M., 241, *251*

Moxley, R. T., 197, 198, *210*

Mukherjee, S., 189, *192*

Mulcahy, K., *88*

Mullarkey, S., 256, *269*

Mullins, L., *249*

Muntoni, F., 197, *210*

Murata, T., 223, *232*

Muris, P., 222, *233*

Murray, J. A., 117, *121*

Murray, J. C., *65*

Murray, T., *53*

Muter, V., 142, *153*

Muzik, O., *170*

Myles, B. S., 217, 218, 221, *230, 233*

Naar-King, S., 276, *284*

Nabors, L. A., 34, *38*

Naidu, S., 220, *233*

Naimon, D., 248, *249*

Nakazawa, T., 114, *122*

Nanao, K., *209*

Narhi, V., *137*

Nash, D. R., 243, *250*

Nash, L. B., 63, *65*

Nassau, J. H., 9, *22*, 48, *54*, 176, *192*

Nathanson, R., *267*

National Digestive Diseases Information Clearinghouse, 114, *121*

National Eye Institute, 273, *284*

National Heart, Lung, & Blood Institute, 238, *250*

National Institute of Mental Health, 214, *233*

National Institute of Neurological Disorders and Stroke, 158, 164, 165, *171, 172*

National Institutes of Health, 128, 130, *136*

SUBJECT INDEX

Chiari malformation, 179
chronic kidney disease, 134
common cold, 240–241
craniofacial anomalies, 60, 63
for designing educational plans, 34–35, 36–37
diabetes, 75
ecological, 15, 19
of eligibility for federal educational assistance, 26, 27–31, 35–36
endocrine disorders, 85–86
fragile X syndrome, 261
growth failure, 69
health-related quality of life, 134
hyperthyroidism, 76–77
hypothyroidism, 76
Lesch–Nyhan disease, 262, 263
for level of intervention, 15–16, 19
Lowe syndrome, 265
neurocutaneous syndromes, 166, 167–168, 169
neurofibromatosis, 158
neurological impairments, 176–177
otitis media, 146
pain, 48
posttraumatic stress disorder, 47
pubertal advancement, 79, 80
seizures and seizure disorders, 91, 92–95, 104
tuberous sclerosis, 163
vision problems, 275–276
vision screening, 280–281
Assistive devices
classroom accommodation for children with neuromuscular diseases, 206
IDEA benefits, 32
Asthma, 238, 241, 242–243, 247–248
Astrocytomas, 44
Athyreosis, 75, 77, 78
Atonic seizures, 95
Atropine eyedrops, 276–278
Attachment, 11
Attention-deficit/hyperactivity disorder, 256
Aura, epileptic, 94
Autism, 214–217
associated neurologic abnormalities, 216–217
epidemiology, 216
etiology, 216
fragile X syndrome and, 260
manifestations, 214–216
tuberous sclerosis and, 165

See also Pervasive developmental disorders
Autism spectrum disorders, 213–214
Autoimmune disorders
associated hyperthyroidism, 76
chronic kidney disease, 126
myasthenia gravis, 201
Automatisms, 93–94
Autonomy
diabetes and, 73
epilepsy and, 99
Autosomal recessive muscular dystrophy of childhood, 197

Barbiturates, 100
Becker muscular dystrophy, 195, 203
Benign juvenile muscular dystrophy, 195
Biofeedback, 188
Biologic response modifiers, 49
Body image
diabetes and, 73
neurocutaneous syndrome and, 168
Bone marrow transplantation, 49
Botulism, 201
Brain abscesses, 184
Brain imaging, 177
visual impairment studies, 273–274
Brain tumors, 44
Breast-feeding child with craniofacial anomalies, 62
Bronchitis, 238, 243
Bronchodilators, 242–243
Bulimia, 116
Busperidone, 225

Cancer, children with
alternative therapies, 50–51
causal attributions, 48
classification and staging, 43
clinical features of disease, 41
cure rate, 42
etiology, 41, 48
family functioning, 45
incidence, 42, 43, 44
mortality, 41, 42, 52
outcomes, 41–42, 45–48, 52
pain management, 46, 47–49
peer relations, 45
psychopathology risk, 45–47, 52
psychosocial considerations, 42
psychosocial interventions, 50
quality of life concerns, 41–42

research needs, 52
school functioning, 45
school reintegration, 51–52
survival patterns, 41–42
treatment side effects and complications, 46, 47, 48, 50
treatment strategies, 49, 52
trends, 42
types of cancers, 43–44
See also specific location of tumor: specific type of cancer
Carbamazepine, 100–101
Cardiac disease, in muscular dystrophy, 195, 196
Carnitine deficiency, myopathic, 198
Carnitive palmityl transferase deficiency, 197
Cataracts, 273, 278, 280
Celiac disease, 111, 117
Central nervous system. *See* Neurological impairment
Cerebral artery dissection, 185
Cerebral palsy, 274
Charcot–Marie–Tooth syndrome, 199
CHARGE syndrome, 59
Chemotherapy, 49
Chiari malformation, 178, 179
Child abuse, growth hormone deficiency and, 68
Children's Visual Function Questionnaire, 275–276
Chronic illness in children, generally
academic implications, 8
ecological model, 9–15
family functioning and, 9
peer relationships and, 8–9
prevalence, 3
trends, 3
See also specific disorder
Cleft lip/palate, 60–61. *See also* Craniofacial anomalies
Clonic seizures, 95
Clonidine, 225
Clozapine, 224
Coenzyme Q10, 182
Cognitive–behavioral therapy
in cancer treatment, 50
with child with craniofacial abnormalities, 63
for neurological impairment symptoms, 188
for recurrent abdominal pain, 118–119
Cognitive functioning

antiepileptic drug side effects, 100
Asperger's syndrome manifestations, 218
cancer treatment side effects, 47
Chiari malformation effects, 179
craniofacial abnormalities and development of, 59
diabetes complications, 74
encephalitis complications, 182–183
epilepsy effects, 97–98
fragile X syndrome manifestations, 260
growth hormone deficiency effects, 70
head injury-related deficits, 186
in Huntington's disease, 181
hydrocephalus effects, 180
hypothyroidism complications, 77
kidney disease effects, 130
Klinefelter syndrome manifestations, 258
in Lesch–Nyhan disease, 263
in Lowe syndrome, 264
neurofibromatosis effects, 159–160
neurological impairments and, 176
neuromusuclar disease outcomes, 203
pervasive developmental disorders, 221
pubertal development and, 81
Rett's disorder manifestations, 219
seizure classification, 93, 95
specific language impairment etiology, 140
speed of information processing, 140
in Sturge–Weber syndrome, 162
tuberous sclerosis complications, 164–165
Turner syndrome manifestations, 255–256
visual impairment and, 272
Collaborative practice
chronic kidney disease management, 135
Individualized Education Plan development, 31–32
intervention challenges, 17–20
neurocutaneous syndrome management, 166
neurological impairment interventions, 186–187, 189
pain management, 17
pharmacotherapy role, 18–19
to promote adherence, 17–18
rationale, 25
for school reintegration, 18

scope of, 7
seizure disorder management, 104–105
student assistance teams, 30–31
systems model, 7–8
treatment of craniofacial abnormalities, 63
Common cold, 240–241, 242, 245–246
Communication problems
in Asperger's syndrome, 217–218
autism manifestations, 214–215, 226
fragile X syndrome manifestations, 260
See also Speech problems
Community-based health delivery, 13
Complementary and alternative therapies, 50–51
for pervasive developmental disorders, 227–229
Confidentiality of educational records, 34
Congenital muscular dystrophies, 197
Contingency management, 149
Coping Cat program, 188
Corticosteroid therapy, 242–243, 244
Cortisol, 82
replacement therapy, 84
Craniofacial anomalies
assessment, 60, 63
associated disorders, 58
associated feeding problems, 62
associated speech problems, 59, 61–62
cognitive functioning and, 59
craniosynostosis, 180–181
definition, 57
dental care and, 61
effects on peer relationships, 9
etiology, 57–58
incidence, 57
medical treatment, 60–62
outcomes, 58–59
psychosocial considerations, 62–63, 64
treatment team, 63
types of, 57
Craniosynostosis, 180–181
Creatine, 204
Cretinism, 76
Crohn's disease, 112, 113
Croup, 239–240, 244
Crouzon syndrome, 57. *See also* Craniofacial anomalies
Curschmann–Batten–Steinert syndrome, 196
Cyanosis, 94–95
Cystic fibrosis, 111, 116–117, 240, 245, 248

Dejerine–Sottas disease, 199
Dental care, 61
Depression
in children with cancer, 45–46
in child with asthma, 241
diabetes and, 73
in neurocutaneous syndromes, 168
pervasive developmental disorder and, 221–222
risk in neuromusuclar disorders, 205
Dermatomyositis syndrome, 198
Development
caregiver role, 11
congenital adrenal hyperplasia and, 83–84
craniofacial abnormalities and, 58–59
ecological model, 10–15, 19
growth hormone deficiency manifestations, 68
health system role, 12–13
hypothyroidism effects, 77–78
kidney disease effects, 130
muscular dystrophy effects, 195
school role, 12
sociocultural context, 14
vision, 272–273
See also Pervasive developmental disorders; Puberty
Dexamethasone, 83
Diabetes mellitus
alcohol use in, 73
assessment, 75
autonomy issues, 73
classification, 72
clinical features, 72
epidemiology, 72
etiology, 72
group interventions, 75
medical management, 74
medical outcomes, 73
neurocognitive effects, 74
physical exercise effects, 74–75
psychoeducational interventions, 74–75
psychosocial risks, 73–74
renal complications, 126
self-image issues, 73
treatment adherence, 73
trends, 72
Dialysis, 125, 127, 130–131
Diplopia, 201, 274
Discrimination
against child with epilepsy, 98

in educational services, 35, 36
protections for persons with neurocutaneous syndrome, 167
Dopamine blockers, 181–182
Dopaminergic system, in Lesch–Nyhan disease, 262
Down syndrome, 59
Drop attacks, 95
Drug resistant bacteria, 239, 243
Duchenne muscular dystrophy, 194–195, 202, 203–204
Dyshormonogenesis, 75
Dysphasia, developmental. *See* Specific language impairment
Dystrophin, 194

E. coli, 124
Eating disorders, 116
diabetes and, 73, 75
Echolalia, 215
Ecological model of development, 19
assessment in, 15, 19
cross-system interactions, 13–14
distinguishing features of, 9–10
environmental systems, 11–13
levels of intervention, 15–16, 19
person–environment interaction, 10–11, 19
sociocultural system, 14–15
Electroencephalography, 93, 94, 176–177
Emery–Dreifuss muscular dystrophy, 196
Encephalitis, 182–183
Endocrine disorders
causes of associated psychosocial problems, 67
clinical features, 67
types of, 67. *See also specific disorder*
variable presentation, 85–86
Endorphins, 181
End-stage renal disease, 125
Enkephalin, 181
Epilepsy, 105–106
academic performance and, 97, 98
adolescent development, 99
age of onset, 92
associated psychosocial problems, 98–99
auras, 94
cognitive functioning and, 97–98, 100
comorbid psychiatric disorder, 93, 97, 98
definition, 91–92

epidemiology, 92, 106
group interventions, 105
ketogenic diet to control, 103–104
morbidity, 96
mortality, 96, 102
motor vehicle operations and, 99
pharmacotherapy, 97–98, 99–102
psychosocial/psychoeducational interventions, 104–105
quality of life effects, 96–97
refractory, 102
seizure classification, 92–95
social costs, 96
Sturge–Weber syndrome and, 160–161
surgical treatment, 102–103
vagus nerve stimulation therapy, 103
Esoptropia, 274
Ethanol, 58
Ethosuximide, 100
Evidence-based interventions, 4
Ewing's sarcoma, 44
Exotropia, 274

Facioscapulohumeral muscular dystrophy, 195–196, 203
Family
in adherence promotion, 17–18
of child with cancer, 45
in ecological model of development, 11
effects of chronic illness, 9
health system linkage, 13
in neurological impairment interventions, 187
psychoeducational interventions for epilepsy management, 105
resilience-promoting factors, 9, 11
rituals, 9
role in chronic care, 7
in school reintegration, 18
school system linkage, 13–14
trust in health professionals, 13
universal preventive intervention, 15–16
See also Parental expectations; Parental role in interventions; Parental stress; Parenting skills
Family Educational Rights and Privacy Act (1974), 34
Fatigue, cancer treatment-related, 46
Fetal development
alcohol exposure, 58
causes of craniofacial anomalies, 58

in congenital adrenal hyperplasia, 82, 84–85

delayed puberty, 71, 80

See also Endocrine disorders

Human leukocyte antigen, 127

Humeroperoneal dystrophy, 196

Huntington's disease, 181–182

Hydrocephalus, 178, 179, 180, 216

Hydroxylase CAH, 82

Hyperglycemia, 72, 73

Hyperthyroidism

assessment, 76–77

clinical features, 76, 78

incidence, 77

medical management, 78–79

treatment adherence, 79

Hypoglycemia, 72, 73

Hypogonadism, 80

Hyponatremia, 101

Hypothalamus, in growth hormone deficiency, 68

Hypothyroidism

acquired, 76, 77–78

age at onset, 77, 78

assessment, 76

clinical features, 75, 76, 77

congenital, 75–76, 77, 78

etiology, 76

incidence, 76

medical management, 77, 78

medical outcomes, 76, 77–78

neurocognitive effects, 77

screening, 76, 77

treatment adherence, 79

types of, 75, 76

Hypoxia, 94

IDEA. *See* Individuals With Disabilities Education Improvement Act

Immune function, stress and, 246

Immunoglobulin-A nephropathy, 126

Immunotherapy, 49

Incidence

AIDS/HIV, 3

bronchitis, 238

cancer, 42, 43, 44

Chiari malformation, 179

congenital adrenal hyperplasia, 82

craniofacial anomalies, 57

croup, 240

cystic fibrosis, 240

Duchenne muscular dystrophy, 194

epilepsy, 92

growth hormone deficiency, 68

Guillain–Barré syndrome, 183

hydrocephalus, 180

kidney failure, 123

Lesch–Nyhan disease, 262

Lowe syndrome, 264

microcephaly, 181

neural tube defects, 177

neurofibromatosis, 158

otitis media, 146

peptic ulcer disease, 113

pervasive developmental disorders, 214

polymyositis and dermatomyositis syndromes, 198

recurrent abdominal pain, 115

seizures, 92

thyroid disorders, 76, 77

tuberous sclerosis, 163

See also Prevalence

Individualized Education Plan

for child with visual impairment, 282

goals, 31–32

initiation, 31

least restrictive environment provisions, 32

needs assessment, 34–35, 36–37

parent's participation in development of, 33–34

purpose, 26–27

Individualized Family Service Plan, 26–27

Individuals With Disabilities Education Improvement Act (IDEA), 25, 133

benefits, 26–27

disagreement over eligibility findings, 31

disease-specific provisions, 34–35

dispute resolution provisions, 34

eligibility, 27–31

extended school year services under, 32

Individualized Education Plan development, 31–32, 34–35, 36–37

least restrictive environment provisions, 32

neurocutaneous syndrome eligibility under, 166

No Child Left Behind Act and, 36

parental participation in programs of, 33–34

procedural safeguards, 34

reevaluations for eligibility, 31

referral for eligibility evaluation, 30

Rehabilitation Act and, 35–36

neurological impairments related to head injury, 186
neuromuscular diseases, 193–194
otitis media, 145–146
Rett's disorder, 219
specific language impairment, 139–140
strabismus, 274
stuttering, 143
tuberous sclerosis, 163–164
Turner syndrome, 255
visual impairments, 272
See also Incidence
Preventive intervention
common cold, 245–246
congenital adrenal hyperplasia, 83
hypothyroidism screening, 76, 77
indicated level, 16
Lowe syndrome, 265
respiratory disorders, 241–242
universal level, 15–16
Primary care
barriers to care, 12
psychoeducational service delivery, 4
Progressive tardive juvenile muscular dystrophy, 195
Protective factors
assessment, 15
causal attributions for cancer, 48
family factors, 9, 11
psychoneuroimmunology, 246–247
Psychoeducational interventions
cancer, 42
celiac disease, 117
child with craniofacial anomalies, 62–63
cystic fibrosis, 117
diabetes, 74–75
epilepsy, 104–105
fragile X syndrome, 261–262
genital reconstruction surgery implications, 85
growth hormone deficiency-related, 70–71
inflammatory bowel disease, 113
irritable bowel syndrome, 114–115
kidney disease, 129–135
Klinefelter syndrome, 258–259
neurocutaneous syndromes, 166–169
neurological impairments, 188–189
neuromuscular disease, 203–204, 205–206
otitis media treatment, 147

pediatric treatment trends, 3–4
pervasive developmental disorder, 225–227
precocious or delayed puberty, 81
psychogenic vomiting, 116
recurrent abdominal pain, 115, 118–119
respiratory disorders, 246–248
rumination, 115–116
selective mutism, 148–149
specific language impairment, 141
spina bifida, 178–179
stuttering, 144–145
training for medical professionals, 14
tuberous sclerosis, 165, 166
Turner syndrome, 257
Psychoneuroimmunology, 246
Ptosis, 201, 273
Puberty
congenital adrenal hyperplasia and, 83
definition, 79
delayed onset, 71, 80, 81
developmental assessment, 79
intellectual development and, 81
interventions in developmental onset, 81
parental expectations, 80–81
precocious, 79–80, 81, 83

Quality of life
assessment, 134
cancer treatment considerations, 41–42

Race/ethnicity
cancer risk, 42
pneumonia risk, 239
pubertal advancement, 79
Radiation therapy, 49
for hyperthyroidism, 78–79
Rehabilitation Act. *See* Section 504 of Rehabilitation Act (1973)
Relaxation training
diabetes management, 75
for neurological impairment symptoms, 188
Renal insufficiency, chronic, 68
Reserpine, 182
Respiratory disorders
asthma, 238, 242–243, 247–248
bronchitis, 238, 243
common cold, 240–241, 242, 245–246
croup, 239–240, 244
cystic fibrosis, 111, 116–117, 240, 245, 248

ABOUT THE EDITOR

LeAdelle Phelps, PhD, is professor and director of the Combined Counseling Psychology/School Psychology PhD Program accredited by the American Psychological Association (APA), and associate dean for Academic Affairs in the Graduate School of Education at the State University of New York at Buffalo. Between 1987 and 1989, she was chief psychologist at the Traumatic Head Injury Clinic located at Still Hospital in Jefferson City, Missouri. She is a fellow of APA Division 16 (School Psychology) and a member of Divisions 40 (Clinical Neuropsychology) and 54 (Society of Pediatric Psychology). She has published more than 100 journal articles and book chapters on such diverse health-related topics as eating disorders, prenatal alcohol and cocaine exposure, and lead poisoning. She developed the Phelps Kindergarten Readiness Scale II, a nationally standardized assessment tool evaluating learning readiness aptitudes predictive of later school achievement (revised in 2003); edited the book *Health-Related Disorders in Children and Adolescents: A Guidebook for Understanding and Educating* (APA, 1998); and coauthored *Pediatric Psychopharmacology: Combining Medical and Psychosocial Interventions*, which was published by APA in 2002. She has been identified as the most published female in the field of school psychology. She is editor of *Psychology in the Schools* and serves on the editorial boards of *School Psychology Quarterly*, *School Psychology Review*, and *Journal of Psychoeducational Assessment*. National leadership roles include membership on the APA Committee on Accreditation (2006 COA Associate Chair) and the APA Council of Chairs of Training Councils, chairing the Council of Directors of School Psychology Programs, chairing the APA Division 16 Task Force on Training Standards in School Psychology, and serving as a liaison to the APA Board of Educational Affairs. She teaches graduate courses such as Psychopathology and Evidence-Based Interventions and Advanced Personality Assessment. She maintains a private practice specializing in neuropsychological assessment and therapeutic interventions with children and adolescents.